MOSBY'S Workbook for

Long-Term Care Assistants

FOURTH EDITION

RELDA T. KELLY, RN, MSN
Professor Emeritus
Kankakee Community College
Kankakee, Illinois
Parish Nurse, Wesley United Methodist Church
Bradley, Illinois

Procedure checklists by
HELEN CHIGAROS, RN, BS, MSN, CRRN, CNS
Professor
Kankakee Community College
Kankakee, Illinois
Parish Nurse, St. Teresa Roman Catholic Church
Kankakee, Illinois

M Mosby

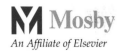

Mosby

An Affiliate of Elsevier

11830 Westline Industrial Drive
St. Louis, Missouri 63146

MOSBY'S WORKBOOK FOR LONG-TERM CARE ASSISTANTS   ISBN 0-323-01920-X

International Standard Book Number 0-323-01920-X

Executive Vice President, Nursing and Health Professions: Sally Schrefer
Acquisitions Editor: Susan R. Epstein
Senior Developmental Editor: Maria Broeker
Publishing Services Manager: John Rogers
Senior Project Manager: Kathy Teal
Designer: Dana Peick, GraphCom Corporation
Cover Art: Kathi Gosche
Design Manager: Kathi Gosche

GC/QWK

Printed in the United States of America

Last digit is the print number: 9 8 7 6 5 4 3 2

This workbook is dedicated to my family—
my husband Earl,
my children Scott and Kelly, and Elisabeth,
and my beautiful grandchildren,
Samuel, Michela, and Ian.
I love them all.

REVIEWERS

ILLUSTRATION CREDITS

PREFACE

This *Workbook* is written to be used with the Sorrentino, Gorek textbook *Mosby's Textbook for Long-Term Care Assistants,* 4th edition. Students will not need other resources to complete the exercises in this *Workbook.* The answer key for the *Workbook* is found at the back of the *Instructor's Guide.*

The *Workbook* is designed to help students apply what they have learned in each chapter of the textbook. Students are encouraged to use this book as a study guide. Each chapter is thoroughly covered in the multiple-choice questions, which will give students practice to take the NAACEP test. In addition, other exercises such as fill-in-the-blank, matching, and crossword puzzles are used in many chapters. **Independent Learning Activities** at the end of each chapter may be used to apply the information learned in a practical setting. In addition, **Procedure Checklists** that correspond with the procedures of the textbook are provided. These checklists are designed to help students become skilled at performing procedures that affect quality of care.

Two new sections are included in this edition. The section titled **Optional Learning Activities** may be used as an alternative exercise to give students more practice in studying the materials. Questions related to *Mosby's Nursing Assistant Skills Videos* have been added to the appropriate chapters. These questions will help students focus on the videos as they watch them.

Assistive personnel are important members of the health team. Completing the exercises in this *Workbook* will increase the student's knowledge and skills. The goal is to prepare students to provide the best possible care and to encourage pride in a job well done.

Relda T. Kelly

CONTENTS

Unit I: Working in Long-Term Care Settings

1. Introduction to Long-Term Care, *1*
2. The Nursing Assistant in Long-Term Care, *11*
3. Work Ethics, *20*
4. Communicating With the Health Team, *26*

Unit II: Focusing on the Person

5. Understanding the Resident, *35*
6. Body Structure and Function, *43*
7. The Older Person, *57*
8. Sexuality, *63*

Unit III: Protecting the Person

9. Safety, *67*
10. Restraint Alternatives and Safe Restraint Use, *75*
11. Preventing Infection, *81*
12. Body Mechanics, *93*

Unit IV: Assisting With Activities of Daily Living

13. The Resident's Unit, *104*
14. Bedmaking, *111*
15. Hygiene, *116*
16. Grooming, *127*
17. Urinary Elimination, *133*
18. Bowel Elimination, *144*
19. Nutrition and Fluids, *153*
20. Exercise and Activity, *167*
21. Comfort, Rest, and Sleep, *176*
22. Oxygen Needs, *183*
23. Assisted Living, *190*

Unit V: Assisting With Assessment

24. Measuring Vital Signs, *195*
25. Assisting With the Physical Examination, *205*

Unit VI: Assisting With Care Needs

26. Admitting, Transferring, and Discharging Persons, *211*
27. Wound Care, *227*
28. Heat and Cold Applications, *231*
29. Common Health Problems, *235*
30. Mental Health Problems, *248*
31. Confusion and Dementia, *252*
32. Developmental Disabilities, *257*
33. Rehabilitation and Restorative Care, *262*
34. Basic Emergency Care, *266*
35. The Dying Person, *272*

Procedure Checklists, 277

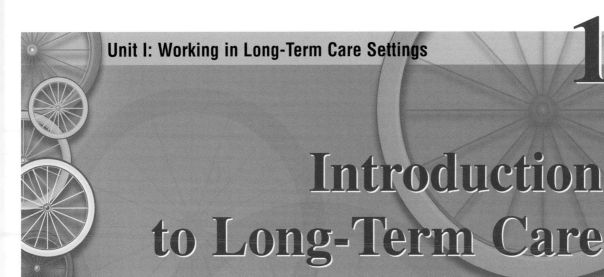

Introduction to Long-Term Care

Acute illness	Licensed practical nurse (LPN)	Omnibus Budget Reconciliation Act
Alzheimer's disease	Licensed vocational nurse (LVN)	of 1987 (OBRA)
Assisted living facility	Medicaid	Primary nursing
Board and care home	Medicare	Private insurance plan
Case management	Nurse practitioner (NP)	Registered nurse (RN)
Chronic illness	Nursing assistant	Residential care facility
Deconditioning	Nursing center	Skilled nursing facility (SNF)
Functional nursing	Nursing facility (NF)	Subacute care
Group insurance	Nursing home	Supportive care
Hospice	Nursing team	Team nursing
Interdisciplinary health care team	Ombudsman	

Fill in the Blanks: Key Terms

Select your answers from the Key Terms listed above.

1. _____

   is the process of becoming weak from illness or lack

   of exercise.

2. An _____

   is an individual who has completed a 1-year nursing

   program and passed a licensing examination.

3. A _____ is

   an insurance plan bought by a group for individuals.

4. A facility that provides health care services to resi-

   dents who require regular or continuous care is a

   _____.

5. Another name for a nursing center or an NF is a

   _____.

6. A _____ is

   an RN with additional education in physical

   examination and assessment.

7. A sudden illness from which the person is expected

   to recover is an _____.

8. A facility that provides nursing care for residents who need complex care but do not need hospital services is a _____.

9. A _____ is an illness, slow or gradual in onset, for which there is no known cure.

10. An _____ provides housing, personal care, supportive services, health care, and social activities in a homelike setting.

11. In _____, a nurse is responsible for the total care of specific residents on a 24-hour basis.

12. RNs, LPNs/LVNs, and nursing assistants provide nursing care as part of the _____.

13. _____ is a disease that affects the brain tissue.

14. The nursing staff performs specific tasks for all assigned residents in a method of organizing nursing care called _____ .

15. _____ is a federal health insurance for persons 65 years of age or older and younger people with certain disabilities.

16. A _____ provides custodial care to a few independent residents, often in a home setting.

17. A nursing center or nursing home may be called a _____.

18. A _____ is a plan bought by an individual.

19. _____ is a federal law concerned with the quality of life, health, and safety of residents.

20. In _____, a nurse serves as a leader and assigns other nurses and nursing assistants to care for certain residents.

21. _____ provides complex medical care or rehabilitation.

22. An individual who has studied nursing for 2, 3, or 4 years and who has passed a licensing examination is a _____.

23. An _____ is an advocate—someone who supports or promotes the needs and interests of another person.

24. Another name for a board and care home is a _____.

25. A method of organizing nursing care whereby an RN coordinates the person's care from admission through discharge and into the home setting is _____.

26. A _____ gives basic nursing care under the supervision of a nurse.

27. Another name for an LPN is _____.

28. A variety of health care workers who work together to provide health care for residents are the _____.

29. _____

   provides care on a 24-hour basis that meets the

   person's basic physical needs.

30. _____

   is a health care payment program sponsored by state

   and federal governments.

31. A health care agency for persons dying is a

   _____.

Circle the BEST Answer

32. Residents who live in a board and care home:
    A. Receive supportive care on a 24-hour basis
    B. Stay there for a short time while recovering from an illness or surgery
    C. Are in a program for persons who are dying
    D. Are in a closed unit that provides a safer environment

33. Assisted living facilities can be part of
    A. A hospital
    B. Retirement communities or nursing centers
    C. A hospice
    D. An SNF

34. SNFs provide
    A. Supportive care
    B. An increased level of complex care for residents with severe health problems
    C. A closed unit for residents who have Alzheimer's disease or other dementia
    D. Rehabilitation for persons who no longer need hospital care

35. Most residents in nursing centers require care
    A. Only when recovering from acute illnesses
    B. That is continuous for chronic problems
    C. Because of communicable diseases
    D. For emotional problems

36. Colds and influenza can cause major health problems for older and disabled persons. These conditions are called
    A. Chronic illnesses
    B. Communicable diseases
    C. Emotional illnesses
    D. Disabilities

37. What is the aim of restorative or rehabilitative care?
    A. A complete return of all functions
    B. Supportive care that meets basic physical needs
    C. To keep the person safe
    D. To help residents return to their highest possible level of physical and mental functioning

38. Children and pets can usually visit at any time when a dying person is in
    A. An Alzheimer's unit
    B. A hospital
    C. A hospice
    D. A subacute care center

39. An Alzheimer's unit is a closed unit that provides
    A. A safer environment for these special residents to wander freely
    B. A program for persons who are dying
    C. A place for residents who are deconditioned after an acute illness
    D. A program for residents with a communicable disease

40. The Joint Commission on Accreditation of Healthcare Organizations (JCAHO)
    A. Is a required accreditation for all health care centers
    B. Determines whether staff members are adequately trained to give care
    C. Develops standards and practices for hospitals, nursing centers, and home health care agencies
    D. Accredits only acute care facilities

41. The nursing assistant is part of the nursing service department in a nursing center. The nursing assistant reports to
    A. The center administrator
    B. The director of nursing (DON)
    C. The nurse supervising his or her work
    D. The nurse manager

42. Who is responsible for coordinating care on each shift in the nursing center?
    A. Physician
    B. Staff nurse
    C. Shift supervisor
    D. DON

43. Which of the following describes an RN?
    A. Completes 1 year of study in a hospital-based program, community college, vocational school, or technical school
    B. Completes additional education in physical examination and assessment
    C. Has formal training to give care and passes a competency examination
    D. Studies for 2 years at a community college, 2- or 3-year hospital-based diploma program, or 4 years at a college or university

44. Which of these workers or areas in a health care center is *not* under the DON in the organizational chart?
    A. Nursing assistants
    B. Medical records
    C. Case managers
    D. Social workers

45. Medicare is a health insurance plan that has benefits for
    A. Persons 65 years of age and older
    B. Families with low incomes
    C. Individuals and families who buy the insurance
    D. Groups of individuals who buy the insurance

46. Part B of Medicare
    A. Pays for hospital costs and some SNF costs
    B. Benefits only persons 65 years of age and older
    C. Is administered by the Social Security Administration
    D. Pays for physician's visits, ambulance service, laboratory fees, and equipment and supplies

47. Under a diagnosis-related group (DRG) plan
    A. Only persons 65 years of age and older receive care.
    B. Payment is determined before the person receives hospital care.
    C. A decision is made about how much to pay for care in an SNF.
    D. For a prepaid fee, persons receive all needed services offered.

48. Under a resource utilization group (RUG) plan
    A. Only persons 65 years of age and older receive care.
    B. Payment is determined before the person receives hospital care.
    C. A decision is made about how much to pay for care in a SNF.
    D. For a prepaid fee, persons receive all needed services offered.

49. If a person has a health maintenance organization (HMO) or preferred provider organization (PPO) insurance contract, who decides where the person goes for services?
    A. The insured person
    B. The physician
    C. The government
    D. The insurance company

50. Under OBRA, a resident has all of the following rights *except*
    A. The right to have a private room in which to live
    B. The right to have personal choice as to what to wear and how to spend his or her time
    C. The right to personal privacy
    D. The right to refuse treatment

51. Under OBRA, if a resident is incompetent (not able) to exercise his or her rights, who can exercise these rights for the resident?
    A. Physician
    B. Spouse or adult child
    C. Nurse
    D. Neighbor

52. If a resident refuses treatment, what should you do?
    A. Avoid giving any care to the person and go on to other duties.
    B. Report the refusal to the nurse.
    C. Tell the resident that the treatment must be done and continue to carry out the treatment.
    D. Tell his or her family so they can make the resident take the treatment.

53. A student wants to observe a treatment, but the resident does not want the student to be present. What is the correct action?
    A. The student cannot watch because this violates the resident's right to privacy.
    B. The student may observe from the doorway where the resident cannot see the student.
    C. The staff nurse tells the resident that he or she must allow the student to watch.
    D. The nurse calls the resident's spouse to get permission.

54. The resident should be given personal choice whenever it
    A. Is safely possible
    B. Does not interfere with scheduled activities
    C. Is approved by the DON
    D. Is ordered by the physician

55. If a resident voices concerns about care and the center promptly tries to correct the situation, this action meets the resident's right to
    A. Participate in a resident group
    B. Voice a dispute or grievance
    C. Personal choice
    D. Freedom from abuse, mistreatment, and neglect

56. A resident volunteers to take care of house plants at the center. This gesture is an acceptable part of the following *except*
    A. The care plan
    B. A requirement to receive care or care items
    C. The resident's regular activity
    D. Rehabilitation

57. When residents and their families plan activities together, this action meets the resident's right to
    A. Privacy
    B. Freedom from restraint
    C. Freedom from mistreatment
    D. Participate in resident and family groups

58. The resident for whom you are caring has many old holiday decorations covering her nightstand. If you throw away these items without her permission, you are denying her right to
    A. Privacy
    B. Work
    C. Care and security of personal possessions
    D. Freedom from abuse

59. A staff member tells a resident that he cannot leave his room because he talks too much. This action denies the resident
    A. Freedom from abuse, mistreatment, and neglect
    B. Freedom from restraint
    C. Care and security of personal possessions
    D. Personal choice

60. When a resident is given certain drugs that affect his mood, behavior, or mental function, it may deny his right to
    A. Freedom from abuse, mistreatment, and neglect
    B. Personal choice
    C. Privacy
    D. Freedom from restraint

61. Which of these actions will promote dignity and privacy?
    A. Calling the resident by a nickname that he does not choose
    B. Helping him dress in clothing appropriate to the time of day
    C. Changing the resident's hairstyle without his permission
    D. Leaving the bathroom door open so you can see the person

62. An ombudsman would carry out which of the following activities?
    A. Organize activities for a group of residents.
    B. Accompany residents to a religious service at a house of worship.
    C. Investigate and resolve complaints made by a resident.
    D. Assist a resident in choosing friends.

63. You ask a resident if you may touch him. This request is an example of
    A. Courteous and dignified interaction
    B. Courteous and dignified care
    C. Providing privacy and self-determination
    D. Maintaining personal choice and independence

64. Assisting a resident to ambulate without interfering with his independence is an example of
    A. Courteous and dignified interaction
    B. Courteous and dignified care
    C. Providing privacy and self-determination
    D. Maintaining personal choice and independence

65. You provide privacy and self-determination for a resident when you
    A. Knock on the door before entering and wait to be asked in.
    B. Allow the resident to smoke in designated areas.
    C. Listen with interest to what the person is saying.
    D. Groom his beard as he wishes.

66. You allow the resident to maintain personal choice and independence when you
    A. Obtain her attention before interacting with her.
    B. Provide extra clothing for warmth, such as a sweater or lap robe.
    C. Assist the resident in taking part in activities according to her interests.
    D. Use curtains or screens during personal care and procedures.

Fill in the Blanks

Write out the meaning of each abbreviation.

67. RN _____

68. LPN/LVN _____

69. NP _____

70. NF _____

71. SNF _____

72. OBRA _____

73. JCAHO _____

74. DON _____

75. FNP _____

76. GNP _____

77. DRG _____

78. RUG _____

79 HMO _____

80. PPO _____

81. List six abbreviations that are titles of people who work in nursing centers.

_____   _____

_____   _____

_____   _____

82. List four abbreviations that are related to methods of payment for services.

_____   _____

_____   _____

83. List the two abbreviations that have regulations related to operating a nursing center.

_____   _____

84. List two abbreviations that refer to a nursing center.

_____   _____

Matching

Match the types of health care service with the correct example.

85. _____ Provides nursing care for residents who need complex care but do not need hospital services

86. _____ Provides supportive care on a 24-hour basis to meet the resident's basic physical needs

87. _____ Provides a closed unit to give residents with certain types of dementia a safer environment in which they can wander freely

88. _____ Health care facility or program for people dying from a terminal illness

89. _____ Residential setting that provides personal care, supportive services, health care, and social activities in a homelike setting

A. SNF

B. Hospice unit

C. Board and care home

D. Alzheimer's unit

E. Assisted living facilities

Match the types of nursing care pattern with the correct examples.

90. _____ Leader (RN) delegates care of certain persons to other nurses and nursing assistants.

91. _____ Primary nurse (RN) is responsible for total care of specific residents on a 24-hour basis.

92. _____ Manager (RN) coordinates resident's care from admission through discharge and into home setting.

93. _____ Each team member does certain tasks or functions.

A. Functional nursing

B. Team nursing

C. Primary nursing

D. Case management

Optional Learning Exercises

Comparing long-term care centers.

94. A board and care home provides _____

_____.

Eight services that are provided include:

_____

_____

_____.

What is not provided?

_____.

95. An assisted living facility provides _____

_____,

_____

in a homelike setting. Six services that are provided

include _____

_____

_____

_____

_____.

96. A nursing center provides health care to residents

_____

_____.

Members of the _____

_____ provide services.

97. An SNF is reserved for residents with _____

_____.

98. What are the purposes and goals of long-term care

centers?

A. _____

B. _____

C. _____

D. _____

99. A hospice is an agency or program for _____

_____.

What needs are met by a hospice?

_____

_____

_____

100. An Alzheimer's unit is designed for persons with

_____

_____.

An Alzheimer's unit is closed off from the rest of the center because these residents often

_____

_____.

101. _____

is provided for persons who no longer need hospital care.

Interdisciplinary Health Care Team
(Table 1-1)

Name the member of the interdisciplinary health care team who provides the service described.

102. Mr. Williams needs assistance to regain skills to dress, shave, and feed himself (activities of daily living [ADLs]). He is assisted by the

_____.

103. The nurse has concern about a drug action, so he or she calls the _____.

104. Mrs. Young needs the corns on her feet treated. The nurse notifies the _____.

105. Ms. Stewart has the responsibility of doing physical examinations, health assessments, and health educations for the center in which she works. She is a

_____.

106. Mr. Gomez keeps turning up the volume of his television. His hearing is tested by the

_____.

107. The _____

meets with a new resident and his family to discuss his nutritional needs.

108. Mr. Fox had a stroke and has weakness on his left side. The _____

assists him by developing a plan that focuses on restoring function and preventing disability from his illness.

109. The physician orders x-rays after Mr. Jackson falls. The x-rays are done by the

_____.

110. Mr. Ling has chronic lung disease and needs respiratory treatments. These treatments are given by the

_____.

111. Ms. Walker plans the recreational needs of a nursing center. She is an _____.

112. After a stroke, Mr. Stubbs has difficulty swallowing. He is evaluated by the

_____.

113. When the physician orders blood tests, the samples are collected by the

_____.

OBRA Actions to Promote Dignity and Privacy *(Box 1-2)*

Match the action to promote dignity and privacy with the example.

114. _____ File fingernails and apply polish as resident requests.

115. _____ Cover the resident with a blanket during a bath.

116. _____ Ask permission before giving care to a resident.

117. _____ Show interest when a resident tells stories about his past.

118. _____ Open containers and arrange food at mealtimes to assist the resident.

119. _____ Close the door when the person asks for privacy.

120. _____ Allow a resident to smoke in a designated area.

121. _____ Make sure the resident is wearing his dentures when he goes to the dining room.

122. _____ Take the resident to his weekly card game.

A. Courteous and dignified interaction

B. Courteous and dignified care

C. Privacy and self-determination

D. Maintain personal choice and independence

Independent Learning Activities

Gather the following information about long-term centers in your area. How many board and care facilities are located in your area? Choose one facility and answer the following questions:

1. Is this facility attached to a nursing center, or is it a separate center?
   - What services are provided?
   - How many residents are in the facility?
   - How many staff members work there? How many staff members are: RNs? LPNs? Nursing assistants? What care is provided by nursing assistants?

2. How many nursing centers are located in your area? Choose one center and answer the following questions.
   - What types of residents are accepted in the center? (For example, does the center consider level of care needed, the resident's disease, or method of payment?)
   - How many residents live in the center?
   - How many staff members work there? How many staff members are: RNs? LPNs? Nursing assistants? What care is provided by nursing assistants?

3. How many nursing centers in your area provide skilled nursing care? Choose one center and answer these questions.
   - How many residents live in the center?
   - How many staff members work there? How many staff members are: RNs? LPNs? Nursing assistants? What care is provided by nursing assistants?

4. How many assisted living facilities are located in your area? Choose one center and answer the following questions.
   - Is this facility independent or part of a long-term care center?
   - How many residents live in the facility?
   - What kind of living quarters do the residents have? (For example, does each resident have an apartment or studio? Do they share kitchen facilities, or does each person have a kitchen?)
   - How many staff members work there? How many staff members are: RNs? LPNs? Nursing assistants? What care is provided by nursing assistants?

5. Find a nursing center that has an Alzheimer's unit and answer the following questions.
   - How is the unit identified? Is it a separate wing? Separate floor? Is the unit closed off?
   - How is the unit different from other units in the center?
   - Do the staff members who work on this unit receive special training? If so, what extra training are they given? What duties are assigned to nursing assistants on this unit?

6. Does your area have a hospice program? If so, answer the following questions about the program.
   - Is this program located within a center, or does it provide care in the person's facility?
   - What type of care is provided?
   - What special training is given to the staff? What duties can a nursing assistant perform?

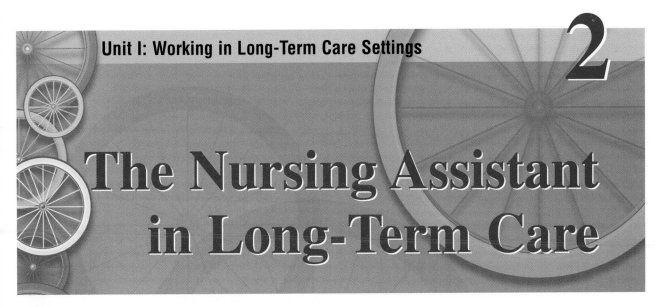

The Nursing Assistant in Long-Term Care

2

Abuse	Criminal law	Invasion of privacy	Responsibility
Accountable	Defamation	Job description	Slander
Assault	Delegate	Law	Standard of care
Battery	Ethics	Libel	Task
Civil law	False imprisonment	Malpractice	Tort
Crime	Fraud	Negligence	Will

Fill in the Blanks: Key Terms

Select your answers from the Key Terms listed above.

1. A _____ is a function, procedure, activity, or work that does not require an RN's professional knowledge or judgment.

2. _____ is negligence by a professional person.

3. Saying or doing something to trick, fool, or deceive another person is _____.

4. _____ is concerned with offenses against the public and society in general.

5. A _____ is a legal statement of how a person wishes to have property distributed after death.

6. Being responsible for one's actions and the actions of others who perform delegated tasks is called being _____.

7. A rule of conduct made by a government body is a _____.

8. _____ is the unauthorized touching of a person's body without the person's consent.

9. The intentional mistreatment or harm of another person is _____.

10. _____ is defamation through oral statements.

11. Injuring a person's name and reputation by making false statements to a third person is

    _____.

12. _____

    is a knowledge of what is right and wrong conduct.

13. Intentionally attempting or threatening to touch a person's body without the person's consent is

    _____.

14. A _____

    is a wrong committed against a person or the

    person's property.

15. _____

    is concerned with relationships between people.

16. A _____

    is a listing of responsibilities and functions the

    agency expects you to perform.

17. The duty or obligation to perform some act or function is called _____.

18. Violating a person's right not to have his or her

    name, photograph, or private affairs exposed or

    made public without giving consent is

    _____.

19. _____

    is the skills, care, and judgment required by the

    health team member under similar circumstances.

20. To _____

    means authorizing another person to perform a task.

21. An act that violates a criminal law is a

    _____.

22. _____ is the un-

    lawful restraint or restriction of a person's movement.

23. Defamation through written statements is

    _____.

24. _____

    is an unintentional wrong in which a person fails to

    act in a reasonable and careful manner and causes

    harm to a person or to the person's property.

Circle the BEST Answer

25. Until the 1980s, nursing assistants
    A. Attended nursing assistant classes approved by the state
    B. Were not used in giving basic nursing care
    C. Received on-the-job training from nurses
    D. Worked only in hospitals

26. What major political issues in 1990s caused hospital closings, hospital mergers, and changes in health care systems?
    A. Nursing shortages
    B. Changes made by OBRA
    C. Rising health care costs
    D. Changes in nurse practice acts

27. Hospitals are now hiring an increasing number of nursing assistants because of
    A. Nursing shortages
    B. An effort to reduce costs
    C. Changes in nurse practice acts
    D. Changes made in insurance payments

28. State laws that regulate nursing assistants' roles and functions are determined by
    A. OBRA
    B. The Nurse Practice Act
    C. The state medical society
    D. Insurance companies

29. If you perform a task beyond the legal limits of your role, you may be
    A. Protected by the Nurse Practice Act
    B. Practicing nursing without a license
    C. Protected by the nurse who supervises your work
    D. Accused of a criminal act

30. OBRA requires that the nursing assistant training and competency evaluation program have at least _____ hours of instruction.
    A. 16
    B. 75
    C. 120
    D. 200

31. Which of these areas of study is *not* included in a training program for nursing assistants?
    A. Communication
    B. Elimination procedures
    C. Resident rights
    D. Phlebotomy (drawing blood)

32. The competency evaluation for nursing assistants has two parts
    A. A written test and a skills test
    B. A multiple choice test and a true-false test
    C. A skills test and a complete bed-bath demonstration
    D. A written test and an oral question and answer test

33. If you fail the competency evaluation the first time it is taken, you
    A. Can retest one more time
    B. Must repeat your training program
    C. Can retest two more times (for a total of three times)
    D. Can retest as often as is necessary free of charge

34. All of the following information is contained in the nursing assistant registry information, *except*
    A. Information about findings of abuse, neglect, of dishonest use of property
    B. Date of birth
    C. Number of dependents
    D. Date the competency examination was passed

35. OBRA requires that retraining and a new competency evaluation test must be taken if you have not worked as a certified nursing assistant for
    A. 2 consecutive years
    B. 5 years
    C. 1 year
    D. 6 months

36. Your work as a nursing assistant is supervised by
    A. An RN or LPN/LVN
    B. The physician
    C. The director of nursing
    D. A nursing assistant with more experience

37. You are alone in the nurses' station and you answer the phone. Dr. Smith begins to give verbal orders to you. You should
    A. Hang up the phone.
    B. Politely give him your name and title and ask him to wait while you get the nurse.
    C. Quickly write down the orders and give them to the nurse.
    D. Politely give him your name and title and ask him to call back later when the nurse is there.

38. As a nursing assistant, you *never* give medications unless
    A. The nurse is busy and asks you to give them.
    B. The resident is in the shower and the nurse leaves the medications at the bedside.
    C. You have completed a state-required medication and training program about giving medications.
    D. You are feeding the resident and the nurse asks you to mix the medications with the food.

39. The nurse asks you to carry out a task that you do not know how to do. You should
    A. Ignore the order because it is something you cannot do.
    B. Perform the task as well as you can.
    C. Ask another nursing assistant to show you how to carry out the task.
    D. Promptly explain to the nurse why you cannot carry out the task.

40. The nurse asks you to assist him as he changes sterile dressings. You should
    A. Assist him as needed.
    B. Tell him you cannot assist in performing any sterile procedures.
    C. Tell him that this is something you cannot do.
    D. Report his request to the supervisor.

41. Who can tell the person or the family a diagnosis or prescribe treatments?
    A. The director of nursing
    B. The RN
    C. The physician
    D. An experienced nursing assistant

42. When you read a job description, you should not take a job if it requires you to
    A. Carry out duties you do not like to do.
    B. Maintain required certification.
    C. Attend in-service training.
    D. Function beyond your training limits.

43. Which of the following is *not* acceptable?
    A. An RN delegates a task to an LPN/LVN.
    B. An LPN/LVN delegates a task to a nursing assistant.
    C. An RN delegates a task to a nursing assistant.
    D. A nursing assistant delegates a task to another nursing assistant.

44. When a nurse considers delegating tasks, the decision
    A. Should always result in the best care for the person
    B. Depends on whether the nurse likes the nursing assistant
    C. Depends on how busy the nurse is that day
    D. Depends on how well the nurse likes the person

45. You have been caring for Mr. Watson for several weeks. The nurse tells you that she will give his care today. Her delegation decision is based primarily on
    A. How well you performed his care yesterday
    B. Changes in Mr. Watson's condition
    C. Whether the nurse knows you or not
    D. How much supervision you need

46. Which of the following is *not* a right of delegation?
    A. The right task
    B. The right person
    C. The right time
    D. The right supervision

47. You agree to perform a task the nurse delegates to you. Which of these statements tells you the circumstance is right for you to do this?
    A. You understand the purpose of the task for this person.
    B. You are comfortable performing the task.
    C. You have reviewed the task with the nurse.
    D. You were trained to do the task.

48. You may refuse to carry out a task for all of the following reasons *except*
    A. The task is not in your job description.
    B. You do not know how to use the supplies or equipment.
    C. You are too busy.
    D. The person might be harmed if you carry out the task.

49. It is unethical if you
    A. Refuse to give care to a person who has different beliefs than you have.
    B. Refuse to carry out a task because you do not know how to do it.
    C. Refuse to perform a task that is against your religious or moral beliefs.
    D. Refuse to carry out a task beyond the legal limits of your role.

50. Which of the following is *not* good conduct for a nursing assistant?
    A. Carry out any assignment that the nurse has given to you.
    B. Take only drugs that have been prescribed by your physician.
    C. Recognize limits of your role and your knowledge.
    D. Consider the needs of the residents to be more important than your own needs.

51. A nurse has failed to do what a reasonable and careful nurse would have done. Legally, this failure is
    A. A crime
    B. A tort
    C. Negligence
    D. Malpractice

52. If you fail to identify a person properly and perform a treatment on him that is intended for another, you are
    A. Committing a crime
    B. Legally responsible for your actions
    C. Not legally responsible but unethical
    D. Guilty of an intentional tort

53. A nursing assistant writes a note containing false statements to a friend that injures the name and reputation of a person. This action is called
    A. Libel   C. Malpractice
    B. Slander   D. Negligence

54. A nursing assistant tells a resident that she is a nurse. The nursing assistant has committed
    A. Fraud   C. Slander
    B. Libel   D. Negligence

55. When a resident is confined to his room by a caregiver, he is a victim of
    A. Physical abuse
    B. False imprisonment
    C. Invasion of privacy
    D. Battery

56. If a resident tells you that he does not want you to dress him and you go ahead and touch him, you can be accused of
    A. Fraud   C. Assault
    B. Battery   D. False imprisonment

57. If you are asked to obtain a resident's signature on an informed consent, you should
    A. Make sure the resident is mentally competent.
    B. Refuse. You are never responsible for obtaining a written consent.
    C. Make sure the resident understands what the resident is signing.
    D. Ask a family member to witness the signed consent.

58. If a person is confused or unconscious, informed consent
    A. Is not necessary
    B. Cannot be obtained and therefore no treatments can be given
    C. Can be given by a husband, wife, son, daughter, or legal representative
    D. Can be given by the director of nursing

59. You can refuse to sign a will if
    A. You are named in the will.
    B. You do not believe the person is of sound mind.
    C. Your nursing center has policies that do not allow employees to witness wills.
    D. All of the above are true.

60. Which of the following is not an element of abuse?
    A. Willful causing of injury
    B. Intimidation
    C. Expecting a person to feed and dress himself within his abilities
    D. Depriving a person of food as punishment

61. What kind of abuse occurs when an elderly person is left to sit in urine or feces?
    A. Physical
    B. Involuntary seclusion
    C. Mental
    D. Sexual

62. An example of verbal abuse can be
    A. Failing to answer a signal light
    B. Locking a person in a room
    C. Oral or written statements that speak badly of a person
    D. Making threats of punishment

63. Depriving a person of needs such as food, clothing, or a place to sleep is
    A. Verbal abuse
    B. Involuntary seclusion
    C. Physical or mental abuse
    D. Sexual abuse

64. Which of the following may be a sign of elder abuse?
    A. The person answers questions openly.
    B. The family makes sure the hearing aides have new batteries.
    C. A caregiver is present during all conversations.
    D. All medications are taken as scheduled.

65. A sign of sexual abuse can be
    A. Small, circle-like burns on the body
    B. Bleeding or bruising in the genital area
    C. Weight loss and signs of poor nutrition
    D. Inadequate personal hygiene

66. If you suspect that an elderly person is being abused, you should
    A. Call the police.
    B. Discuss the situation and your observations with the nurse.
    C. Discuss the situation with the family.
    D. Notify community agencies that investigate elder abuse.

67. What happens to a nursing assistant who is found taking money from a resident's purse?
    A. The amount of money taken will be deducted from the next paycheck.
    B. The nursing assistant can lose his or her job, and the state nursing assistant registry will be notified.
    C. The nursing assistant will be transferred to another unit.
    D. The nursing assistant will be expected to apologize to the resident.

68. Which of these persons might be a child abuser?
    A. A person with little education
    B. A person with a high income
    C. A person who was abused as a child
    D. All of the above

69. Children who are deprived of food, clothing, shelter, and medical care are victims of
    A. Physical neglect
    B. Emotional neglect
    C. Physical abuse
    D. Sexual abuse

70. Children who are molested are victims of
    A. Physical neglect
    B. Emotional neglect
    C. Physical abuse
    D. Sexual abuse

71. If you suspect a child is being abused, you should
    A. Share your concerns with the nurse.
    B. Talk with the child.
    C. Inform the physician.
    D. Call a child protection agency.

72. A husband does not allow his wife to use the car, to leave the home, or to visit with family and friends. This pattern is a form of domestic violence called
    A. Verbal abuse
    B. Social abuse
    C. Physical abuse
    D. Economic abuse

Matching

Match the examples with the correct tort.

73. _____ While cleaning a resident's dentures, the nursing assistant drops and breaks them.

74. _____ A nursing assistant opens a resident's mail and reads it without permission.

75. _____ Instead of allowing the resident a choice, the nursing assistant tells him that he will get a shower whether he wants one or not.

76. _____ An individual touches a person's body without the person's consent.

77. _____ An individual tricks or fools another person.

78. _____ An individual restrains or restricts a resident's freedom of movement without a physician's order.

79. _____ A nurse gives a treatment to the wrong person.

80. _____ A nursing assistant injures the name and reputation of a resident by making false statements to a third person.

81. _____ A nursing assistant writes notes, falsely accusing another nursing assistant of stealing her purse.

A. Negligence

B. Malpractice

C. Libel

D. Defamation

E. False imprisonment

F. Assault

G. Battery

H. Fraud

I. Invasion of privacy

Nursing Assistant Skills Video Exercise

View the **Basic Principles** *video to answer these questions.*

82. Federal and state laws and _____ policies define the roles and responsibilities of the nursing team.

83. The nursing team is responsible for meeting four needs of the patient or resident and of the family members. These needs are _____, _____, _____, and _____.

84. An _____ identifies nursing care problems, develops and implements nursing care plans, and evaluates the effectiveness of care.

85. An _____ can give simple care to a person whose condition is stable.

86. A _____ helps the nurse with bedside care.

87. What four things do you need to know before you carry out a procedure?

    A. _____

    B. _____

    C. _____

    D. _____

88. An RN _____

    tasks, activity, or work that does not require an RN's

    professional judgment.

89. What are the five rights of delegation?

    A. _____

    B. _____

    C. _____

    D. _____

    E. _____

Optional Learning Exercises

OBRA requirements related to the nursing assistant

90. The nursing assistant must meet federal and state

    training and competency requirements to work in

    _____.

91. OBRA requires _____ hours of instruction. _____

    hours must be supervised practical training. Where

    can the practical training take place?

    _____

    or _____.

92. OBRA requires 15 areas of study. Write the area of

    study where you learn the skill in each example.

    A. You make a bed:

       _____

    B. You close Mr. Smith's door to give him privacy:

       _____

    C. You tell Mrs. Forbes the time of day and the day
       of week frequently during the day:

       _____

D. You apply lotion to a resident's dry skin:

   _____

E. You assist a resident in putting on his shirt:

   _____

F. When assigned to a new unit, you check to find
   the location of the fire alarm:

   _____

G. You wash your hands before and after giving
   care:

   _____

H. You get help to move a resident from his bed to
   the chair.

   _____

I. When speaking to Mr. Jackson, you maintain
   good eye contact.

   _____

J. The nurse tells you to exercise a resident's
   extremities (limbs).

   _____

K. You shave Mr. Stewart.

   _____

L. You position a urinal for a resident in bed.

   _____

M. You assist Mrs. Young in walking in the hall.

   _____

N. You notice that Mrs. Peck has an elevated
   temperature and her skin is warm.

   _____

O. You cut up the meat on Mr. Johnson's plate
   before helping him eat.

   _____

The National Nursing Assistant Assessment Program (NNAAP) *(Appendix)*

93. The NNAAP written test has _____ questions. List the percentage of questions in each area.

    A. _____ Activities of daily living

    B. _____ Basic nursing skills

    C. _____ Restorative skills

    D. _____ Emotional and mental health needs

    E. _____ Spiritual and cultural needs

    F. _____ Communications

    G. _____ Client rights

    H. _____ Legal and ethical behavior

    I. _____ Members of the health care team

94. List the skills that are tested on the NNAAP.

    A. _____

    B. _____

    C. _____

    D. _____

    E. _____

    F. _____

    G. _____

    H. _____

    I. _____

    J. _____

    K. _____

    L. _____

    M. _____

    N. _____

    O. _____

    P. _____

    Q. _____

    R. _____

    S. _____

    T. _____

    U. _____

    V. _____

    W. _____

    X. _____

    Y. _____

Position Description

95. During admission, transfer, and discharge procedures, the nursing assistant may be assigned to _____ and _____ the residents.

96. If the nursing assistant observes reddened areas or skin breakdown, the nursing assistant should _____.

97. When a nursing assistant tells the resident the date, day of the week, and time of day during daily care, he or she is meeting the job responsibility of providing _____.

98. When the nursing assistant attends in-service education programs as required, he or she will learn _____.

99. The nursing assistant is expected to attend at least _____ of staff meetings.

100. Current Basic Cardiac Life Support certification must be completed in _____ of the hire date.

Independent Learning Activities

1. Make a list of tasks that would conflict with your moral or religious beliefs.
   - How would you feel about performing these tasks in your job?
   - What would you say to your employer or co-workers?

2. Role-play a situation in which you are asked to perform one of the tasks you identified in the previous activity. Have one student play the person asking you to perform the task. Have a second student observe and answer these questions:
   - What was your reaction when asked?
   - In what way did you communicate your discomfort?
   - What suggestions did you offer to make sure the task was done?

3. Identify agencies in your community that help victims of abuse (for example, elder, child, domestic). Visit one of the agencies and ask these questions:
   - How do you find out about the victim?
   - What services do you offer?
   - What happens to the victim after you identify a problem?
   - Do you have a place where they can be protected?

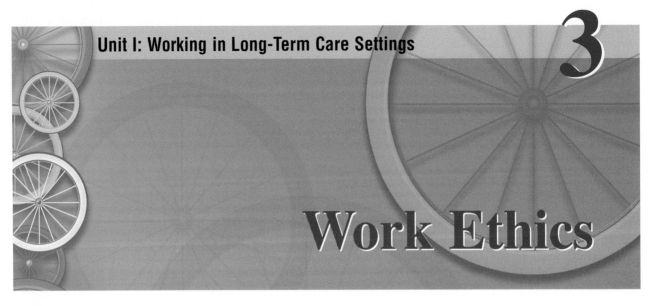

Work Ethics

Confidentiality	Preceptor
Courtesy	Stress
Gossip	Stressor
Harassment	Work ethics

Fill in the Blanks: Key Terms

Select your answers from the Key Terms listed above.

1. A staff member who guides is a

   _____ .

2. A _____

   is the event or factor that causes stress.

3. Trusting others with personal and private informa-

   tion is _____ .

4. _____

   is behavior in the workplace.

5. _____

   is to spread rumors or talk about the private matters

   of others.

6. The response or change in the body caused by any

   emotional, physical, social, or economic factor is

   _____ .

7. _____

   is a polite, considerate, or helpful comment or act.

8. _____

   means to trouble, torment, offend, or worry a person

   by one's behavior or comments.

Circle the BEST Answer

9. Work ethics involve
   A. How well you do your skills
   B. What religion you practice
   C. How you treat and work with others
   D. Cultural beliefs and attitudes

10. Your diet will maintain your weight if
    A. You avoid salty and sweet foods.
    B. You take in fewer calories than your energy
       needs require.
    C. It includes foods with fats and oils.
    D. The number of calories taken in equals your en-
       ergy needs.

11. Adults need about _____ hours of sleep daily.
    A. 7
    B. 10
    C. 4
    D. 12

12. Exercise is needed for:
    A. Rest and sleep
    B. Muscle tone and circulation
    C. Good body mechanics
    D. Good nutrition

13. Smoking odors
    A. Disappear quickly when the person finishes smoking
    B. Can be covered up by chewing gum
    C. Are noticed only by the smoker
    D. Stay on the person's breath, hands, clothing, and hair

14. The most important reason a person should not work under the influence of alcohol or drugs is that
    A. Resident safety is affected.
    B. The person becomes disorganized.
    C. Co-workers become angry.
    D. Your nursing center does not allow the practice.

15. Which of the following is *not* part of good personal hygiene for work?
    A. Bathe daily and use a deodorant.
    B. Practice good hand washing.
    C. Cut toenails straight across.
    D. Keep fingernails long and polished.

16. Tattoos should be covered when working because they
    A. May offend residents, families, and co-workers
    B. Can become infected
    C. May confuse residents
    D. Increase the risk of skin injuries

17. When working, the nursing assistant may wear
    A. Jewelry in pierced eyebrow, nose, lips, or tongue
    B. Wedding and engagement rings
    C. Multiple earrings in each ear
    D. Nail polish

18. When working, the nursing assistant should *not* wear
    A. A beard or mustache that is clean and trimmed
    B. Hair that is off the collar and away from the face
    C. Perfume, cologne, or aftershave
    D. A wristwatch with a second hand

19. Displaying good work ethics at your clinical experience site may help you find a job because
    A. You will pass the course.
    B. It will show you care.
    C. You will get better grades.
    D. The staff always looks at students as future employees.

20. You should be well groomed when looking for a job because it
    A. Shows you are cooperative
    B. Makes a good first impression
    C. Shows you are respectful
    D. Shows you have values and attitudes that fit with the center

21. How does an employer know that you can perform required job skills?
    A. They will request proof of training and will check your record in the state nursing assistant registry.
    B. They will have you give a demonstration of your skills.
    C. You will be asked many questions about performing certain skills.
    D. You will be required to take a written test.

22. You can get a job application from
    A. The personnel office or the human relations office
    B. A friend who works at the center
    C. From the director of nursing
    D. The receptionist in the lobby of the center

23. You should take a dry run to a job interview to
    A. Show you follow directions well
    B. Show you listen well
    C. Make sure you will be on time for the interview
    D. Look over the center to see if you want to work there

24. When you are interviewing, it is correct to
    A. Have a glass of wine before going
    B. Look directly at the interviewer
    C. Wear a sweat suit and athletic shoes
    D. Shake hands very gently

25. What is a good way to share your list of skills with the interviewer?
    A. Tell the person verbally what you can do.
    B. Ask for a list of skills and check the ones that you know.
    C. Bring a list of your skills and give it to the interviewer.
    D. Tell the interviewer you will send a list as soon as possible.

26. It is important for you to ask questions at the end of the interview because it
    A. Will show the interviewer that you are interested in the job
    B. Will help you to decide if the job is right for you
    C. Shows that you have good communication skills
    D. Shows that you are dependable

27. If you are assigned a preceptor, the person may be
    A. An RN
    B. Another nursing assistant
    C. An LPN/LVN
    D. Any of the above

28. What is a common reason for losing a job?
    A. Not knowing how to perform a task
    B. Frequent absences or excessive tardiness
    C. Being disorganized
    D. Lacking self-confidence

29. If you are scheduled to begin work at 3:00 PM, you should arrive
    A. At 3:00 PM
    B. At 2:30 PM
    C. Early enough to be ready to work at 3:00 PM
    D. As close to 3:00 PM as you can

30. You can avoid being part of gossip by
    A. Remaining quiet when you are in a group in which gossip is occurring
    B. Talking only about residents and family members to co-workers
    C. Repeating comments only in writing
    D. Removing yourself from a group or situation in which gossip is occurring

31. Privacy and confidentiality for residents are rights protected by
    A. Your job description
    B. Resident rights under OBRA
    C. An agreement between the resident and the nurse
    D. A doctor's orders

32. When you are working, you should not wear
    A. Jeans
    B. A loose-fitting shirt
    C. A shirt with the top button open
    D. White socks

33. Slang or swearing should not be used at work because:
    A. Words used with family and friends may offend residents and their family members.
    B. The resident may not understand you.
    C. The resident may have difficulty hearing.
    D. Co-workers may overhear it.

34. You should say "please" and "thank you" to others because
    A. Courtesies mean so much to people; it can brighten someone's day.
    B. It shows respect to the person.
    C. It is required by your job.
    D. It shows that you like the person.

35. It is acceptable at work if you
    A. Take a pen to use at home.
    B. Sell cookies for your child's school project.
    C. Use a pay telephone on your break to call your child.
    D. Make a copy of a letter on the copier in the nurse's station.

36. When you leave and return to the unit for breaks or lunch you should
    A. Tell each resident.
    B. Tell any family members who are present.
    C. Tell the nurse.
    D. All of the above are true.

37. Safety practices are important to follow because
    A. They help you be more organized.
    B. Negligent behavior affects the safety of others.
    C. They save the center money.
    D. You will get promoted more quickly.

38. Care should be planned around
    A. Your break and lunch time
    B. Resident mealtimes, visiting hours, activities, and therapies
    C. Co-workers' schedules
    D. The time scheduled by the nurse

39. Stress occurs
    A. Only when you have unpleasant situations in your life
    B. Because you do not handle your problems well
    C. Because you are in the wrong job
    D. Every minute of every day and in everything you do

40. What physical effects of stress can be life threatening?
    A. High blood pressure, heart attack, strokes, and ulcers
    B. Increase heart rate and faster and deeper breathing
    C. Anxiety, fear, anger, and depression
    D. Headaches, insomnia, and muscle tension

41. Which of these actions is harassment?
    A. Offending others with gestures or remarks
    B. Offending others with jokes or pictures
    C. Making a sexual advance or requesting sexual favors
    D. All of the above

42. If you resign from a job, it is good practice to give
    A. 1-week notice   C. 4-week notice
    B. 2-week notice   D. No notice

43. Good work ethics help residents
    A. Feel safe, secure, loved, and cared for
    B. Receive adequate care
    C. Recover from their illnesses
    D. Have more freedom to go to activities

Crossword

Use the terms in Box 3-2: **Qualities and Characteristics for Good Work Ethics** *to complete the crossword puzzle.*

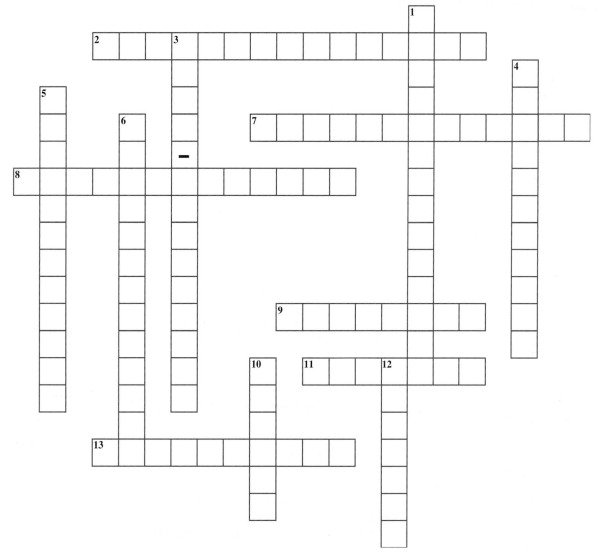

Across

2. Residents and staff members have confidence in you
7. Be careful, alert, and exact in following instructions
8. Report to work on time and when scheduled
9. Be polite and courteous to residents, families, visitors, and co-workers
11. Accurately report the care given, your observations, and any errors
13. Be eager, interested, and excited about your work

Down

1. Treat the person with respect and dignity at all times; also show respect for the health team
3. Know you own feelings, strengths, and weaknesses
4. Willingly help and work with others
5. Do not be moody, bad tempered, or unhappy at work
6. Respect the person's physical and emotional feelings
10. Have concern for the person
12. Seeing things from the person's point of view; putting yourself in the person's position

Optional Learning Exercises

44. List six places that you can find out about job openings.

_____

_____

_____

_____

_____

_____

Job Application *(Box 3-3)*

45. If a job application asks you to print in black ink, why is it a poor idea to use blue ink?

_____

_____.

46. How can writing illegibly on a job application affect getting a job?

_____

_____.

47. Why is it important to give information about employment gaps or leaving a job?

_____

_____.

48. If you lie on a job application, it is

_____. If you

commit this offense, what can happen?

_____

_____.

Qualities and Characteristics of Good Work Ethics *(Box 3-2)*

Match the qualities and characteristics of good work ethics with the examples.

49. _____ While working with Mr. Smith, you try to understand and feel what it must be like to be paralyzed on one side.

50. _____ You realize that you are good at giving basic care. You know that you need to improve your communication skills.

51. _____ When caring for elderly residents, you try to do small things that will make them happy or to find ways to ease their pain.

52. _____ You thank co-workers when they help you and remember to wish residents happy birthday as appropriate.

53. _____ When Mrs. Gibson is upset and angry, you remember to respect her feelings and to be kind.

54. _____ You report the blood pressure and temperature readings accurately to the nurse.

55. _____ You realize giving care to residents is important, and you are excited about your work.

56. _____ Your supervisor tells you that she knows she can count on because you are always on time and perform delegated tasks as assigned.

57. _____ Even though Mr. Acevado has different cultural and religious views than you have, you value his feelings and beliefs.

58. _____ Before you left home today, you had an argument with your child. When you get to work, you make every effort to put that encounter aside and be pleasant and happy.

59. _____ The nurse discusses a resident's problem with you and states that she knows you will keep the information confidential.

60. _____ When you are assigned to give care to a resident, you make sure his care is done thoroughly and exactly as instructed.

61. _____ Your co-worker says she needs help to turn her resident and you cheerfully offer to help.

A. Caring
B. Dependability
C. Consideration
D. Cheerfulness
E. Empathy
F. Trustworthiness
G. Respectfulness
H. Courtesy
I. Conscientiousness
J. Honesty
K. Cooperation
L. Enthusiasm
M. Self-awareness

Independent Learning Activities

1. How well do you take care of your own health? What can you do to improve your health practices?
   - Do you maintain a healthy weight by eating calories adequate for your energy needs? What can you do to improve your diet?
   - How much sleep do you get each night?
   - How do you practice good body mechanics at all times, not just at work?
   - How many hours do you exercise each week? What type of exercise do you do?
   - When did you last have your eyes checked? Do you wear glasses if they were prescribed?
   - Do you smoke? How much? Have you considered any smoking-cessation programs?
   - Are you taking any drugs that affect your thinking, feeling, behavior, and function? Did a doctor prescribe them, or are you self-medicating? Have you talked with your doctor about the effect of any drugs you are taking?
   - Do you drink alcohol? How much? Have you been told that it affects your behavior? Have you considered finding a program to help you to quit drinking alcohol?

2. Have you ever applied for a job? How did you feel when you were being interviewed? After reading this chapter, how would you handle a future interview?
   - Role-play a job interview with a classmate. Take turns playing the interviewer and the job applicant. Use the lists in this chapter to ask questions. Practice answers that you can use in a real interview.
   - Think of three people who you might use as references when applying for a job. Ask their permission to use them as references. If they agree, make a list of the people and their titles, addresses, and telephone numbers to use when you apply for a job.

Communicating With the Health Team

Abbreviation	Medical diagnosis	Recording
Assessment	Medical record	Reporting
Chart	Nursing diagnosis	Root
Communication	Nursing intervention	Signs
Comprehensive care plan	Nursing process	Subjective data
Conflict	Objective data	Suffix
Evaluation	Observation	Symptoms
Goal	Prefix	Triggers
Implementation	Progress note	Word element
Kardex		

Fill in the Blanks: Key Terms

Select your answers from the Key Terms listed above.

1. A written guide giving directions about the nursing care that a person should receive is a

   _____.

2. A _____ is a word element placed at the beginning of a word to change the meaning of the word.

3. An _____ is a shortened form of a word or phrase.

4. Clues for the resident assessment protocols are

   _____.

5. A _____ is an action or measure that the nursing team takes to help the person reach a goal.

6. _____ is the exchange of information; a message sent is received and interpreted by the intended person.

7. Collecting information about the person is

   _____.

8. Information that can be seen, heard, felt, or smelled by another person is _____, also called signs.

9. A _____ is a clash between opposing interests and ideas.

10. A type of card file that summarizes information found in the medical record is a

    _____.

11. _____ is that which is reported by a person and cannot be observed by using the senses, also called symptoms.

12. A part of a word is a _____.

13. A _____ is that which is desired in or by the person as a result of nursing care.

14. The method used by RNs to plan and deliver care is called the _____.

15. Subjective data is also called

    _____.

16. Using the senses of sight, hearing, touch, and smell to collect information about a person is

    _____.

17. Measuring if the goals in the planning step of the nursing process were met is

    _____.

18. Objective data is also called

    _____.

19. The _____ is the medical record.

20. The identification of a disease or condition by a doctor is a _____.

21. _____ is a verbal account of resident care and observations.

22. A written description of the care given and the person's response and progress is the

    _____.

23. A word element placed at the end of a root word to change the meaning of the word is a

    _____.

24. A _____ is a statement describing a health problem that can be treated by nursing measures.

25. A word element containing the basic meaning of the word is the _____.

26. _____ is performing or carrying out nursing measures in the care plan.

27. A _____ is a written account of a person's illness and response to the treatment and care given by the health team, also called a chart.

28. Writing or charting resident care and observations is

    _____.

Circle the BEST Answer

29. For communication to be effective:
    A. Use words that have the same meaning for the sender and the receiver.
    B. Use terms that are unfamiliar to residents and families.
    C. Add unrelated information to the message.
    D. Answers should not be specific.

30. The medical record will include all of the following *except*
    A. Physical examination results
    B. Graphic sheet
    C. Change-of-shift reports
    D. X-ray examination reports

31. To prevent errors and improper placement of records, the medical record is
    A. Kept in the resident's room
    B. Placed in a locked cabinet
    C. Stamped with the person's name, room number, and other identifying information on each page
    D. Printed on colored paper

32. Before a nursing assistant reads a resident's chart, he or she should
    A. Know the center's policy.
    B. Ask the nurse for permission.
    C. Ask the doctor's permission.
    D. Sign a sheet to get permission.

33. If a resident asks to see the chart, you should:
    A. Give it to the resident because the person always has a right to see the chart.
    B. Read the chart and tell the person what it says.
    C. Report the request to your supervisor.
    D. Tell the person that residents are not allowed to see the chart.

34. The admission sheet is used to
    A. Find out the resident's physical condition.
    B. Help the resident become familiar with the center.
    C. Learn background information about a person.
    D. Carry out a physical examination.

35. Progress notes are usually written
    A. Every shift
    B. When there is a change in the resident's condition
    C. Each day
    D. Once a year

36. OBRA requires that summaries of care be written
    A. Once a day
    B. Once every month
    C. At least every 3 months
    D. Once a year

37. What information is *not* included on the activities of daily living flow sheet?
    A. Temperature, pulse, and respirations
    B. Activity
    C. Bowel movements
    D. Amount of food consumed

38. The nursing process includes all of the following *except*
    A. Assessment
    B. History
    C. Implementation
    D. Evaluation

39. You can assist the RN to assess a person's body systems and mental status by
    A. Performing a physical examination
    B. Making observations as you give care and talk to the resident
    C. Giving physical care
    D. Taking a history

40. Objective data are
    A. Seen, heard, felt, or smelled
    B. Written information
    C. Things a person tells you that you cannot observe through the senses
    D. A weekly evaluation

41. Subjective data are
    A. Seen, heard, felt, or smelled
    B. Written information
    C. Things a person tells you that you cannot observe through the senses
    D. A weekly evaluation

42. A minimum data set (MDS) is
    A. Completed when the resident is admitted to the center
    B. Updated before each care conference
    C. Renewed and completed once a year or when a change occurs
    D. All of the above

43. Who has the final responsibility for information on the MDS?
    A. The RN responsible for resident care
    B. The LPN/LVN who is caring for the resident
    C. The director of nursing
    D. The doctor who is caring for the resident

44. A nursing diagnosis
    A. Is the identification of a disease or condition by the doctor
    B. Is a health problem that can be treated by nursing measures
    C. Is a physical assessment
    D. Are the priorities and goals set during planning care

45. Clues in the MDS are called
    A. Signs   C. Symptoms
    B. Triggers   D. Diagnosis

46. Resident assessment protocols (RAP) are
    A. Health problems that can be treated by nursing measures
    B. Activities of daily living
    C. Guidelines used to develop the resident care plan
    D. Problems identified on the MDS

47. An interdisciplinary care planning (IDCP) conference is held regularly to
    A. Identify the medical diagnosis
    B. Review and update care plans
    C. Share end-of-shift report information
    D. Chart day-to-day care of the person

48. Care plan suggestions are welcomed from
    A. Nurses
    B. Nursing assistants
    C. Other health team members
    D. All of the above

49. The nursing care plan
    A. Changes only at the IDCP conference
    B. Is revised as the person's needs change
    C. Stays the same after being developed at admission
    D. Changes daily for every resident

50. If you make an error when recording, you should
    A. Erase it.
    B. Use correction fluid to cover it.
    C. Throw away the page and start over.
    D. Cross out the incorrect part and write "error" over it.

51. Assignment sheets
    A. List information from the care plan
    B. Communicate tasks delegated to you
    C. Record vital signs
    D. Give the days that the nursing assistant is scheduled to work

52. The resident and family can
    A. Attend the IDCP conference
    B. Attend problem-focused conferences
    C. Refuse actions suggested by the health team at a conference
    D. All of the above

Circle the word that is spelled correctly for each of the following definitions (Questions #53 through #62)..

53. Slow heart rate
    A. Bradecardia   C. Bradacordia
    B. Bradycardia   D. Bradicardia

54. Difficulty in urinating
    A. Dysuria   C. Dysuira
    B. Dysurya   D. Disuria

55. Paralysis on one side of the body
    A. Hemyplegia   C. Hemoplega
    B. Hemaplegia   D. Hemiplegia

56. Opening into the ileum
    A. Ileostomie   C. Ileastoma
    B. Ileostomy   D. Illiostomy

57. Blue color or condition
    A. Cyonosis   C. Cyanosis
    B. Cyinosis   D. Cianosys

58. Opening into trachea
    A. Tracheastomy   C. Tracheostome
    B. Trachiostomy   D. Tracheostomy

59. Pain in a nerve
    A. Neuralgia   C. Nourealgia
    B. Neuroalgia   D. Neurilegia

60. Examination of a joint with a scope
    A. Arthoscopie   C. Arethroscopy
    B. Arthroscopy   D. Artheroscope

61. Rapid breathing
    A. Tachepnea   C. Tachypnea
    B. Tachypinea   D. Tachypnia

62. Removal of gallbladder
    A. Cholecystectomy   C. Cholicystetomy
    B. Cholcystectomy   D. Cholecistectomy

63. When you are given a computer password, you
    A. Must never change it
    B. Can share it with a co-worker
    C. Should never tell anyone your password
    D. Can use another person's password when entering the computer

64. Computers should not be used to
    A. Send messages and reports to the nursing unit
    B. Store resident records and care plans
    C. Send e-mails that require immediate reporting
    D. Monitor blood pressure, temperatures, and heart rates

65. When you answer the telephone, do not place callers on hold if
    A. The person has an emergency.
    B. It is a doctor.
    C. The call needs to be transferred to another unit.
    D. You are too busy to find the nurse.

66. If you have a conflict with a co-worker, you should
    A. Ask the nurse in charge to schedule you at different times.
    B. Ignore the person.
    C. Identify the cause of the conflict and try to resolve it.
    D. Talk to other co-workers to explain your side of the story.

67. When a conflict occurs, what is the first step you should take?
    A. Talk with other co-workers to see if they also have a conflict with the person.
    B. Confront the person and demand that the person meet with you.
    C. Identify the real problem.
    D. Assume the conflict will resolve itself if you ignore it.

68. Why is it important to resolve a conflict at work?
    A. Unkind words or actions may occur.
    B. The work environment becomes unpleasant.
    C. Resident care is affected.
    D. All of the above are true.

Matching

Match the word with the correct definition.

69. _____ Neuralgia

70. _____ Gastrostomy

71. _____ Cholecystectomy

72. _____ Dysuria

73. _____ Gastritis

74. _____ Enteritis

75. _____ Bacteriogenic

76. _____ Glossitis

77. _____ Cyanotic

78. _____ Dermatology

79. _____ Oophorectomy

80. _____ Colostomy

81. _____ Nephritis

82. _____ Bronchoscope

83. _____ Proctoscopy

A. Difficulty urinating

B. Inflammation of kidneys

C. Pertaining to blue coloration

D. Caused by bacteria

E. Study of the skin

F. Incision into large intestine

G. Instrument used to examine bronchi

H. Inflammation of the tongue

I. Nerve pain

J. Examination of rectum with instrument

K. Excision of gallbladder

L. Excision of ovary

M. Incision into stomach

N. Inflammation of stomach

O. Inflammation of intestine

Fill in the Blanks

84. What are the four senses you use to obtain information about a patient?

_____

_____

_____

_____

85. Each of the following is either subjective or objective data. In the blank next to each statement, place an "S" for subjective and an "O" for objective.

A. _____ Sleepy

B. _____ Chest pain

C. _____ Skin cool

D. _____ Cyanosis of nails

E. _____ Labored breathing

F. _____ Gas pain

G. _____ Pain when urinating

H. _____ Productive cough

I. _____ Breath has fruity odor

J. _____ Pulse rapid

86. Next to each time, write the time using the 24-hour clock.

A. _____ 11:00 AM   G. _____ 3:00 AM

B. _____ 8:00 AM   H. _____ 4:50 AM

C. _____ 4:00 PM   I. _____ 5:30 PM

D. _____ 7:30 AM   J. _____ 10:45 PM

E. _____ 6:45 PM   K. _____ 11:55 PM

F. _____ 12 noon   L. _____ 9:15 PM

Write the definition of each prefix.

87. Auto-: _____

88. Brady-: _____

89. Dys-: _____

90. Ecto-: _____

91. Leuk-: _____

92. Macro-: _____

93. Neo-: _____

94. Supra-: _____

95. Uni-: _____

Write the definition of each root word.

96. Adeno: _____

97. Angio: _____

98. Broncho: _____

99. Cranio: _____

100. Duodeno: _____

101. Entero: _____

102. Gyneco: _____

103. Masto: _____

104. Pyo: _____

Write the definition of each suffix.

105. -asis: _____

106. -genic: _____

107. -oma: _____

108. -phasia: _____

109. -ptosis: _____

110. -plegia: _____

111. -megaly: _____

112. -scopy: _____

113. -stasis: _____

Write the correct abbreviations.

114. Before meals: _____

115. After meals: _____

116. With: _____

117. Cancer: _____

118. Discontinued: _____

119. Lower left quadrant: _____

120. Every day: _____

121. Range-of-motion: _____

Labeling

Convert the times from military to standard time and from standard to military time. Use the chart as a guide.

122. 2:00 AM: _____

123. 10:30 AM: _____

124. 5:00 AM: _____

125. 9:30 AM: _____

126. 5:45 PM: _____

127. 10:45 PM: _____

128. 0600 hrs: _____ AM/PM

129. 1145 hrs: _____ AM/PM

130. 1800 hrs: _____ AM/PM

131. 2200 hrs: _____ AM/PM

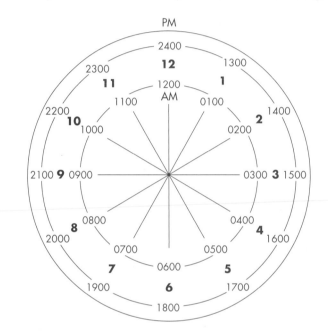

Label the four abdominal regions in the drawing. Use RUQ, LUQ, RLQ, and LLQ to label.

132. A. _____

B. _____

C. _____

D. _____

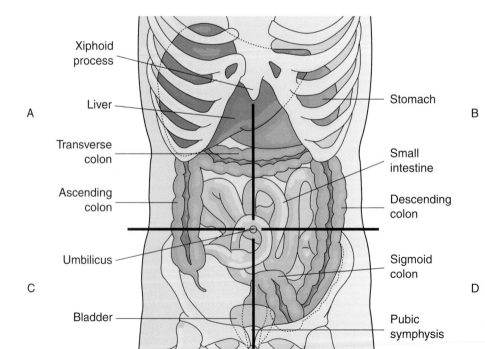

Nursing Assistant Skills Video Exercise

*View the **Basic Principles** video to answer these questions.*

133. Basic rules of communication

A. _____

B. _____

C. _____

D. _____

E. _____

F. _____

134. When you communicate with the person, you should

A. _____

B. _____

C. _____

D. _____

E. _____

135. When recording, what should you record, and what rules are important?

A. _____

B. _____

C. _____

D. _____

E. _____

F. _____

G. _____

H. _____

136. What are the five steps in the nursing process?

A. _____

B. _____

C. _____

D. _____

E. _____

Optional Learning Exercises

Class Experiment

Describing fluids in a clear and precise manner is often difficult. Set up the following examples that imitate situations in which you need to describe intake, output, or drainage. Describe as accurately as possible what you see in terms of amounts, colors, and textures. Compare your notes with classmates to see if you are using words that all have the same meaning. What words were used that were clear to understand? What words were used that had more than one meaning?

- Bloody drainage: Mix a teaspoon of ketchup and a teaspoon of water. Pour onto the center of a paper napkin.
- Urine: Pour a tablespoon of tea into the center of a paper towel.
- Bleeding: Smear a teaspoon of red jelly in the center of a paper towel.
- Broth: Pour 4 ounces of tea into a bowl.

Class Experiment

Substance	Observations
Bloody drainage	
Urine	
Bleeding	
Broth	

Case Study

Mr. Larsen was admitted to a subacute care center after his abdominal surgery 1 week ago. This morning, the nursing assistant gave Mr. Larsen a shower and assisted him in sitting in a comfortable chair. The nursing assistant noticed that he sat there very still and held his arms across his abdomen. He asked for a pillow and held it tightly against his abdomen.

Imagine that you are the patient and answer these questions.
- What would you like the nursing assistant to ask you?
- How would you communicate your feelings to the nursing assistant?
- How might you let the nursing assistant know that you had pain without telling her?

Imagine that you are the nursing assistant and answer these questions.
- What observations would be important to make about Mr. Larsen?
- What questions might you ask Mr. Larsen?
- What nonverbal communication would give you information about Mr. Larsen?

Case Study

Mrs. Miller was admitted to the health care center since you began working 3 days ago. You have just started your shift and have been assigned to Mrs. Miller.
- What information would you need to know before giving care? Why?
- What information would be important to provide to the oncoming shift?
- What methods would you use to communicate this information?

Independent Learning Activities

1. Answer these questions about situations in which you may need to communicate with others.
   - When have you had a problem with communicating?
   - Why was it difficult to communicate?
   - How did you handle this problem?

2. Think about a situation in which you believed that you communicated your point well.
   - What made the communication successful? How might you use a similar technique in caring for residents?
   - How would you communicate with a person who speaks a language that you do not speak or understand? What methods might you use to explain what you are going to do?
   - How would you communicate with a person from a different culture?

3. Make flash cards of the prefixes, suffixes, and root words in Chapter 4. Place the meaning of each one on the back of the appropriate card. Work alone or with a partner, and, by looking at the cards, practice identifying the correct meaning of each term.

4. The next time you or a member of your family visits the doctor and are instructed to fill a prescription, look at what the doctor has written. Do you see any abbreviations that you learned in this chapter? What do they mean? How did this chapter help you understand what was written?

5

Understanding the Resident

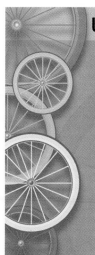

Body language	Holism	Religion
Comatose	Need	Self-actualization
Culture	Nonverbal communication	Self-esteem
Disability	Optimal level of function	Verbal communication
Esteem	Paraphrasing	

Fill in the Blanks: Key Terms

Select your answers from the Key Terms listed above.

1. Experiencing one's potential is called

   _____.

2. _____

   is thinking well of oneself, seeing oneself as useful,

   and being well thought of by others.

3. A person's highest potential for mental and physical

   performance is the _____.

4. A _____

   is that which is necessary or desirable for main-

   taining life and mental well-being.

5. Communication that uses the written or spoken word

   is called _____.

6. _____ is lost,

   absent, or impaired physical or mental function.

7. _____

   is communication that does not involve words.

8. The characteristics of a group of people—language,

   values, beliefs, habits, likes, dislikes, customs—

   passed from one generation to the next is called

   _____.

9. The worth, value, or opinion that one has of a person

   is _____.

10. _____

    is spiritual beliefs, needs, and practices.

11. A person who is _____

    has an inability to respond to verbal stimuli.

12. Restating the person's message in your own words is

    called _____.

13. _____

    sends messages through facial expressions, gestures,

    posture, and body movements.

14. _____

    is a concept that considers the whole person.

Circle the BEST Answer

15. Who is the most important person in the nursing
    center?
    A. The director of nursing
    B. The resident
    C. The doctor
    D. The nurse

16. Which of these losses may have happened to an
    older resident?
    A. Loss of home and family members
    B. Loss of the person's role in the family or
       community
    C. Loss of body functions
    D. All of the above

17. When speaking about the resident, which of these
    statements is best?
    A. "Mrs. Jones in 135 needs a pain pill."
    B. "Granny Jones needs something for pain."
    C. "135 needs a pain pill."
    D. "Janie is complaining of pain."

18. What is the main reason you call a resident by a title
    such as Mr., Mrs., or Miss?
    A. It best identifies the person.
    B. It gives the person dignity and respect.
    C. It is polite.
    D. It shows the person that you are in charge.

19. When is it acceptable to call a person by his or her
    first name or another name?
    A. You have cared for the person for several months.
    B. The person is confused.
    C. The person asks you to use the name.
    D. The person has difficulty hearing.

20. Which of these needs is affected when the person is
    ill or is an older adult?
    A. Physical   C. Psychologic
    B. Social   D. All of the above

21. What needs are most important for survival?
    A. Physical   C. Love and belonging
    B. Safety and security   D. Self-esteem

22. It is important for the person to know what to expect
    when care is given because the person will
    A. Be combative
    B. Feel safer and more secure
    C. Have a more meaningful relationship
    D. Experience his or her potential

23. What need is rarely, if ever, totally met?
    A. Physiological   C. Self-esteem
    B. Safety and security   D. Self-actualization

24. Mrs. Young is a new resident. All of the following
    will help her feel more secure *except*
    A. Giving her explanations of routines and proce-
       dures only one time
    B. Treating her with kindness and patience
    C. Making sure she understands how a procedure is
       to be done
    D. Listening to her concerns and explaining all rou-
       tines and procedures as often as is needed

25. Mrs. Peck never has visitors and is becoming weaker
    and unable to care for herself. What need is not
    being met?
    A. Physiological   C. Love and belonging
    B. Safety and security   D. Self-esteem

26. Which of these practices may relate to both religion
    and culture?
    A. Language
    B. Hygiene habits
    C. Days of worship
    D. Beliefs about causes and cures of illness

27. When you are caring for a person of a different cul-
    ture, you should
    A. Expect all people in the culture to follow the
       same practices.
    B. Judge the person by your standards.
    C. Remember that each person is unique.
    D. Ignore the cultural practices.

28. A person who is ill and disabled is often angry
    because
    A. The care that the person is receiving is poor.
    B. This response to illness and disability is common.
    C. The person does not like you.
    D. The person has a bad temper.

29. How can you help Mr. Clay maintain his optimal level of functioning?
    A. Give him complete care.
    B. Encourage him to be as independent as is possible.
    C. Avoid staying with him to visit.
    D. Do not respond promptly when he asks for help.

30. Mrs. Nelson is alert and oriented. Why would she require care in a nursing center?
    A. She has trouble remembering where she is.
    B. She cannot tell you what she needs or wants.
    C. She has a disabling disease such as arthritis or multiple sclerosis.
    D. She does not know who she is.

31. Which of the following is a reason that confusion and disorientation may be temporary?
    A. The person has a disabling disease.
    B. The person is newly admitted to the nursing center.
    C. The person needs complete help with all activities of daily living (ADL).
    D. The person is terminally ill.

32. Mrs. Smithers is admitted to the nursing center. The nurse tells you that Mrs. Smithers will be here only short term. You know that the reason for most short-term admissions is to
    A. Provide quality care to dying residents
    B. Give complete care to the resident
    C. Help the resident recover from fractures, acute illness, or surgery
    D. Prevent injury of the resident

33. Respite care provides
    A. Time to recover from surgery or acute illness
    B. Recover from temporary confusion
    C. Care for a dying person
    D. The caregiver a chance to take a vacation, tend to business, or rest

34. A person who needs lifelong care has a disability that occurs
    A. Because of birth defects or childhood illnesses or injuries
    B. Because of mental illness
    C. Because of the aging process
    D. Because the person is dying

35. If a resident were comatose, how would you know whether the person is in pain?
    A. The person cries and lies very still.
    B. The person asks for pain medications.
    C. Pain is shown by grimacing and groaning.
    D. You cannot tell if the person is in pain.

36. Which of these ways to deal with a person with behavior issues would not be helpful?
    A. Argue with the person to show him that he is wrong.
    B. Explain reasons for long waits.
    C. Answer the person's questions clearly and thoroughly.
    D. Stay calm and professional if the anger and hostility is directed at you.

37. Which of the following would *not* help effective communication?
    A. Use words that have the same meaning to both you and the person.
    B. Communicate in a logical and orderly manner.
    C. Give specific and factual information.
    D. Use medical terminology when talking to the person.

38. Mrs. Stevens cannot speak. How does she use verbal communication?
    A. She may use touch.
    B. Her body language sends messages.
    C. She can use gestures to communicate.
    D. She may write messages on a paper pad.

39. When you go to Mrs. Hart's room, you can tell that she is not happy or not feeling well because
    A. Her hair is well groomed.
    B. She has a slumped posture.
    C. She smiles when you come in the room.
    D. She protects an affected body part.

40. All of the following would show that you listen effectively *except* when you
    A. Face the resident and have good eye contact.
    B. Lean back and cross your arms.
    C. Respond to the resident by asking questions.
    D. Use words the person can understand.

41. Which of these statements is paraphrasing?
    A. "You don't know how long you will be here."
    B. "Do you want to take a tub bath or a shower?"
    C. "Tell me about living on a farm."
    D. "Can you explain what you mean?"

42. When you say, "Mr. Davis, have you taken a shower this morning?" you are
    A. Paraphrasing his thoughts
    B. Asking a direct question
    C. Focusing his thoughts
    D. Asking an open-ended question

43. Responses to open-ended questions are generally
    A. Longer and give more information than direct questions
    B. Yes or no answers
    C. Able to make sure you understand the message
    D. Focused on dealing with a certain topic

44. Mr. Parker often rambles and tells long stories during which his thoughts wander. You need to know if he had a bowel movement today, so you will
    A. Make a clarifying statement.
    B. Ask an open-ended question.
    C. Ask a focusing question.
    D. Paraphrase his thoughts.

45. What is best if the person takes long pauses between statements?
    A. Just being there shows you care.
    B. Try to cheer up the person by talking.
    C. Leave the room.
    D. Find another resident to talk with the person.

46. Mrs. Duke has visitors and you need to give care. What would you do?
    A. Give the care while visitors are present.
    B. Politely ask the visitors to leave the room.
    C. Tell the visitors to give the care.
    D. Tell the visitors that they must leave the nursing center.

Basic Needs Exercise

47. Fill in the blanks with the correct needs.

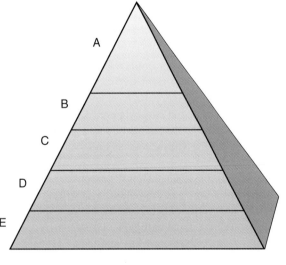

Physical   Safety and security
Love and belonging   Self-esteem
Self-actualization

A. _____

B. _____

C. _____

D. _____

E. _____

Optional Learning Exercises
Basic Needs
Physical Needs

48. What are the six physical needs required for survival?

_____

_____

_____

_____

_____

_____

49. The physical needs must be met before the

_____ needs.

Safety and Security

50. Safety and security needs relate to protection from

_____,

_____, and

_____.

51. Why do many people feel a loss of safety and security when they are admitted to a nursing center?

    A. _____

    B. _____

    C. _____

Love and Belonging

52. The need for love and belonging relates to

_____,

_____,

_____,

_____, and

_____.

53. How can you help a resident feel loved and accepted?

_____

_____

Self-Esteem

54. To what does self-esteem relate?

A. _____

B. _____

C. _____

55. Why is it important to encourage residents to do as much as possible for themselves?

_____

Self-Actualization

56. What does self-actualization involve?

_____

_____

_____

_____

57. What happens if self-actualization is postponed?

_____

_____

Culture and Religion Practices

Religion

58. How can you help a resident observe religious practices if services are held in the nursing center?

_____

_____

59. What should you do if the resident wants to leave the center to attend services or have a visit from a spiritual leader?

_____

_____

60. What should you do if the resident wants a pastor to visit in the room?

_____

_____

_____

Cultural Health Care Beliefs

Mexico and the Dominican Republic

61. What happens when hot and cold imbalances occur?

_____

_____

62. What are "hot" conditions?

_____

_____

_____

_____

_____

63. What are "cold" conditions?

_____

_____

_____

_____

_____

_____

Vietnam

64. How are foods and medications given to restore hot-cold balance?

    _____

    _____

    _____

    _____

Cultural Sick Practices

Vietnam

65. How do Vietnamese folk practices treat the following illnesses?

    A. Common cold:

    _____

    B. Headache and sore throat:

    _____

66. What illnesses do these Russian folk practices treat?

    A. _____:

    an ointment is placed behind the ears and

    temples, and also the back of the neck.

    B. _____:

    place a dough made of dark rye flour and honey

    on the spinal column.

Cultural Touch Practices

67. Why is touch important in the Mexican and Philippine cultures?

    _____

    _____

68. What nonverbal communications using touch is common in Russia?

    _____

    _____

69. If you are caring for a resident from India, what might you notice about his practice of hands?

    _____

    _____

70. Residents from some countries might not like to be touched. Give two examples of these countries.

    _____

    _____

Eye Contact Practices

71. Why would you avoid making direct eye contact with a resident from Mexico?

    _____

    _____

72. If a resident from Vietnam blinks when you explain a

    procedure, it probably means that the message

    _____

    _____.

73. Direct eye contact is practiced among people from

    _____ and

    _____.

Family Roles in Sick Care

74. You are caring for a resident from China. You might expect the family members to

    _____,

    _____, and

    _____

    the person.

75. A man from Mexico is a resident, and his daughter says that she cannot care for him when he goes home. This failure may be because, in Mexico, women cannot give care if

    _____,

    _____.

Communication Techniques

You have completed your duties for the morning and have some free time. Mr. Harry Donal is a resident in the nursing center. He rarely has visitors, and you try to spend time with him when you can. Complete the following statements about communication techniques that you use when you visit with Mr. Donal.

76. You sit in a chair next to Mr. Donal so you can see each other. This position will help you to have better

    _____.

77. You should lean _____

    Mr. Donal to show interest.

78. Mr. Donal says, "I know this is the best place for me, but I miss my flower garden at home." You respond, "You miss your home." This response is an example of _____.

79. You ask Mr. Donal, "You told me you did not sleep well last night. Can you tell me why?" He replies, "There was a lot of noise in the hall." This response is an example of a

    _____.

80. You say to Mr. Donal, "Tell me about your flower garden at home." This statement is an

    _____ statement.

81. When you say, "Can you explain what that means?" you are asking a person to

    _____.

82. Mr. Donal says that he "hurts all over" and then begins to talk about the weather. You say, "Tell me more about where you hurt. You said you hurt all over." This statement helps in _____

    _____ the topic.

83. Mr. Donal begins to cry when he talks about his flower garden. You can show caring and respect for his situation and feelings by _____

    _____.

84. When Mr. Donal begins to cry, you quickly begin to talk about the activities planned this morning. Changing the subject is a

    _____.

Independent Learning Activities

1. Use the section of Chapter 5 that discusses needs to think about how well you are meeting your own needs.
   - Do you smoke? What needs may be affected by smoking?
   - What kinds of foods and fluids do you eat? Is your diet meeting your basic needs for food and water?
   - How much rest and sleep do you get each day? How much do you need to feel well rested?
   - How safe do you feel at home? At school? In your community? How do your feelings affect your ability to hold a job or attend school?
   - Who are the people who make you feel loved? Who helps you when you have problems?
   - What are you doing that helps you meet the need for self-actualization?

2. Answer these questions about your personal health care practices.
   - What health care practices are followed in your family? How are these practices related to your cultural or religious beliefs?
   - How often do you go to the doctor? For regular checkups? Only when ill?
   - When do you go to the dentist? Once or twice a year for cleaning and checkups? Only when you have a toothache?
   - When a family member is in a health care center, how does your family respond? Does someone stay with the person and perform all of the care, or do family members visit for brief periods and let health care workers provide all of the care? Is the family response related to any cultural or religious practices?

3. Look at your answers to both of the previous sets of questions.
   - How well are you meeting your basic needs? How can you improve in meeting these needs? What changes would be the most beneficial?
   - How much influence on your practices comes from cultural or religious traditions in your family? Are these influences helping you or hindering you in meeting needs?

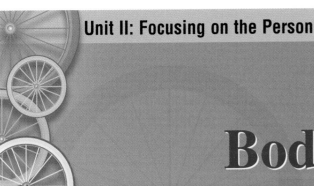

Body Structure and Function

Artery	Hormone	Peristalsis
Capillary	Immunity	Respiration
Cell	Menstruation	System
Digestion	Metabolism	Tissue
Hemoglobin	Organ	Vein

Fill in the Blanks: Key Terms

Select your answers from the Key Terms listed above.

1. The substance in red blood cells that carries oxygen and gives blood its color is

   _____.

2. _____

   is protection against a disease or condition.

3. The process of supplying the cells with oxygen and removing carbon dioxide from them is

   _____.

4. The process of physically and chemically breaking down food so that it can be absorbed for use by the

   cells is _____.

5. _____ is the

   burning of food for heat and energy by the cells.

6. A blood vessel that carries blood away from the

   heart is an _____.

7. _____ is the

   involuntary muscle contractions in the digestive

   system that move food through the alimentary canal.

8. Organs that work together to perform special func-

   tions form a _____.

9. The basic unit of body structure is a

   _____.

10. Groups of tissues with the same function form an

    _____.

11. A _____

    is a tiny blood vessel.

12. A group of cells with similar function is

_____.

13. _____ is the

process by which the lining of the uterus breaks up

and is discharged from the body through the vagina.

14. A chemical substance that the glands secrete into the

bloodstream is a _____.

15. A _____

is a blood vessel that carries blood back to the heart.

Circle the BEST Answer

16. A cell is
    A. Found only in muscles
    B. The basic unit of body structure
    C. Can exist without oxygen
    D. A group of tissues

17. The control center of a cell is the
    A. Membrane   C. Cytoplasm
    B. Protoplasm   D. Nucleus

18. Genes control
    A. Cell division
    B. Tissues
    C. Physical and chemical traits that children inherit
    D. Organs

19. Connective tissue
    A. Covers internal and external body surface
    B. Receives and carries impulses to the brain and
       back to body parts
    C. Anchors, connects, and supports other body tissues
    D. Allows the body to move by stretching and
       contracting

20. Living cells of the epidermis contain
    A. Blood vessels and many nerves
    B. Sweat and oil glands
    C. Pigment that gives skin color
    D. Hair roots

21. Sweat glands help
    A. The body regulate temperature
    B. Keep the hair and skin soft and shiny
    C. Protect the nose from dust, insects, and other
       foreign objects
    D. The skin sense pleasant and unpleasant sensations

22. Long bones
    A. Allow skill and ease in movement
    B. Bear the weight of the body
    C. Protect organs
    D. Allow various degrees of movement and flexion

23. Blood cells are manufactured in
    A. The heart
    B. The liver
    C. Blood vessels
    D. Bone marrow

24. Joints move smoothly because of
    A. Cartilage
    B. Synovial fluid
    C. Muscle
    D. Ligaments

25. A joint that moves in all directions is a
    A. Ball and socket
    B. Hinge
    C. Pivot
    D. All of the above

26. Voluntary muscles are
    A. Found in the stomach and intestines
    B. Attached to bones
    C. Cardiac muscles
    D. Tendons

27. Muscles produce heat by
    A. Contracting
    B. Relaxing
    C. Maintaining posture
    D. Working automatically

28. The central nervous system consists of
    A. A myelin sheath
    B. Nerves throughout the body
    C. The brain and spinal column
    D. Cranial nerves

29. The medulla controls
    A. Muscle contraction and relaxation
    B. Heart rate, breathing, blood vessel size, and
       swallowing
    C. Reasoning, memory, and consciousness
    D. Hearing and vision

30. Cerebrospinal fluid
    A. Cushions shocks that can injure structures of the
       brain and spinal cord
    B. Controls voluntary muscles
    C. Lubricates movement
    D. Controls involuntary muscles

31. Cranial nerves conduct impulses between the
    A. Brain and the head, neck, chest, and abdomen
    B. Brain and the skin and extremities
    C. Brain and internal body structure
    D. Spinal cord and lower extremities

32. Which nervous system is stimulated when you are frightened?
    A. Sympathetic
    B. Parasympathetic
    C. Central
    D. Cranial

33. Receptors for vision and nerve fibers of the optic nerve are found in the
    A. Sclera
    B. Choroids
    C. Retina
    D. Cornea

34. What structure of the ear is involved in balance?
    A. Malleus
    B. Auditory canal
    C. Tympanic membranes
    D. Semicircular canals

35. Hemoglobin in red blood cells gives blood its red color and carries
    A. Oxygen
    B. Food to cells
    C. Waste products
    D. Water

36. Red blood cells remain viable for
    A. Approximately 9 days
    B. 3 or 4 months
    C. 4 days
    D. 1 year

37. White blood cells or leukocytes
    A. Protect the body against infection
    B. Are necessary for blood clotting
    C. Carry food, hormone, chemicals, and waste products
    D. Pick up carbon dioxide

38. The left atrium of the heart
    A. Receives blood from the lungs
    B. Receives blood from the body tissues
    C. Pumps blood to the lungs
    D. Pumps blood to all parts of the body

39. Arteries
    A. Return blood to the heart
    B. Pass food, oxygen, and other substances into the cells
    C. Pick up waste products, including carbon dioxide, from the cells
    D. Carry blood away from the heart

40. In the lungs, oxygen and carbon dioxide are exchanged
    A. In the epiglottis
    B. Between the right bronchus and the left bronchus
    C. By the bronchioles
    D. Between the alveoli and capillaries

41. The lungs are protected by
    A. The diaphragm
    B. The pleura
    C. A bony framework of the ribs, sternum, and vertebrae
    D. The lobes

42. Food is moved through the alimentary canal (gastrointestinal [GI] tract) by
    A. Chyme
    B. Peristalsis
    C. Swallowing
    D. Bile

43. Water is absorbed from chyme in the
    A. Small intestine
    B. Stomach
    C. Esophagus
    D. Large intestine

44. Digested food is absorbed through tiny projections called
    A. Jejunum
    B. Ileum
    C. Villi
    D. Colon

45. A function of the urinary system is to
    A. Remove waste products from the blood
    B. Rid the body of solid waste
    C. Rid the body of carbon dioxide
    D. Burn food for energy

46. A person feels the need to urinate when the bladder contains about
    A. 1000 ml of urine
    B. 500 ml of urine
    C. 250 ml of urine
    D. 125 ml of urine

47. Testosterone is needed for
    A. Male secondary sex characteristics
    B. Female secondary sex characteristics
    C. Sperm to be produced
    D. Ova to be produced

48. The prostate gland lies
    A. In the scrotum
    B. In the testes
    C. Just below the bladder
    D. In the penis

49. The ovaries secrete progesterone and
    A. Estrogen
    B. Testosterone
    C. Ova
    D. Semen

50. When an ovum is released from an ovary, it travels first through the
    A. Uterus
    B. Fallopian tubes
    C. Endometrium
    D. Vagina

51. Menstruation occurs when
    A. The hymen is ruptured
    B. The ovary releases an ovum
    C. The endometrium breaks up
    D. Fertilization occurs

52. A fertilized cell implants in the
    A. Ovary
    B. Fallopian tubes
    C. Endometrium
    D. Vagina

53. The master gland is the
    A. Thyroid gland
    B. Parathyroid gland
    C. Adrenal gland
    D. Pituitary gland

54. Thyroid hormone regulates
    A. Growth
    B. Metabolism
    C. Proper functioning of nerves and muscles
    D. Energy produced during exercise

55. If the pancreas produces too little insulin, the person has
    A. Tetany
    B. Slow growth
    C. Diabetes mellitus
    D. Slowed metabolism

56. When antigens enter the body, they are attacked and destroyed by
    A. Antibodies
    B. Lymphocytes
    C. B cells
    D. T cells

Matching

Match the terms with the description.

Musculoskeletal

57. _____ Connective tissue at the end of long bones

58. _____ Skeletal muscle

59. _____ Membrane that covers bone

60. _____ Connects muscle to bone

61. _____ Point at which two or more bones meet

62. _____ Heart muscle

63. _____ Involuntary muscle

64. _____ Acts as a lubricant so the joint can move smoothly

A. Periosteum

B. Joint

C. Cartilage

D. Synovial fluid

E. Striated muscle

F. Smooth muscle

G. Cardiac muscle

H. Tendons

Nervous System

65. _____ Contains eustachian tubes and ossicles

66. _____ Has 12 pairs of cranial nerves and 31 pairs of spinal nerves

67. _____ White of the eye

68. _____ Outside of cerebrum; controls highest function of brain

69. _____ Inner layer of eye that contains receptors for vision

70. _____ Controls involuntary muscles, heart beat, blood pressure, and other functions

71. _____ Structure through which light enters the eye

72. _____ Contain midbrain, pons, and medulla

73. _____ Waxy substance secreted in auditory canal

74. _____ Contains semicircular canal and cochlea

A. Sclera

B. Cornea

C. Retina

D. Cerumen

E. Middle ear

F. Inner ear

G. Brainstem

H. Cerebral cortex

I. Autonomic nervous system

J. Peripheral nervous system

Circulatory System

75. _____ Liquid part of blood

76. _____ Thin sac covering the heart

77. _____ Very tiny blood vessels

78. _____ Substance in blood that picks up oxygen

79. _____ Carry blood away from heart

80. _____ White blood cells

81. _____ Carry blood toward heart

82. _____ Red blood cells

83. _____ Thick, muscular portion of heart

84. _____ Platelets; necessary for clotting

85. _____ Membrane lining the inner surface of heart

A. Plasma

B. Erythrocytes

C. Hemoglobin

D. Leukocytes

E. Thrombocytes

F. Pericardium

G. Myocardium

H. Endocardium

I. Arteries

J. Veins

K. Capillaries

Respiratory System

86. _____ Into which air passes from larynx

87. _____ A two-layered sac that covers the lungs

88. _____ Piece of cartilage that acts as a lid over the larynx

89. _____ Separates lungs from the abdominal cavity

90. _____ The voice box

91. _____ Several small branches that divide from the bronchus

92. _____ Tiny one-celled air sacs

A. Epiglottis

B. Larynx

C. Bronchiole

D. Trachea

E. Alveoli

F. Diaphragm

G. Pleura

Digestive System

93. _____ Structure that adds extra digestive juices to chyme

94. _____ Semiliquid food mixture formed in stomach

95. _____ Portion of the GI tract that absorbs food

96. _____ Stores bile

97. _____ Portion of the GI tract that absorbs water

98. _____ Produces bile

99. _____ Moistens food particles in the mouth

100. _____ Produces digestive juices

A. Liver

B. Chyme

C. Colon

D. Duodenum

E. Jejunum

F. Saliva

G. Pancreas

H. Gallbladder

Urinary System

101. _____ Basic working unit of the kidney

102. _____ Bean-shaped structure that produces urine

103. _____ A cluster of capillaries in Bowman's capsule

104. _____ Structure that allows urine to pass from the bladder

105. _____ A tube that is attached to the renal pelvis of the kidney

106. _____ Hollow muscular sac that stores urine

107. _____ Opening at the end of the urethra

108. _____ Structure in which fluid and waste products form urine

A. Bladder

B. Glomerulus

C. Kidney

D. Meatus

E. Nephrons

F. Tubules

G. Ureter

H. Urethra

Reproductive System

109. _____ Male or female sex organs

110. _____ Two folds of tissue on each side of the vagina

111. _____ Sac between thighs that contains testes

112. _____ External genitalia of female

113. _____ Testicles; produces sperm

114. _____ Attached to uterus; ovum travels through this structure

115. _____ Stores sperm and produces semen

116. _____ Tissue lining the uterus

A. Scrotum

B. Testes

C. Seminal vesicle

D. Gonads

E. Fallopian tubes

F. Endometrium

G. Labia

H. Vulva

Endocrine System

117. _____ Released by pancreas: regulates sugar in blood

118. _____ Sex hormone secreted by testes

119. _____ Sex hormone secreted by ovaries

120. _____ Regulates metabolism

121. _____ Regulates calcium levels in the body

122. _____ Stimulates to produce energy during emergencies

A. Epinephrine

B. Estrogen

C. Insulin

D. Parahormone

E. Testosterone

F. Thyroxine

Immune System

123. _____ Normal body substances that recognize abnormal or unwanted substances

124. _____ Type of cell that destroys invading cells

125. _____ Type of white blood cell that digests and destroys microorganisms

126. _____ Type of cell that causes production of antibodies

127. _____ An abnormal or unwanted substance

128. _____ Types of white blood cells that produce antibodies

A. Antibodies

B. Antigens

C. Phagocytes

D. Lymphocytes

E. B cells

F. T cells

Labeling

129. Label the parts of the cell.

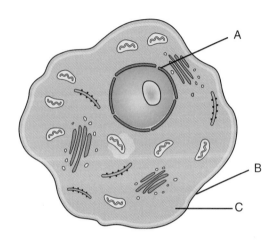

A. _____

B. _____

C. _____

130. Label each type of joint.

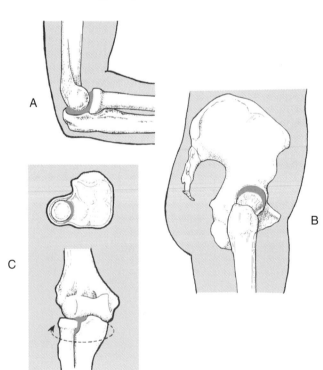

A. _____

B. _____

C. _____

131. Label the parts of the brain.

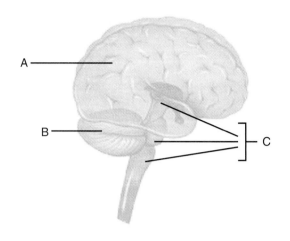

A. _____

B. _____

C. _____

132. Label the four chambers of the heart.

A. _____

B. _____

C. _____

D. _____

133. Label the structures of the respiratory system.

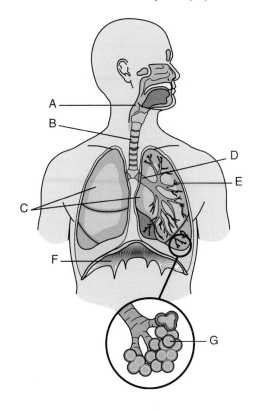

134. Label the structures of the digestive system.

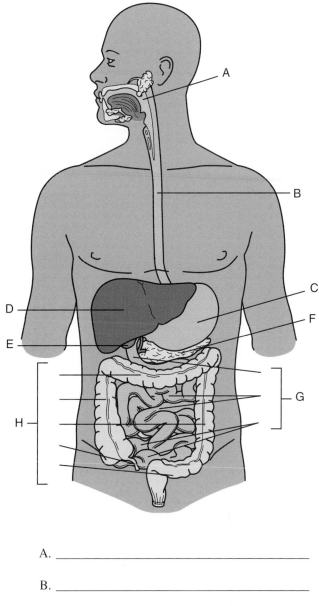

A. _____

B. _____

C. _____

D. _____

E. _____

F. _____

G. _____

A. _____

B. _____

C. _____

D. _____

E. _____

F. _____

G. _____

H. _____

135. Label the structures of the urinary system.

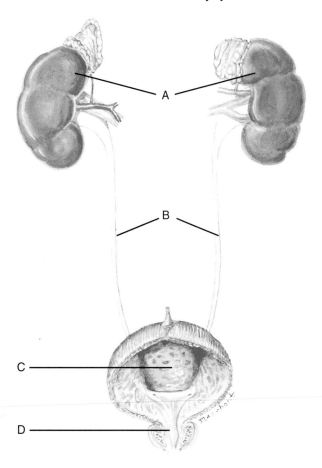

136. Label the structures of the male reproductive system.

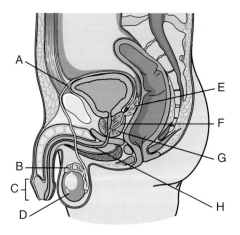

A. _____

B. _____

C. _____

D. _____

A. _____

B. _____

C. _____

D. _____

E. _____

F. _____

G. _____

H. _____

137. Label the external female genitalia.

A. _____

B. _____

C. _____

D. _____

E. _____

F. _____

Optional Learning Exercises

138. Explain the function of each part of the cell.

A. Cell membrane: _____

_____

B. Nucleus: _____

_____

C. Cytoplasm: _____

_____

D. Protoplasm: _____

_____

E. Chromosomes: _____

_____

F. Genes: _____

_____

139. List the structures that are contained in the two skin layers.

A. Epidermis: _____

_____

B. Dermis: _____

_____

140. Explain the function of the types of bone.

A. Long bones: _____

_____

B. Short bones: _____

_____

C. Flat bones: _____

_____

D. Irregular bones: _____

_____

141. Describe how each type of joint moves, and give an example of each type.

A. Ball and socket: _____

_____

_____

Ex: _____

B. Hinge: _____

_____

_____

Ex: _____

C. Pivot: _____

_____

_____

Ex: _____

142. Explain what happens when muscles contract.

_____

_____

_____

_____

143. Explain the function of the three main parts of the brain. Include the function of the cerebral cortex and the midbrain, pons, and medulla.

A. Cerebrum: _____

_____

Cerebral cortex: _____

_____

B. Cerebellum: _____

_____

C. Brainstem: _____

_____

Midbrain and pons: _____

_____

_____

Medulla: _____

_____

_____

144. Explain how the sympathetic and parasympathetic nervous systems balance each other.

_____

_____

_____

_____

_____

_____

145. Explain what happens to each of these structures when light enters the eye.

A. Choroid: _____

_____

B. Cornea: _____

_____

C. Lens: _____

_____

D. Retina: _____

_____

146. Explain how each of these structures help carry sound in the ear.

A. Ossicles: _____

_____

B. Cochlea: _____

_____

C. Auditory nerve: _____

_____

147. Where are red blood cells destroyed as they wear out?

_____

_____

148. When an infection occurs, what do white blood cells do?

_____

_____

149. Explain the function of the four atria of the heart.

    A. Right atrium: _____

    _____

    B. Left atrium: _____

    _____

    C. Right ventricle: _____

    _____

    D. Left ventricle: _____

    _____

150. Explain where each of these veins carries blood.

    A. Inferior vena cava: _____

    _____

    B. Superior vena cava: _____

    _____

151. Explain what happens in the alveoli.

    _____

    _____

    _____

152. After food is swallowed, explain what happens in each of these parts of the digestive tract.

    A. Stomach: _____

    _____

    B. Duodenum: _____

    _____

    C. Jejunum and ileum: _____

    _____

    D. Colon: _____

    _____

    E. Rectum: _____

    _____

    F. Anus: _____

153. Explain what happens in these structures of the kidney.

    A. Glomerulus: _____

    _____

    B. Collecting tubules: _____

    _____

    C. Ureters: _____

    _____

    D. Urethra: _____

    _____

    E. Meatus: _____

154. Sperm is produced in the testicles. What happens to the sperm in each of these structures?

    A. Testes: _____

    _____

    B. Vas deferens: _____

    _____

    C. Seminal vesicle: _____

    _____

    D. Ejaculatory duct: _____

    _____

    E. Prostate gland: _____

    _____

    F. Urethra: _____

155. What is the function of the endometrium?

_____

_____

156. Menstruation occurs about every _____

days. Ovulation usually occurs on or about day

_____ of the cycle.

157. What is the function of each of these pituitary hormones?

  A. Growth hormone: _____

  _____

  B. Thyroid-stimulating hormone: _____

  _____

  C. Adrenocorticotropic hormone: _____

  _____

  D. Antidiuretic hormone: _____

  _____

  E. Oxytocin: _____

  _____

158. What is the function of insulin?

_____

_____

_____

What happens if too little insulin is produced?

_____

_____

_____

159. What happens when the body senses an antigen?

_____

_____

Independent Learning Activities

1. Using your own body, move joints of each type to see how they move.
   - What joint is a ball and socket? How many ways were you able to move it?
   - What joint moves like a hinge? How does it work differently than the ball and socket?
   - What joint is a pivot joint? Compare its movement with the other two joints.

2. Listen to a friend's chest with a stethoscope.
   - What sounds do you hear?
   - What body systems are making the sounds?
   - Are you able to count any of the sounds you hear? What are you counting?

3. Listen to your lower abdomen with a stethoscope.
   - What sounds can you hear?
   - What causes sound in the abdomen? What body system is involved in this activity?
   - What is occurring when you hear your "stomach growl?" What is the term for this activity that you learned in this chapter?

4. Look at a friend's eyes in a dimly lighted area and observe the size of the pupils.
   - What size are the pupils? Are they both the same?
   - Shine a flashlight in the eye. What happens to the pupil?
   - What happens when you move the light away? If you see a change, how quickly does it occur?

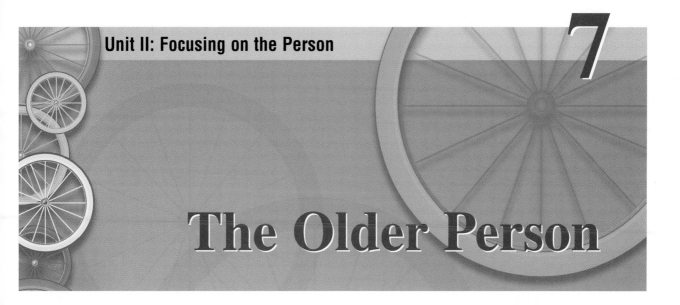

The Older Person

Dysphagia
Dyspnea
Geriatrics

Gerontology
Old
Old-old

Presbyopia
Young-old

Fill in the Blanks: Key Terms

Select your answers from the Key Terms listed above.

1. _____:

   difficult, labored, or painful breathing

2. _____:

   people over the age of 85

3. _____:

   difficulty swallowing

4. _____:

   people between the ages of 65 and 74

5. _____:

   the care of aging people

6. _____:

   people between the ages of 75 and 84

7. _____:

   the study of the aging process

8. _____:

   age-related farsightedness

Circle the BEST Answer

9. How many people today are over 65?
   A. 1 in 10
   B. 1 in 100
   C. 1 in 8
   D. 1 in 4

10. Most older people live
   A. In a nursing center
   B. Alone
   C. In a family setting
   D. With nonrelatives

11. The old-old age range is
    A. 65 to 74 years
    B. 75 to 84 years
    C. 60 to 65 years
    D. Over 85 years

12. As aging occurs
    A. Disability always results.
    B. Changes are gradual.
    C. Most people adapt poorly.
    D. All of the above are true.

13. Psychologic and social changes include
    A. Graying hair
    B. Disabilities
    C. The need for retirees to replace work with activities
    D. Decreased physical strength

14. It may be difficult to meet all self-esteem needs when retired because
    A. The person can do whatever he or she wants.
    B. Work brings fulfillment and usefulness.
    C. A retired person develops new relationships.
    D. Physical strength decreases.

15. Retired people may promote usefulness and well-being by
    A. Traveling
    B. Working part-time or doing volunteer work
    C. Living alone
    D. Developing new friends and relationships

16. Money problems can result with retirement because
    A. Income is reduced.
    B. Expenses increase.
    C. The person is unable to work.
    D. The person plans for retirement.

17. Loneliness may be a bigger problem for foreign-born persons because
    A. Families from other cultures do not care about older persons.
    B. The person is not accepted by native-born persons.
    C. They may not have anyone with whom to talk in their native language.
    D. They have more chronic illnesses.

18. An older person can adjust to social relationship changes by doing all of the following *except*
    A. Find new friends.
    B. Develop hobbies and church and community activities.
    C. Have regular contact with family.
    D. Stay at home alone to save money.

19. When children care for older parents
    A. The older person may feel unwanted and useless.
    B. The older person may feel more secure.
    C. Tension may develop among the children and the family.
    D. All of the above are true.

20. What causes wrinkles to appear on an older person?
    A. Decreases in oil and sweat gland secretions
    B. Fewer nerve endings
    C. Loss of elasticity, strength, and fatty tissue layer
    D. Poor circulation

21. Healing in older people is delayed as a result of
    A. Poor nutrition
    B. Decreased number of blood vessels
    C. Fewer nerve endings
    D. Loss of fatty tissue

22. Older persons can prevent bone loss and loss of muscle strength by
    A. Activity, exercise, and diet
    B. Taking hormones
    C. Resting with feet elevated
    D. Taking vitamins

23. Dizziness may increase in older people because
    A. They have difficulty sleeping.
    B. Blood flow to the brain is decreased.
    C. Nerve cells are lost.
    D. Brain cells are lost.

24. Bones may break easily because
    A. Joints become stiff and painful.
    B. Joints become slightly flexed.
    C. Bones lose strength and become brittle.
    D. Vertebrae shorten.

25. Painful injuries and disease may go unnoticed because
    A. The person is confused.
    B. Touch and sensitivity to pain are reduced.
    C. Memory is shorter.
    D. The blood flow is reduced.

26. Eyes become irritated easily because
    A. The lens yellows.
    B. The eye takes longer to adjust to changes in light.
    C. Tear secretion is less.
    D. The person becomes farsighted.

27. If circulatory changes occur, the person
    A. May be encouraged to walk long distances
    B. May need rest periods during the day
    C. May not do any kind of exercise
    D. Should exercise only once a week

28. A person with dyspnea can breathe easier when
    A. Lying flat in bed
    B. Covered with heavy bed linens
    C. Allowed to be on bed rest
    D. Resting in the semi-Fowler's position

29. Dulled taste and smell decreases
    A. Peristalsis
    B. Appetite
    C. Saliva
    D. Swallowing

30. Older persons need
    A. Fewer calories
    B. Fewer fluids
    C. More calories
    D. Low-protein diets

31. Many older persons have to urinate several times during the night because
    A. Bladder infections are common.
    B. Urine is more concentrated.
    C. Bladder muscles weaken and bladder size decreases.
    D. Urinary incontinence may occur.

32. Which of the following is *not* an advantage of an older person living with family?
    A. It provides companionship.
    B. The family can provide care.
    C. Living expenses can be shared.
    D. Sleep arrangements may change.

33. Adult day care centers
    A. Provide meals, supervision, and activities for older persons
    B. Accept only self-care persons and those who can walk without help
    C. Provide complete care
    D. Provide respite care

34. Meals are not usually provided when an older person lives in
    A. An apartment
    B. Senior citizen housing
    C. Board and care homes
    D. Adult foster care

35. Assisted living facilities provide the following *except*
    A. Nursing care
    B. Help with meals
    C. Health care
    D. Social contact with other residents

36. Continuing care retirement communities (CCRC)
    A. Have independent living units
    B. Have food service and help nearby
    C. Add services as the person's needs change
    D. All of the above

37. Nursing centers are housing options for older persons who
    A. Need only companionship
    B. Cannot care for themselves
    C. Need care during the daytime while their family works
    D. Are developmentally disabled

38. Moving to a nursing center
    A. Is an exciting change for the older person
    B. Can cause feelings of loneliness and isolation
    C. Is always a permanent move
    D. Allows the person to have more personal freedom

39. A quality nursing center must be certified
    A. By the medical society
    B. For Medicare and Medicaid
    C. By the state board of nursing
    D. By the local health department

40. A quality nursing center would *not* be required to have
    A. An activity area for the resident's use
    B. Halls wide enough so two wheelchairs can pass with ease
    C. Toilet facilities that can be accessed by people in wheelchairs
    D. Private rooms for each resident

41. Sufficient space and equipment requirements by OBRA include
    A. Halls with handrails and other safety needs
    B. Private bathrooms for each resident
    C. Expecting residents to provide furniture for their rooms
    D. Using tablecloths and cloth napkins in the dining room

42. "Quality of Life" requirements of OBRA include all of the following *except*
    A. Acceptable noise level
    B. Individual televisions for each resident
    C. Paint or wallpaper that is appealing to residents
    D. Clean, soft, adequate linens for residents

Matching

Match physical changes during the aging process with the affected body system.

43. _____ Reduced blood flow to kidneys

44. _____ Decreased elasticity and narrowing of the arteries

45. _____ Forgetfulness

46. _____ Gradual loss of height

47. _____ Decreased strength for coughing

48. _____ Decreased secretion of oil and sweat glands

49. _____ Difficulty digesting fried and fatty foods

50. _____ Decreased pumping force of the heart

51. _____ Decreased strength of bladder muscles

52. _____ Difficulty seeing green and blue colors

53. _____ Difficulty swallowing

54. _____ Decreased elasticity of lung tissue

55. _____ Decreased bone mass

56. _____ Decreased ability to feel heat and cold

57. _____ Hair thins or loses color

A. Integumentary

B. Musculoskeletal

C. Nervous

D. Circulatory

E. Respiratory

F. Digestive

G. Urinary

Optional Learning Exercises

Nursing concerns with physical changes

58. When bathing an older person, what kind of soap should be used?

_____

_____

Often, no soap is used on the

_____.

59. What can happen if a nick or cut occurs on the feet?

_____

_____

Why can this result happen?

_____

_____

60. What types of skin growths are common in older persons?

A. _____

B. _____

61. Why are these skin growths dangerous if untreated?

_____

_____

62. When bone mass decreases, why is it important to turn an older person carefully?

63. Why does an older person often have a gradual loss of height?

64. What types of exercise help prevent bone loss and loss of muscle strength?

65. Older people have change in the nervous system. When the following changes happen, what physical problems occur?

   A. Nerve conduction and reflexes are slower:

   B. Blood flow to brain is reduced:

   C. Progressive loss of brain cells:

66. When you are eating with an older person, you notice that she puts salt on vegetables that taste fine to you? What may be a reason she does this?

67. A female nurse has a high-pitched voice, and several residents seem to have difficulty hearing her. They do not complain about hearing the male charge nurse. What may be a reason for the difference?

68. How can you help the circulation of persons confined to bed?

   What other body system will be helped by this activity?

69. What can the nursing assistant do to prevent respiratory complications from bed rest?

70. The stomach and colon empty slower, and flatulence and constipation are common in the older person. What causes all of these problems?

71. How does good oral hygiene and denture care improve food intake?

72. Why should you plan to give most fluids to the older person before 1700 (5:00 PM)?

Independent Learning Activities

1. Interview an older person who lives independently. Use these questions to find what concerns the person has about remaining independent.
    *   What physical problems does the person have, if any?
    *   What activities are more difficult than they were when the person was younger?
    *   What does the person use to provide safety (walkers, canes, alarms, daily telephone calls)?
    *   What comfort measures are needed to decrease pain or help the person sleep?
    *   What are the person's transportation needs? Does the person drive? How does the person shop for groceries? Visit with family, friends? Attend social functions?
    *   How are social needs met? How often does the person go to socialize? How often does the person have visitors?

2. Interview an older person and talk about life when the person was young.
    *   Observe facial expression and tone of voice when the person talks about events remembered. What changes do you see?
    *   Compare how well the person remembers events of long ago with that which happened recently.
    *   How do you feel differently about the person after hearing about the person's youth?

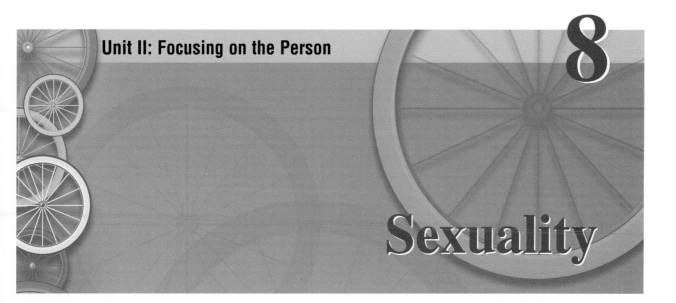

Sexuality

Bisexual	Menopause
Erectile dysfunction	Sex
Heterosexual	Sexuality
Homosexual	Transsexual
Impotence	Transvestite

Fill in the Blanks: Key Terms

Select your answers from the Key Terms listed above.

1. _____

    is the time when menstruation stops; it marks the

    end of a woman's reproductive years.

2. Another name for impotence is _____

    _____.

3. _____

    is the physical, psychologic, social, cultural, and

    spiritual factors that affect a person's feelings and

    attitudes about his or her sex.

4. A _____

    is a person who becomes sexually excited by

    dressing in the clothes of the other sex.

5. A person attracted to both sexes is _____

    _____.

6. A _____

    is a person who believes that he or she is really a

    member of the other sex.

7. A _____

    is a person who is attracted to members of the

    same sex.

8. The physical activities involving the organs of reproduction is _____.

9. A person who is attracted to members of the other sex is _____.

10. The inability of the male to have an erection is erectile dysfunction or _____ .

Circle the BEST Answer

11. Sexuality
    A. Involves the personality and the body
    B. Is the physical activities involving reproductive organs
    C. Is unimportant in old age
    D. All of the above

12. A woman who is attracted to men is
    A. Homosexual
    B. Heterosexual
    C. Lesbian
    D. Bisexual

13. Transvestites are often
    A. Homosexual
    B. Transsexual
    C. Married and heterosexual
    D. Bisexual

14. Diabetes, spinal cord injuries, and multiple sclerosis may cause
    A. Impotence
    B. Menopause
    C. Sexual aggression
    D. Heterosexuality

Fill in the Blanks

20. Sexuality develops when the baby is _____.

21. Children know their own sex at age _____.

22. Homosexuality has existed for _____.

23. Sexual ability may be affected by:

    A. _____

    B. _____

    C. _____

    D. _____

15. Which of the following is *not* true about sexuality and older persons?
    A. An orgasm is less forceful than it is in younger persons.
    B. Arousal takes longer.
    C. Hormone production increases in men and women.
    D. Love, affection, and intimacy are needed throughout life.

16. When older adult couples are living in a nursing center, they
    A. Can share the same room
    B. Are placed in separate rooms
    C. Are not encouraged to be intimate
    D. Cannot share a bed

17. When a person in a nursing center is sexually aggressive, it may be a result of
    A. Confusion
    B. Using a way to gain your attention
    C. Genital soreness or itching
    D. All of the above

18. If a person touches you in the wrong way, you should
    A. Ignore it and realize the person is not responsible.
    B. Tell the person you do not like him or her.
    C. Tell the person that these behaviors make you uncomfortable.
    D. Refuse to give care to the person.

19. If you do not share a person's sexual attitudes, values, practices, or standards, you should
    A. Avoid judging or gossiping about the person.
    B. Avoid the person.
    C. Tell him or her your feelings.
    D. Discuss the person's relationships with other staff members.

24. As aging occurs, hormones decrease. These hormones are:

    A. _____ (in men)

    B. _____ (in women)

25. Some older people do not have intercourse. They may express their sexual needs or desires by

    _____

    _____.

26. When you are assisting persons, what grooming practices will promote sexuality for residents?

    A. Men: _____

    B. Women: _____

27. What can you do to allow privacy for a person and a partner?

    A. Close _____

    B. Remind the person about _____

    C. Tell other _____

    D. Knock _____

28. Masturbation is a normal _____

Optional Learning Exercises

Mr. and Mrs. Davis are 78-year-old residents in a nursing center where they share a room. They need assistance with activities of daily living (ADL) but are mentally alert. They are affectionate people who care deeply for each other. Answer these questions about meeting their sexuality needs.

29. Mr. Davis has diabetes and high blood pressure. What effect can these disorders have on sexuality?

    _____

    _____

30. Mrs. Davis tells you that she and her husband are still sexually active, but that "it is not the same" as it was when they were younger. What changes occur with aging that can affect sexual performance?

    A. Men:

    _____

    _____

    _____

    B. Women:

    _____

    _____

    _____

31. Because of the changes, what do you think would be an important thing that you can do when they ask for privacy?

    _____

    _____

Independent Learning Activities

1. Consider this situation about a sexually aggressive person and answer the questions about how you would respond.

   SITUATION: John James is 72 years of age and has paraplegia because of an accident several years ago. His care-givers report that John has recently begun to make sexually suggestive remarks. While you are giving his morning care, he touches you several times in private areas and makes frequent sexually suggestive remarks. The other nursing assistants tell you to just ignore him or joke around with him about the actions.

   - What would you say to Mr. James when he touched you in private areas?
   - How would you respond to his suggestive remarks?
   - What would you say to your colleagues who suggest that you ignore or joke with Mr. James?
   - Has this type of situation ever occurred to you? How did you handle it? What would you do differently after studying this chapter?

2. Consider this situation about caring for a person who is gay. Answer the questions about how you would respond.

   SITUATION: Bobbie Freeman is 45 years of age and has had gall bladder surgery. While assisting her to ambulate, Bobbie begins to talk about her friend, Judy. She tells you that they have been lovers for 15 years.

   - What would you say to a person who tells you that she is gay?
   - What effect would this information have on the care you provide for the person?
   - Has this type of situation ever occurred when you were caring for a person? How did you respond? How would you respond after studying this chapter?

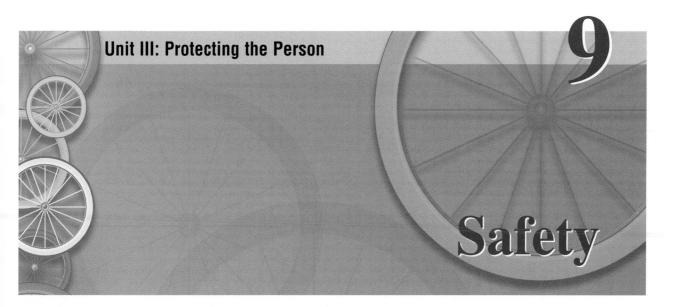

Coma	Hazardous substance
Dementia	Hemiplegia
Disaster	Paraplegia
Electrical shock	Quadriplegia
Ground	Suffocation

Fill in the Blanks: Key Terms

Select your answers from the Key Terms listed above.

1. A set of chronic signs and symptoms in which a person loses memory and the ability to think and reason is _____.

2. Paralysis from the neck down is

   _____.

3. _____ is any chemical that presents a physical hazard or a health hazard in the workplace.

4. A _____ is a sudden catastrophic event in which many people are injured and killed and property is destroyed.

5. _____ occurs when breathing stops resulting from the lack of oxygen.

6. Paralysis on one side of the body is

   _____.

7. A _____ is a state of being unaware of one's surroundings and being unable to react or respond to people, places, or things.

8. That which carries leaking electricity to the earth and away from an electrical item is a

   _____.

9. _____

is paralysis from the waist down.

10. _____ occurs

when electrical current passes through the body.

Circle the BEST Answer

11. To protect the person from harm, you need to
    A. Use restraints.
    B. Follow the person's care plan.
    C. Limit mobility.
    D. Lock all doors.

12. Age is an accident risk factor for all but one of the following
    A. Balance is affected and they fall easily.
    B. They may have poor vision or hearing problems.
    C. They are less sensitive to heat and cold.
    D. They are more sensitive to hazardous materials.

13. People with dementia are at risk of injury because they
    A. No longer know what is safe and what is dangerous
    B. Are in a coma
    C. Have problems sensing heat and cold
    D. Have poor vision

14. Medications can be a risk factor because they
    A. Affect hearing
    B. Reduce the ability to sense heat and cold
    C. Can cause loss of balance or lack of coordination
    D. Can cause hemiplegia

15. Identifying residents is most important because
    A. You need to give the right care to the right person.
    B. Visitors may ask your help to find someone.
    C. You need to call the person by the right name.
    D. You will have to give care to two people if you give it to the wrong person first.

16. Which of the following is *not* a reliable way to identify the person?
    A. Check the identification bracelet.
    B. Use the person's picture to compare with the person.
    C. If resident is alert and oriented, follow the center policy to identify.
    D. Call the person by name.

17. Falls may occur at shift change because
    A. Residents become restless when new caregivers come on duty.
    B. Confusion can occur about who is giving care and answering signal lights.
    C. Residents require more care at that time.
    D. No staff members are available at that time.

18. Which of the following is *not* a factor that increases the risks of falling?
    A. Medication side effects
    B. Dizziness on standing
    C. Elimination needs
    D. High blood pressure

19. You will find a list of measures for the person's specific risk factors of falls in the
    A. Nurse's notes
    B. Flow sheet
    C. Care plan
    D. Physician's orders

20. Bed rails
    A. Are used for all residents
    B. Are safe for confused and disoriented persons
    C. Are raised when the nurse and the care plan tells you
    D. Can be used when you think the resident needs them

21. Gaps should be 4 inches or less
    A. Between the mattress and the headboard
    B. Between the bed rail and the mattress
    C. From the bed controls to the bed rails
    D. Between the mattress and the footboard

22. If you raise the bed and the resident does not use bed rails, you should
    A. Raise the far bed rail if you are working alone.
    B. Raise both rails if you leave the bedside.
    C. Tell the person to lie still if you need to leave the bedside.
    D. Ask a co-worker to stand on the far side of the bed.

23. Which of the following would be a safety measure to prevent falls?
    A. Allow the person to walk to the bathroom in his socks.
    B. Place a scatter rug next to the bed.
    C. Tie the person's robe belt securely.
    D. Turn out all lights at night.

24. Bed rails *cannot* be used
    A. When the bed is in the lowest position
    B. When the bed is in the highest position
    C. Unless the resident or the legal representative gives consent for raised bed rails
    D. When the person is alert

25. Handrails or grab bars
    A. Provide support for persons who are weak or unsteady when walking
    B. Provide support when sitting down or getting up from a toilet
    C. Are used in getting in and out of a bathtub
    D. All of the above

26. Wheels on beds, wheelchairs, or stretchers are locked to
    A. Keep the equipment properly positioned
    B. Prevent injury to you or the person
    C. Keep the person from moving the furniture
    D. Keep your body in alignment

27. Accidental poisoning is a problem in nursing centers because
    A. Poor vision and confusion are major risk factors with residents.
    B. Safely storing poison is difficult.
    C. Many items that are used in a nursing center are poisonous.
    D. Residents have free access to all areas of a nursing center.

28. A leading cause of death, especially among children and older persons is(are)
    A. Falls
    B. Burns
    C. Accidental poisoning
    D. Suffocation

29. Resident-owned electrical items are safety checked by the
    A. Nurse
    B. Maintenance department
    C. Fire department
    D. Director of nursing

30. Food should be cut in small, bite-sized pieces to
    A. Make it easier for residents to feed themselves
    B. Make the food more appealing
    C. Increase the amount of food eaten
    D. Prevent choking and suffocation

31. You can help prevent the spread of infection by
    A. Keeping residents from touching each other
    B. Thorough hand washing
    C. Sterilizing all equipment
    D. Placing all residents in isolation

32. An electrical shock is especially dangerous because it can
    A. Start a fire
    B. Damage equipment
    C. Affect the heart and cause death
    D. Violate OBRA regulations

33. If you are shocked by electric equipment, you should
    A. Immediately report the shock.
    B. Try to see what is wrong with the equipment.
    C. Make sure it has a ground prong.
    D. Test the equipment in a different outlet.

34. Wheelchair brakes should be locked when
    A. Transporting the person
    B. Taking a wheelchair up or down stairs
    C. A person is moving to or from the wheelchair
    D. Storing the wheelchair

35. When moving a person on a stretcher, which of the following practices is *not* correct?
    A. Safety straps or side rails are used only when the person is confused.
    B. Lock the stretcher before transferring the person.
    C. Do not leave the person unattended.
    D. Stand at the head of the stretcher. Your co-worker stands at the foot.

36. Which one of the following organizations requires that health care employees understand the risks of hazardous substances and how to handle them safely.
    A. OBRA
    B. Occupational Safety and Health Administration (OSHA)
    C. Joint Commission on Accreditation of Healthcare Organizations (JCAHO)
    D. Material safety data sheets (MSDS)

37. Warning labels may include all of the following *except*
    A. Physical hazards and health hazards
    B. What protective equipment to wear
    C. The telephone number of the local emergency system
    D. Storage and disposal information

38. Where would you find the MSDS for hazardous materials?
    A. Attached to the substance
    B. In the administrator's office
    C. In a binder at a specified location on each unit
    D. On the Internet

39. A resident who is receiving oxygen is at special risk for
    A. Burns
    B. Suffocation
    C. Poisoning
    D. Electrical shock

40. All of the following are needed for a fire *except*
    A. Spark or flame
    B. Electrical equipment
    C. Materials that will burn
    D. Oxygen

41. If a fire occurs, what should you do first?
    A. Rescue people in immediate danger.
    B. Sound the nearest fire alarm and call the switchboard operator.
    C. Close doors and windows to confine the fire.
    D. Use a fire extinguisher on a small fire that has not spread to a larger area.

42. If evacuation is necessary, residents who are
    A. Closest to the outside door are rescued first
    B. Able to walk are rescued last
    C. Closest to the danger are evacuated first
    D. Helpless are rescued last

43. If there is a disaster, you
    A. Are expected to go to your nursing center immediately
    B. May be called into work if you are off duty
    C. Should stay away or leave to get out of the way
    D. May go home to check on your family

44. Why is workplace violence a big concern in health care?
    A. According to OSHA, more assaults occur in health care settings than they do in other industries.
    B. Acutely disturbed and violent persons may seek health care.
    C. Agency pharmacies are a source of drugs and are therefore a target for robberies.
    D. All of the above are true.

45. Which of the following would *not* be effective in preventing or controlling workplace violence?
    A. Stand away from the person.
    B. Know where to find panic buttons, call bells, and alarms.
    C. Sit quietly with the person in his room. Hold his hand to calm him.
    D. Tell the person you will get a nurse to speak to him or her.

46. When you are filling out a valuables list or envelope, which of the following would be the best description?
    A. "A diamond in a gold setting"
    B. "A one-carat diamond in a 14K gold setting"
    C. "A white stone in a yellow setting"
    D. "A white diamond-like stone in a gold-like setting"

47. Which of the following would *not* be reported as an accident or error?
    A. Forgetting to give care
    B. Giving the wrong care
    C. Assisting a co-worker to give care
    D. Losing a resident's dentures

Matching

Match each safety measure with the risk of injury that it prevents.

48. _____ Do not use electric blankets.

49. _____ Keep resident room free of clutter.

50. _____ Be sure residents smoke only in smoking areas.

51. _____ Keep electrical items away from water.

52. _____ The person is assisted with elimination needs at regular times and whenever a request is made.

53. _____ Do not give the resident a shower or tub bath when there is an electrical storm.

54. _____ Never leave residents unattended in the bathtub.

55. _____ Report loose teeth or dentures to the nurse.

56. _____ Use correct equipment to move and transfer residents from beds and chairs.

57. _____ Do not touch a person who is experiencing an electrical shock.

58. _____ Move all residents from the area if you smell gas or smoke.

59. _____ Do not allow smoking near oxygen tanks or concentrators.

A. Burns

B. Suffocation

C. Falls

D. Equipment

Optional Learning Exercises

60. What does the abbreviation RACE mean when a fire occurs?

    R: _____

    A: _____

    C: _____

    E: _____

In questions 61 through 66, which risk of falling can occur with these examples? (Box 9-1)

61. The resident is wearing bedroom slippers that are a size too big.

    _____

    _____

62. The person falls when he tries to go to the bathroom without assistance.

    _____

    _____

63. The resident is lying in bed, stands up too quickly, and falls.

    _____

    _____

64. A new resident gets out of bed and trips going the wrong direction to the bathroom.

    _____

    _____

65. The person cannot find his glasses and falls over a chair.

_____

_____

66. The person trips on his intravenous pole while walking down the hall.

_____

_____

In questions 67 through 73, which safety measure to prevent falls is practiced in each example? (Box 9-2)

67. The nursing assistant picks up newspapers that are lying next to the bed.

_____

_____

68. A bathmat is placed in the tub.

_____

_____

69. The person wears rubber-soled shoes with Velcro closures.

_____

_____

70. The nursing assistant takes the resident to the bathroom at 8:00 AM, 10:00 AM, and 2:00 PM.

_____

_____

71. The nursing assistant gives the resident a back massage and a warm drink at bedtime.

_____

_____

72. The nursing assistant checks the name label on the walker before giving it to the resident.

_____

_____

73. Visitors leave and the nursing assistant notices the signal light has fallen on the floor.

_____

_____

In questions 74 through 81, read the following examples and write the related guideline. (Boxes 9-3, 9-4)

74. The nursing assistant tells the resident that his shower will be delayed until the storm passes.

_____

_____

75. The nursing assistant tells the nurse that she has never used the portable footbath before.

_____

_____

76. The nursing assistant dries her hands carefully before plugging in an electric razor.

_____

_____

77. An electric fan will not work, and the staff member follows the correct procedure to have it repaired.

_____

_____

78. The nursing assistant moves an electrical cord that is lying across a heat vent.

_____

_____

79. The nursing assistant makes sure that the person has both feet on the wheelchair footrests.

_____

_____

80. The nursing assistant notices that one wheel is flat on a wheelchair and reports it to the nurse.

_____

_____

81. The nursing assistant locks the wheelchair when the person is sitting in it next to his bed.

_____

_____

In questions 82 through 85, what should you do when handling hazardous materials in these situations? (Box 9-5)

82. When cleaning up a hazardous material, how do you know what equipment to wear?

_____

_____

83. When a spill occurs, what is the correct way to wipe it up?

_____

_____

84. The nurse tells the nursing assistant that the resident is having an x-ray done in her room.

_____

_____

85. The staff opens the windows when cleaning up a hazardous material.

_____

_____

In questions 86 through 88, what fire-prevention measure is being practiced? (Box 9-6)

86. The resident is taken to the smoking area in his wheelchair.

_____

_____

87. When cleaning the smoking area, the staff uses a metal can that is partially filled with sand.

_____

_____

88. When heating food for a resident, the nursing assistant remains in the kitchen.

_____

_____

In questions 89 through 93, what measures to prevent or control workplace violence are being used or should be used? (Box 9-7)

89. What type of jewelry can serve as a weapon?

_____

_____

90. Why is long hair worn up?

_____

_____

91. Why are pictures, vases, and other items removed from certain areas?

_____

_____

92. What type of glass protects nurses' stations, reception areas, and admitting areas?

_____

_____

93. What clothing items should be worn by staff to assist the ability to run?

_____

_____

In questions 94 through 101, list personal safety practices that apply. (Box 9-8)

94. Parking your car in a parking garage:

_____

_____

95. What items should you keep in the car for safety?

_____

_____

96. Why is "dry run" important?

_____

_____

97. If you think someone is following you, what should you do?

_____

_____

98. If someone wants your wallet or purse, what should you do?

_____

_____

99. How can you use your car keys as a weapon?

_____

_____

100. How can you use your thumbs as a weapon?

_____

_____

101. What part of the body can you attack on either a man or woman?

_____

_____

Independent Learning Activities

1. Safety is important to everyone and needs to be practiced at all times. Check the following items or areas in your own home to determine how safe it is.
   - What areas are adequately lighted for safety? What areas need improved lighting?
   - Check electrical cords and plugs on appliances and lamps. How many have frayed cords? Ungrounded plugs? What are other problems that make them unsafe to use?
   - How many smoke detectors do you have in your home? When were the batteries last replaced? How can you check the smoke detector to make sure it is working correctly?
   - How many scatter rugs are used on slippery surfaces? How many have some type of backing to prevent slipping?
   - Where are hazardous materials (medications, cleaning solutions, painting supplies) stored? Which of these materials can children reach? What can be done to store them more safely?
   - Make a list of good safety practices in your home. Make a list of safety practices that can be improved.

2. Develop a plan for your home and family that helps everyone know how to escape if a fire occurs.
   - Make sure every person knows at least two escape routes from the sleeping area.
   - Practice how to check a door for heat before opening.
   - Arrange a place to meet once you are outside the building.

10

Restraint Alternatives and Safe Restraint Use

Active physical restraint
Passive physical restraint
Restraint

Fill in the Blanks: Key Terms

Select your answers from the Key Terms listed above.

1. Any item, object, device, garment, material, or

   chemical that limits or restricts a person's freedom

   of movement or access to one's body is a

   _____.

2. An _____

   is a restraint attached to the person's body and to a

   fixed (nonmovable) object.

3. A _____

   is a restraint near but not directly attached to the

   person's body; it does not totally restrict freedom of

   movement and allows access to certain body parts.

Circle the BEST Answer

4. Restraints are used
   A. Whenever the nurse believes that they are
      necessary
   B. Only as a last resort to protect residents from
      harming themselves or others
   C. To make sure the person does not fall
   D. To decrease work for the staff

5. The decision to use restraints is discussed by the
   A. Nurse and physician
   B. Nurse and family
   C. Interdisciplinary health care team, the resident,
      and family members
   D. Nurse and nursing assistants who are providing
      care

6. Research shows that restraints
   A. Prevent falls
   B. Cause falls
   C. Are used whenever the nurse decides
   D. Are not effective

7. A person's harmful behaviors may be caused by
   A. Being afraid of a new setting
   B. Being too hot or too cold
   C. Being hungry or thirsty
   D. All of the above

8. Guidelines about using restraints are part of the resident rights in
   A. Food and Drug Administration regulations
   B. Occupational Safety and Health Administration rules
   C. OBRA regulations
   D. Joint Commission on Accreditation of Healthcare Organizations (JCAHO) recommendations

9. Restraints are *not* used to
   A. Prevent harm to the person
   B. Discipline the person for behaviors
   C. Prevent a person from pulling at a wound or dressing
   D. Keep an IV from being pulled out

10. Which of the following is a type of restraint?
    A. A soft chair with a footstool to elevate the feet
    B. A bed without side rails
    C. A geriatric chair (Geri-chair)
    D. A drug that helps a person function at his or her highest level

11. The most serious risk from restraints is
    A. Cuts, bruises, and fractures
    B. Death from strangulation
    C. Falls
    D. Depression, anger, and agitation

12. After receiving instructions about the proper use of a restraint, you should
    A. Ask for help to apply it to a resident.
    B. Demonstrate proper application to the nurse before using it on a person.
    C. Watch someone else apply it to a resident.
    D. Apply it to the resident independently.

13. Which of the following is *not* a physical restraint?
    A. A vest restraint
    B. A chair with an attached tray
    C. A drug that affects the person's mental function
    D. Sheets tucked in so tightly, they restrict movement

14. To use a restraint, the nurse must
    A. Get permission from the family.
    B. Obtain a physician's order.
    C. Get permission from the interdisciplinary health care team.
    D. Receive OBRA permission.

15. Which of the following is an active physical restraint?
    A. Vest
    B. Bedrail
    C. Wedge cushion
    D. Pillow

16. OBRA requires informed consent. This consent is obtained by
    A. The resident legal representative
    B. The physician or nurse
    C. The resident
    D. The nursing assistant

17. When restraining a combative and agitated person, it should be done
    A. Slowly by only one person
    B. Only after explaining to the person what will be done
    C. With enough staff to complete the task safely and efficiently
    D. In a public area so the person is distracted

18. The person who is restrained must be observed every
    A. 5 minutes
    B. 15 minutes
    C. Hour
    D. 2 hours

19. Wrist restraints are used when a person
    A. Tries to get out of bed
    B. Moves his or her wheelchair without permission
    C. Pulls at tubes used in medical treatments
    D. Slides out of a chair easily

20. A vest restraint
    A. Always crosses in the front
    B. Is applied next to the skin under clothing
    C. Must be secured very tightly to be safe
    D. May cross in the back

21. A belt restraint
    A. Is more restrictive than are other restraints
    B. Allows the person to turn from side to side
    C. Must be released by the staff
    D. Can only be used in bed

22. When applying wrist restraints
    A. Tie the straps to the bed rail.
    B. Tie firm knots in the straps.
    C. Place the restraints over clothing.
    D. Place the soft part toward the skin.

23. If you are not using padded mitt restraints for the hands, you should
    A. Give the person a hand roll to hold.
    B. Pad the mitt with soft material.
    C. Make sure the mitt is securely tied.
    D. Make sure the mitt is free of wrinkles.

24. When using a vest restraint in bed
    A. The straps are secured at waist level out of the person's reach.
    B. The straps are secured to the bed rail.
    C. The vest crosses in the back.
    D. The person can turn over.

25. How can you improve the quality of life for a person with restraints?
    A. Provide water or other fluids frequently.
    B. Check often to make sure breathing and circulation are normal.
    C. Treat the person with kindness, caring, respect, and dignity.
    D. All of the above are true.

Matching

Match the safety guidelines with the correct example.

26. _____ Injuries and deaths have occurred from improper restraint and poor observation.

27. _____ A restraint is used only when it is the best safety precaution for the person.

28. _____ The nurse gives you the printed instructions about applying and securing the restraint safely.

29. _____ Restrained persons need repeated explanations and reassurance.

30. _____ The physician gives the reason for the restraint, what to use, and how long to use the restraint.

31. _____ Residents in immediate danger of harming themselves or others are restrained quickly.

32. _____ Because they are the least restrictive, passive physical restraints should be used when possible.

33. _____ The goal of this guideline is to meet the person's needs using as little restraint as possible.

34. _____ If told to apply a restraint, you must clearly understand the need.

35. _____ When the restraint is removed, range-of-motion exercises are done, or the person is ambulated.

36. _____ The care plan must include measures to protect the resident and to prevent the person from harming others.

37. _____ The resident must understand the reason for the restraints.

38. _____ The person must be comfortable and able to move the restrained part to a limited and safe extent. Food, fluid, comfort, safety, exercise, and elimination needs must be met.

A. Restraints are used to protect the person. OBRA does not allow restraints for staff convenience or to discipline a person.

B. Restraints require a physician's order.

C. OBRA requires using the least restrictive method.

D. Restraints are used only after trying other methods to protect the person.

E. Unnecessary restraint is false imprisonment.

F. OBRA requires informed consent for restraint use.

G. The manufacturer's instructions are followed.

H. The health team meets the restrained person's basic needs.

I. Restraints are applied with enough help to protect the person and staff from injury.

J. Restraints can increase a person's confusion and agitation.

K. OBRA requires that the resident's quality of life be protected.

L. The resident is observed at least every 15 minutes or more often, as required by the care plan.

M. The restraint is removed, the person repositioned, and basic needs met at least every 2 hours.

Fill in the Blanks

39. When using restraints, what information is reported and recorded?

    A. _____

    B. _____

    C. _____

    D. _____

    E. _____

    F. _____

    G. _____

    H. _____

    I. _____

40. Persons who are restrained in a supine position must

    be monitored constantly because they are at great

    risk for _____.

41. You should carry scissors with you because, in an

    emergency, _____

    _____.

Labeling

42. Explain what is being done. _____

    _____

    _____

43. Draw a belt restraint applied correctly on the person in a wheelchair. What is the correct angle for this belt?

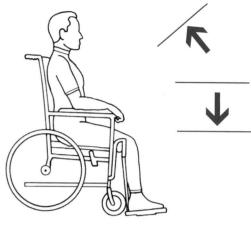

Nursing Assistant Skills Video Exercise

View the **Safety and Restraints** *video to answer these questions.*

44. Where is information about the procedure guidelines obtained?

    _____

    _____

45. How do you check to make sure a vest restraint is applied properly to allow breathing?

    _____

    _____

46. Where is a vest restraint secured on the bed to prevent sliding?

    _____

    _____

47. How do you check a wrist restraint to make sure it is properly applied?

    _____

    _____

48. After the restraints are applied, what procedural guidelines are followed?

    A. _____

    B. _____

    C. _____

    D. _____

49. If the person wearing a vest restraint has respiratory difficulty, you should call

    _____

    _____.

50. If the person wearing a wrist restraint has no pulse and the fingers are cold, blue or pale, you should

    _____

    _____.

51. What information is recorded and reported?

    A. _____

    B. _____

    C. _____

    D. _____

    E. _____

    F. _____

Optional Learning Exercises

52. What type of restraint is a drug?

    _____

53. How can a drug be considered a restraint?

    A. _____

    B. _____

    C. _____

54. How does a restraint increase incontinence?

    _____

    _____

55. What lifelong habits and routines can be included in the nursing care plan as alternatives to restraints?

    _____

    _____

56. Why would a person in restraints be at risk for dehydration?

    _____

    _____

57. Why would video tapes of family and friends or visiting with family be good alternatives to restraints?

    _____

    _____

Independent Learning Activities

1. Role-play with one person as a nursing assistant and one as a person who is restrained. An active physical restraint is applied as the person sits in a chair or wheelchair. When the restraint is in place, the nursing assistant leaves and does not return for 15 minutes. Discuss the following questions with each other after the experiment.
   - How did the person feel when the restraints were applied? What did the nursing assistant tell the person about the restraints?
   - Did the nursing assistant ask the person if toileting was needed? If the person was thirsty?
   - Was the chair comfortable? Was there any padding? Did the nursing assistant check for wrinkles? Was the person able to move around to reposition the body for comfort?
   - How was the person able to get help during the 15 minutes of being alone?
   - What diversions were offered while the person was restrained? Television or radio? Reading materials? A window with a pleasant view? If any of these diversions were provided, who chose the channel, station, book, or view?
   - Was the person told that someone would return in 15 minutes? Was a clock or watch available to see the time? How long did it seem?
   - What was learned from this experience by both people?

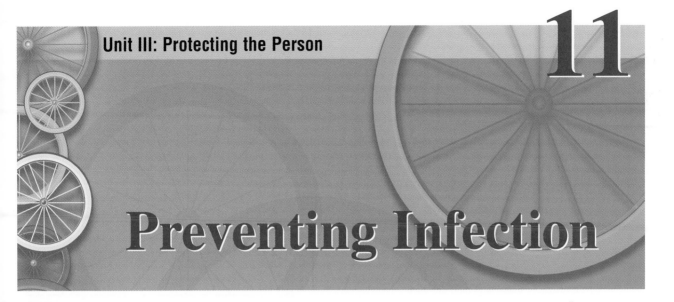

Preventing Infection

11

Asepsis	Germicide	Pathogen
Autoclave	Immunity	Reservoir
Biohazardous waste	Infection	Spore
Carrier	Medical asepsis	Sterile
Clean technique	Microbe	Sterile field
Communicable disease	Microorganism	Sterile technique
Contagious disease	Nonpathogen	Sterilization
Contamination	Normal flora	Surgical asepsis
Disinfection	Nosocomial infection	Vaccine

Fill in the Blanks: Key Terms

Select your answers from the Key Terms listed above.

1. A human or animal that is a reservoir for microbes but does not have signs and symptoms of infection is a

    _____.

2. A _____ is a small living plant or animal seen only with a micro-scope; a microbe.

3. Protection against a certain disease is

    _____.

4. A preparation that contains dead or weakened microbes and is given to produce immunity against an infectious disease is a

    _____.

5. A work area that is free of all pathogens and nonpathogens is a

    _____.

6. _____

   are items contaminated with blood, body fluids,

   secretions, and excretions that may be harmful to

   others.

7. _____

   are practices used to remove or destroy pathogens

   and to prevent their spread from one person or place

   to another person or place; clean technique.

8. A communicable disease is also called a

   _____ .

9. An _____

   is a disease state resulting from the invasion and

   growth of microorganisms in the body.

10. _____

    is the practice that keeps equipment and supplies

    free of all microbes; sterile technique.

11. A _____

    is a disease caused by pathogens that spread easily;

    contagious disease.

12. The process of destroying pathogens is

    _____ .

13. A _____

    is an infection that is acquired after admission to a

    health care agency.

14. _____

    is being free of disease-producing microbes.

15. Another name for a microorganism is a

    _____ .

16. The environment in which microbes live and grow

    is a _____ ;

    host.

17. Medical asepsis is also called

    _____ .

18. The process of being unclean is

    _____ .

19. The absence of all microbes is

    _____ .

20. Surgical asepsis is also called

    _____ .

21. A bacterium protected by a hard shell that forms

    around the microbes is a

    _____ .

22. _____

    are microbes that usually live and grow in a certain

    location.

23. A disinfectant that is applied to skin, tissue, or non-

    living objects is a

    _____ .

24. A microbe that does not usually cause an infection

    is a _____ .

25. _____

    is the process of destroying all microbes.

26. A microbe that is harmful and can cause an infection is a _____.

27. A pressure steam sterilizer is an

_____.

Circle the BEST Answer

28. Germs are a type of microbe called
    A. Protozoa
    B. Fungi
    C. Viruses
    D. Bacteria

29. Rickettsiae are transmitted to humans by
    A. Plants
    B. Other humans
    C. Insect bites
    D. One-celled animals

30. To live and grow, all microbes require
    A. Oxygen
    B. A reservoir
    C. A hot environment
    D. Plenty of light

31. Normal flora
    A. Are always pathogens
    B. Are always nonpathogens
    C. Become pathogens when transmitted from its natural site to another site
    D. Cause signs and symptoms of an infection

32. Which of the following is *not* a sign or symptom of infection?
    A. Rash
    B. Fatigue and loss of energy
    C. Constipation
    D. Sores on mucous membranes

33. The source of infection is
    A. A break in the skin
    B. A human or animal
    C. Nutritional status
    D. A pathogen

34. In the chain of infection, a portal of exit can be
    A. Blood
    B. Humans and animals
    C. General health
    D. A carrier

35. Nosocomial infections occur when
    A. Insects are present.
    B. Hand hygiene is poor.
    C. Medical asepsis is used correctly.
    D. A person is in isolation.

36. The practice that keeps equipment and supplies free of all microbes is
    A. Medical asepsis
    B. Clean technique
    C. Contamination
    D. Surgical asepsis

37. What is the easiest and most important way to prevent the spread of infection?
    A. Sterilize all equipment.
    B. Use only disposable equipment.
    C. Keep all residents in isolation.
    D. Practice good hand hygiene.

38. An alcohol-based hand rub may be used to decontaminate your hands
    A. When the hands are visibly dirty or soiled with blood, body fluids, or secretions and excretions
    B. After using the restroom
    C. After contact with the person's intact skin
    D. After all of the above

39. When washing hands, you should
    A. Use hot water.
    B. Keep hands lower than the elbows.
    C. Turn off faucets after lathering.
    D. Keep hands higher than elbows.

40. Clean under the fingernails by rubbing your fingers against your palms
    A. Each time you practice hand hygiene
    B. If you have long fingernails
    C. For the first handwashing of the day and when your hands are highly soiled
    D. For at least 10 seconds

41. To avoid contaminating your hands, turn off the faucets
    A. After soap is applied
    B. Before drying hands
    C. With clean paper towels
    D. With your elbows

42. When using alcohol-based hand rub
    A. Moisten hands with warm water.
    B. Make certain you cover all surfaces of your hands and fingers.
    C. Rub hands together for 15 seconds.
    D. Dry hands with clean paper towels.

43. When cleaning dirty equipment
    A. Wear protective equipment.
    B. Rinse in hot water.
    C. Use the clean utility room.
    D. Remove any organic materials with a paper towel.

44. Residents with dementia rely on the health team to prevent the spread of infection because
    A. They do not understand aseptic practices.
    B. They are more susceptible to infection.
    C. They resist handwashing and other antiseptic practices.
    D. All of the above.

45. Standard precautions are used
    A. For a person with a respiratory infection
    B. For a person with a wound infection
    C. For a person with tuberculosis
    D. In the care of all residents

46. Gloves worn in standard precautions
    A. Do not need to be changed when performing several tasks for the same person
    B. Can be worn until they tear or are punctured
    C. Should be removed before going to another person
    D. Are worn only if the person has an infection

47. If you are allergic to latex gloves, you should
    A. Wash your hands each time you remove the gloves.
    B. Make sure the gloves have powder inside.
    C. Report the allergy to the nurse.
    D. Never wear any gloves.

48. Hands are decontaminated
    A. Even if you wore gloves
    B. For 5 minutes between residents
    C. Only when moving between residents
    D. Only if gloves were not worn

49. What should be done with reusable equipment when a resident leaves a facility?
    A. Send it home with the family.
    B. Discard it.
    C. It is cleaned, disinfected, or sterilized.
    D. Give it to another resident.

50. If you must handle used needles, you should
    A. Remove needles from disposable syringes by hand.
    B. Place used disposable syringes and needles in plastic bags to discard.
    C. Never recap used needles.
    D. Bend the needles before discarding.

51. A person placed in airborne precautions may have
    A. Meningitis, pneumonia, or influenza
    B. A wound infection
    C. Mumps, rubella, or pertussis
    D. Measles, chickenpox, or tuberculosis

52. You do not need to wear a mask when the person has measles or chickenpox if
    A. They no longer have skin lesions.
    B. You are immune to the disease.
    C. They are not sneezing or coughing.
    D. The skin lesions are covered.

53. A gown is worn when entering a room
    A. That is isolated for airborne precautions
    B. That is isolated for droplet precautions
    C. That is isolated for contact precautions
    D. In which you will have substantial contact with a person in contact precautions

54. Which of these statements about wearing gloves is *true*?
    A. The inside of the glove is contaminated.
    B. Slightly used gloves can be saved and reused.
    C. You may need more than one pair of gloves for a task.
    D. Gloves are easier to put on when hands are damp.

55. When removing gloves
    A. Touch only the outside of the gloves with the other glove.
    B. Pull the gloves off by the fingers.
    C. Reach inside the glove with the gloved hand to pull it off.
    D. Hold the discarded gloves tightly in your hand.

56. When removing a mask, only the ties are touched because
    A. The front of the mask is contaminated.
    B. The front of the mask is sterile.
    C. Your gloves are contaminated.
    D. Your hands are contaminated.

57. When donning a gown, what is tied first?
    A. Strings at the neck
    B. Strings at the back
    C. Mask ties
    D. No preference

58. When removing protective apparel, which of the following is done first?
    A. Remove the mask.
    B. Remove the gloves.
    C. Remove the gown.
    D. Untie the gown.

59. If you wear reusable eyewear and it is contaminated
    A. It should be discarded.
    B. It should be autoclaved.
    C. Wash it with soap and water and then a disinfectant.
    D. Rinse in cool running water.

60. How are contaminated items identified when sent to the laundry or trash collection?
    A. Bags are transparent so materials are visible.
    B. The items are labeled as "contaminated."
    C. The items are always double-bagged.
    D. The items are labeled as "biohazard."

61. How are specimens collected in a contaminated room handled?
    A. All are double-bagged.
    B. It depends on center policy.
    C. Testing must be done in the room.
    D. Special containers are needed.

62. If a resident in isolation precautions must be transported to another area, all of the following would be done *except*
    A. The person wears a mask for any transmission-based precautions.
    B. The staff wears a gown, mask, and gloves as required by the isolation precautions.
    C. The staff in the receiving area is alerted so they can wear protective equipment as needed.
    D. The wheelchair or stretcher is disinfected after use.

63. Which of the following will *not* help a person in isolation meet the need for love, belonging, and self-esteem?
    A. Avoid the room so you do not disturb the person.
    B. Let the person see your face before putting on the mask.
    C. Encourage the person to telephone family and friends.
    D. Provide reading materials.

64. Persons with dementia in isolation may have increased confusion and agitation because
    A. The infection increases confusion.
    B. Personal protective equipment increases these behaviors.
    C. They feel dirty and undesirable.
    D. They do not receive any visitors.

65. What viruses are blood-borne pathogens?
    A. Influenza and pneumococcus
    B. Measles and chickenpox
    C. Acquired immunodeficiency syndrome (AIDS), human immunodeficiency virus (HIV), and hepatitis B virus (HBV)
    D. Staphylococcus and streptococcus

66. Which of these items can transmit bloodborne pathogens?
    A. Suction equipment
    B. Dressings
    C. Needles
    D. All of the above

67. How do staff members know what to do if exposed to a bloodborne pathogen?
    A. Employers must provide yearly training and information.
    B. Information is provided on the Internet.
    C. They may attend classes offered at colleges or hospitals.
    D. The nurse tells them what they need to know.

68. HBV vaccine
    A. Requires only one vaccination
    B. Must be given every year
    C. Involves three injections
    D. Is required by law

69. Which of the following is *not* a work practice control to reduce exposure risks?
    A. Discard contaminated needles and sharp instruments in containers that are closable, puncture-resistant, and leak proof.
    B. Do not store food or drinks where blood or potential infectious materials are kept.
    C. Break contaminated needles before discarding.
    D. Decontaminate hands after removing gloves.

70. Personal protective equipment
    A. Is free to employees
    B. Is purchased by staff members
    C. Must be worn by all employees rather than regular uniforms
    D. Is paid for by deducting the cost from the employee's paycheck

71. If glass is broken
    A. It can be picked up carefully with gloved hands.
    B. It is cleaned up with a brush and dustpan.
    C. A person who is especially trained to remove biohazardous materials is required to clean it up.
    D. It is wiped up with wet paper towels.

72. When discarding regulated waste, the containers are
    A. Plastic bags that are specially labeled
    B. Labeled as "contaminated" in red letters
    C. Melt-away bags
    D. Closable, puncture-resistant, and leak-proof

73. If an exposure incident occurs
    A. Report it at once.
    B. You can have free medical evaluation and follow-up.
    C. You will receive a written opinion of the medical evaluation.
    D. All of the above are true.

74. If a sterile item touches a clean item
    A. It can still be used.
    B. It is no longer sterile.
    C. It should be handled with sterile gloves.
    D. It can be placed on the sterile field.

75. When working with a sterile field, you should
    A. Always wear a mask.
    B. Keep items within your vision and above your waist.
    C. Keep the door open.
    D. Wear clean gloves.

76. When arranging the inner package of sterile gloves
    A. Have the right glove on the left and the left glove on the right.
    B. Have the fingers pointing toward you.
    C. Have the right glove on the right and the left glove on the left.
    D. Straighten the gloves to remove the cuff.

77. When picking up the first glove
    A. Grasp it by the cuff, touching only the inside.
    B. Reach under the cuff with your fingers.
    C. Grasp the edge of the cuff with your hand.
    D. Slide your hand into the glove without touching it with the other hand.

Matching

Match the kind of asepsis being used with each example.

78. _____ An item is placed in an autoclave.

79. _____ Each person has his or her own toothbrush, towel, washcloth, and other personal care items.

80. _____ Hands are washed before preparing food.

81. _____ Boiling water is used to clean items.

82. _____ Single-use or multi-use disposable items reduce the spread of infection.

83. _____ Liquid or gas chemicals are used to destroy microbes.

84. _____ Hands are washed every time you use the bathroom.

A. Medical asepsis (clean technique)

B. Surgical asepsis (sterile technique)

Match the aseptic measures used to control the related chain of infection with the step in the chain.

85. _____ Provide the person with tissues to use when coughing or sneezing.

86. _____ Make sure linens are dry and wrinkle-free to protect the skin.

87. _____ Use leak-proof plastic bags for soiled tissues, linens, and other materials.

88. _____ Wear protective equipment.

89. _____ Hold equipment and linens away from your uniform.

90. _____ Assist with cleaning or clean the genital area after elimination.

91. _____ Clean from the cleanest area to the dirtiest.

92. _____ Label bottles.

93. _____ Follow the care plan to meet the person's nutritional and fluid needs.

94. _____ Make sure drainage tubes are properly connected.

95. _____ Do not use items that are on the floor.

96. _____ Assist the person with cough and deep-breathing exercises as directed.

97. _____ Avoid sitting on a person's bed. You will pick up microorganisms and transfer them.

A. Reservoir (host)

B. Portal of exit

C. Method of transmission

D. Portal of entry

E. Susceptible host

Match the practices with the correct principles for surgical asepsis.

98. _____ Consider any item as contaminated if you are unsure of its sterility.

99. _____ Wear a mask if you need to talk during the procedure.

100. _____ Place all sterile items inside the 1-inch margin of the sterile field.

101. _____ Do not turn your back on a sterile field.

102. _____ Prevent drafts by closing the door and avoiding extra movements.

103. _____ Avoid spilling and splashing when pouring sterile fluids into sterile containers.

104. _____ If you cannot see an item, it is contaminated.

105. _____ You know when you have contaminated an item or a field. Report it to the nurse.

106. _____ Hold wet items down.

A. A sterile item can touch only another sterile item.

B. Sterile items or a sterile field are always kept within your vision and above your waist.

C. Airborne microbes can contaminate sterile items or a sterile field.

D. Fluid flows down, in the direction of gravity.

E. The sterile field is kept dry, unless the area below it is sterile.

F. The edges of a sterile field are contaminated.

G. Honesty is essential to sterile technique.

Labeling

107. These drawings show how to remove gloves. List the procedure steps shown in each drawing.

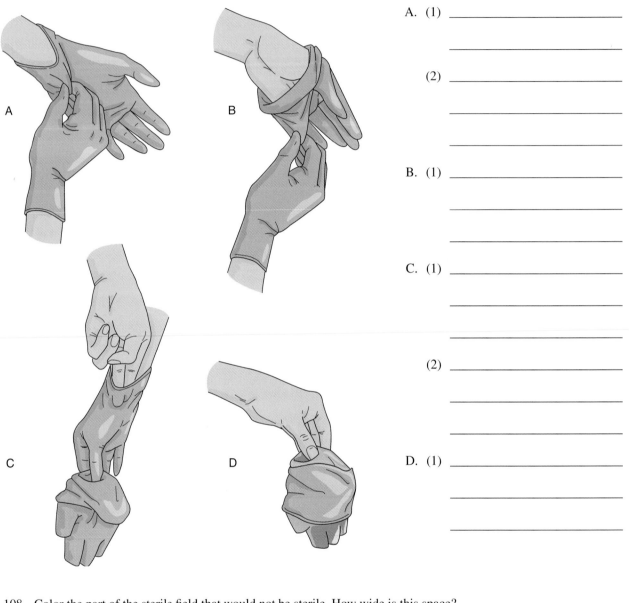

A. (1) _____

         _____

      (2) _____

         _____

B. (1) _____

         _____

         _____

C. (1) _____

         _____

         _____

      (2) _____

         _____

         _____

D. (1) _____

         _____

         _____

108. Color the part of the sterile field that would not be sterile. How wide is this space? _____

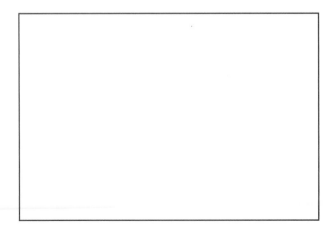

Crossword

Fill in the crossword puzzle by answering the clues with words from this list.

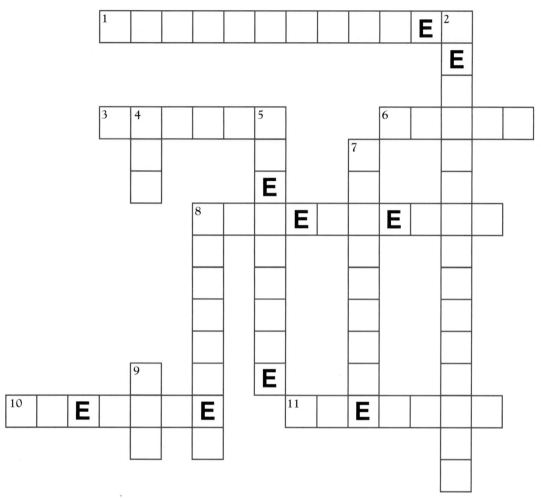

Across

1. The presence or the reasonably anticipated presence of blood or other potentially infectious material on an item or surface.
3. Any object that can penetrate the skin, such as needles, scalpels, broken glass, and broken capillary tubes.
6. Human blood, human blood components and products made from human blood.
8. Piercing mucous membranes or the skin barrier through such events as needlesticks, human bites, cuts, and abrasions.
10. The absence of all microbes.
11. Being free of disease-producing microbes.

Down

2. Use of physical or chemical means to remove, inactivate, or destroy bloodborne pathogens on a surface or item.
4. Hepatitis B virus.
5. The use of a physical or chemical procedure to destroy all microbial life, including highly resistant bacterial spores.
7. A pressure steam sterilizer.
8. A microbe that is harmful and can cause an infection.
9. Human immunodeficiency virus.

Nursing Assistant Skills Video Exercise

View the **Basic Principles Video** *to answer these questions.*

109. When should hands be washed?

_____

_____

110. How do you get a good lather when washing hands?

_____

_____

111. To clean the fingernails, rub them against the

_____ ,

and clean under them with

_____ .

112. When you dry the hands, you should start with

_____ .

Optional Learning Exercises

113. Compare medical asepsis to surgical asepsis. Medical asepsis is _____

_____ .

Surgical asepsis is _____

_____ .

114. Why are hands and forearms kept lower than elbows in hand washing?

_____

_____

115. What is the shortest length of time you should wash your hands?

_____

_____

116. Why is lotion applied after hand hygiene?

_____

117. Hands should be washed with soap and water

A. _____

B. _____

C. _____

118. Alcohol-based hand rub may be used

A. _____

B. _____

C. _____

D. _____

E. _____

F. _____

119. If you do not have alcohol-based hand rub available, you should

_____

120. When are gloves worn in standard precautions?

_____

_____

121. Masks, eye protections, and face shields are worn

during _____ .

122. What information does the nursing assistant need from the nurse or care plan when the resident requires transmission-based precautions?

   A. _____

   B. _____

   C. _____

   D. _____

123. If a person has measles and you are susceptible, what should you do?

   _____

   _____

124. Why is keeping the door closed especially important with airborne precautions?

   _____

   _____

125. If a person who is in airborne precautions must leave the room, the person must wear what?

   _____

126. How is preventing the spread of infection an important part of your job?

   _____

   _____

127. How does wearing gloves protect you and the person? It protects you _____

   _____.

   It protects the person _____

   _____.

128. Why is the gown turned inside out as you remove it?

   _____

   _____

129. If you are wearing gloves, gown, and mask, in what order are they donned?

   _____

   _____

130. When you remove gloves, gown, and mask, in what order are they removed?

   _____

   _____

131. Why is a moist mask or gown changed?

   _____

   _____

132. What basic needs may not be met when a person is in isolation?

   _____

   _____

133. In addition to blood, what body fluids are potentially infectious materials?

   _____

   _____

134. What information is included in training about bloodborne pathogens?

   A. _____

   B. _____

   C. _____

   D. _____

   E. _____

   F. _____

   G. _____

   H. _____

   I. _____

   J. _____

135. How are containers that are used to discard needles and sharp instruments identified?

_____

_____

136. The Occupational Safety and Health Administration (OSHA) requires these measures for safely handling and using personal protective equipment:

A. _____

B. _____

C. _____

D. _____

E. _____

F. _____

G. _____

H. _____

137. If you are asked to assist with a sterile procedure, what information do you need before beginning?

A. _____

B. _____

C. _____

D. _____

E. _____

Independent Learning Activities

1. Hand hygiene practices are important to use wherever you are to prevent the spread of infection. Use this exercise to make yourself aware of your own habits.
   - Make a list of when you decontaminated your hands for 1 day.
     - How did you decontaminate your hands? Did you use the method taught in this chapter?
     - How many times did you decontaminate your hands at work? At home?
     - How many times did you realize that you had forgotten to decontaminate your hands? What was the reason you forgot?
   - How can you improve your hand hygiene practices? What will you change after studying this chapter?

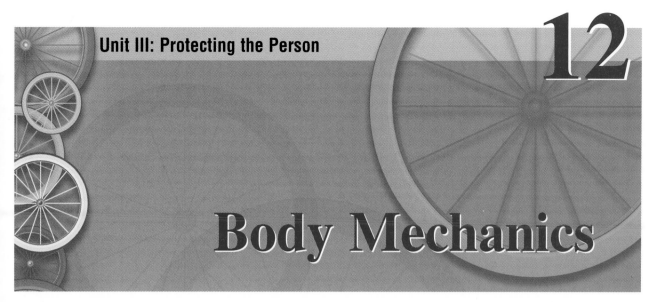

Body Mechanics

Base of support	Friction	Shearing
Body alignment	Gait belt	Side-lying position
Body mechanics	Lateral position	Sims' position
Dorsal recumbent position	Logrolling	Supine position
Ergonomics	Posture	Transfer belt
Fowler's position	Prone position	

Fill in the Blanks: Key Terms

Select your answers from the Key Terms listed above.

1. Another name for the lateral position is

   _____.

2. The way in which the head, trunk, arms, and legs

   are aligned with one another is

   _____

   or posture.

3. A _____

   is used to transfer persons who are unsteady or dis-

   abled. The device is also called a gait belt.

4. The _____

   is also called the side-lying position.

5. Another name for a transfer or safety belt is a

   _____.

6. The _____

   is the same as the back-lying or supine position.

7. _____

   occurs when skin sticks to a surface and muscles

   slide in the direction that the body is moving.

8. The area on which an object rests is the

   _____.

9. Turning the person as a unit, in alignment, with one

   motion is

   _____.

10. _____

    is a left side-lying position in which the upper leg is

    sharply flexed so that it is not on the lower leg, and

    the lower arm is behind the person.

11. A semisitting position with the head of the bed at 45

    to 90 degrees is

    _____.

12. Lying on the abdomen with the head turned to one

    side is

    _____.

13. _____

    is using the body in an efficient and careful way.

14. The back-lying or dorsal-recumbent position is also

    called the

    _____.

15. _____

    is another name for body alignment.

16. The rubbing of one surface against another is

    _____.

17. _____

    is the science of designing the job to fit the worker.

Circle the BEST Answer

18. Using good body mechanics will
    A. Prevent good posture
    B. Cause back injuries
    C. Prevent fatigue, muscle strain, and injury
    D. Cause muscle injury

19. For a wider base of support
    A. Bend your knees and squat to pick up heavy objects.
    B. The head, trunk, arms, and legs are aligned with one another.
    C. Stand with your feet apart.
    D. Make sure you are in good physical condition.

20. When you bend your knees and squat to lift a heavy object, you are
    A. Using poor body mechanics
    B. In danger of injury
    C. Likely to strain your back
    D. Using good body mechanics

21. If you have pain when standing or rising from a seated position, you
    A. May have a back injury
    B. Are using poor body mechanics
    C. Have worked too many hours
    D. Should exercise more

22. Which of these activities will help prevent back injury?
    A. Reposition a person in bed or a chair.
    B. Transfer a person from a wheelchair to the toilet.
    C. Weigh a person.
    D. Have a co-worker help you lift, move, turn, or transfer a person.

23. How many people are needed to move a person?
    A. At least one person
    B. Two or three people
    C. One, if using a mechanic lift
    D. As many as is needed to safely move the person

24. How can you reduce friction and shearing?
    A. Raise the head of the bed to a sitting position.
    B. Roll or lift the person to reposition.
    C. Pull the person up in bed.
    D. Massage the skin.

25. If a resident with dementia resists your effort to move him
    A. You can get help from coworkers to move him.
    B. You should proceed calmly and slowly.
    C. Let the person alone.
    D. Tell him firmly that he must let you move him.

26. Before lifting or moving a person, you need the following information *except*
    A. If special equipment is needed
    B. Any limits in the person's ability to move or be repositioned
    C. If the person is awake
    D. How many staff members are needed to safely lift and move the person

27. For safety and efficiency, you should
    A. Decide how you will move the person before starting the procedure.
    B. Try to move the person alone at first.
    C. Ask for help only after trying to move the person alone.
    D. Always use a mechanical lift.

28. Beds are raised horizontally to
    A. Allow the person to get out of bed with ease
    B. Lift and move persons in bed
    C. Provide safety for the person
    D. Make it easier for the person to breathe

29. When raising a person's head and shoulders
    A. You can always do this alone.
    B. A mechanical lift is needed.
    C. It is best to have help with an older person to prevent pain and injury.
    D. A transfer belt will be needed.

30. When raising the person's head and shoulders
    A. Both hands are placed under the person's back.
    B. Use a lift sheet to raise the person.
    C. The person puts his or her near arm under your near arm and behind your shoulder.
    D. Your free arm rests on the edge of the bed.

31. When assisting a person to move up in bed
    A. You may move lightweight adults up in bed by yourself if they use a trapeze.
    B. You must always use two people to move any person.
    C. Two people grasp the person under the arms and pull the person up in bed as he or she remains still.
    D. You should use a mechanical lift to avoid injury to yourself and the person.

32. What is the position of the bed when moving a person up in bed?
    A. Fowler's
    B. Semi-Fowler's
    C. As flat as comfortable for the person
    D. Trendelenburg's

33. When moving the person up in bed, the pillow is placed
    A. On the bedside table
    B. Against the headboard if the person can be without it
    C. Under the knees to help the person push up
    D. Against the bed rail

34. When moving a person, you move
    A. On the count of "2"
    B. On the count of "3"
    C. When the person says he is ready
    D. As soon as everyone is in position

35. A lift sheet is used to move persons who
    A. Cannot move themselves
    B. Are unconscious
    C. Are recovering from spinal cord surgery
    D. All of the above

36. When using a lift sheet to move a person
    A. The bed must be completely flat.
    B. The sheet is placed under the person from the head to above the knees.
    C. One person may work alone to move the person.
    D. The sheet is placed under the person from the hips to the knees.

37. A person is moved to the side of the bed before turning to
    A. Make sure the person is in the center of the bed after turning on his side.
    B. Make turning the person easier.
    C. Prevent injury to the person.
    D. Prevent skin injuries.

38. If you are moving the person in segments, which of the following would be *incorrect*?
    A. Start the movement with hips first, then move the shoulders and legs.
    B. Place your arms under the person's neck and shoulders, then move the upper part toward you.
    C. Place one arm under the person's waist and one under the thighs, then rock backward.
    D. Rock backward with your arms under the person's thighs and calves.

39. When using a lift sheet to move a person to the side of the bed, you should support the
    A. Back
    B. Knees
    C. Head
    D. Hips

40. After a person is turned for repositioning, the person
    A. Should be given good personal care
    B. Must be positioned in good body alignment
    C. Needs to have the head of the bed elevated
    D. Is at risk for friction or shearing

41. When directed to turn a person, you need to know all of the following *except*
    A. How much assistance the person needs
    B. Which procedure to use
    C. What supportive devices are needed for positioning
    D. Whether the physician has ordered the turning

42. When a person is turned on his side, he lays
    A. On the side of the bed with his back against the bedrail
    B. On the side of the bed with his face close to the bedrail
    C. In the middle of the bed
    D. Wherever he is comfortable

43. To prevent musculoskeletal injuries, skin breakdown, or pressure ulcers when a person is turned, the person must be in
    A. A special bed
    B. Good body alignment
    C. Good body mechanics
    D. All of the above

44. How do you decide whether to turn a person toward you or away from you?
    A. Check the physician's orders.
    B. Check the care plan.
    C. Ask the person whom he prefers.
    D. Use the method you like best.

45. When turning the person away from you, how are your hands placed?
    A. One on the person's far shoulder and the other on the far buttock
    B. One on the person's near shoulder and the other on the near buttock
    C. On the back near the shoulders and at the waist
    D. On the back and at the knees

46. When you position the person on the side, you will commonly do all of the following *except*
    A. Have the person lay on his shoulder and arm.
    B. Position a pillow against the back.
    C. Flex the upper leg in front of the lower leg.
    D. Place a pillow under the head and neck.

47. Logrolling is used to turn
    A. Older persons with arthritic spines or knees
    B. Persons with spinal cord injuries
    C. Persons who are recovering from hip fractures
    D. All of the above

48. When logrolling, all of the following would be correct *except*
    A. One person can work alone to logroll a person.
    B. Two or three staff members are needed to logroll a person.
    C. A turning sheet is sometimes used.
    D. The spine is kept straight throughout the move.

49. When preparing to logroll the person, a pillow is placed
    A. At the head of the bed
    B. Between the knees
    C. Under the head
    D. Under the shoulders

50. What information do you need before dangling a person?
    A. The person's diagnosis
    B. Any areas of weakness
    C. Whether the person likes to dangle
    D. When the person ate last

51. When you have a person sit on the side of the bed (dangle) and the person complains of dizziness, you should
    A. Call the nurse.
    B. Talk to the person to distract him or her.
    C. Lay the person down in bed.
    D. Offer the person a drink of water.

52. When preparing to dangle a person, the head of the bed should be
    A. Flat
    B. Slightly raised
    C. In a sitting position
    D. At a comfortable height for the person

53. When preparing to transfer a person, you should
    A. Arrange the room so there is enough space for a safe transfer.
    B. Keep furniture in the position that the resident desires.
    C. Remove all furniture from the room.
    D. Take the person to another area if you cannot transfer in the room.

54. Nonskid footwear is used to
    A. Protect the person from falling.
    B. Allow the person to bend the foot more easily.
    C. Promote comfort for the person.
    D. Keep the feet warm.

55. When applying a gait belt, which of the following is *incorrect*?
    A. Apply the belt over clothing.
    B. Tighten the belt so you can slide four fingers between the person and the belt.
    C. Place the buckle over the spine.
    D. Make sure a woman's breast is not caught under the belt.

56. When helping a person out of bed to transfer, the person should
    A. Get out of bed on the weak side.
    B. Get out of bed on the strong side.
    C. Get out of bed on the left side.
    D. Get out of bed on the right side.

57. When transferring a person, the nurse may ask you to assess the
    A. Blood pressure before and after the transfer
    B. Pulse before and after the transfer
    C. Respirations before and after the transfer
    D. Temperature before and after the transfer

58. When using a transfer belt to transfer, you grasp it
    A. At each side
    B. In the front
    C. By the buckle
    D. At the back

59. When transferring without a transfer belt, your hands are placed
    A. On the person's waist
    B. Under the person's arms and around the shoulder blades
    C. On the person's wrists
    D. On the person's elbows

60. When transferring a person who is weak on one side back to bed from a chair
    A. Transfer the person into the same side of the bed from which the person was transferred out of bed.
    B. Transfer the person into the opposite side of the bed from which the person was transferred out of bed.
    C. Always use a mechanical lift.
    D. Always have another staff member help.

61. Which of the following is *not* a factor when the nurse decides that a person will be lifted without a mechanical device?
    A. The person's height and weight
    B. The skills and strength of the staff members
    C. The height and weight of the staff members
    D. The amount of room for the transfer

62. If you are standing behind the wheelchair to transfer a person without a mechanical lift, how do you grasp the person?
    A. Grasp the person by the upper arms.
    B. Place your hands under the person's buttocks.
    C. Place your arms under the person's arms and grasp the person's forearms.
    D. Lift the person under the axilla.

63. When using a mechanical lift
    A. You may work by yourself.
    B. At least two staff members are needed.
    C. You know that all lifts are the same and do not require special training.
    D. The person's weight is not considered because the lifts are designed to lift any person.

64. As you lift a person in the sling of a mechanical lift, the person
    A. May hold the swivel bar
    B. May hold the straps or chains
    C. Must keep the arms crossed
    D. Should keep the leg outstretched to prevent injury

65. When transferring a person from a wheelchair to the toilet
    A. The toilet should have an elevated seat.
    B. The toilet seat should be removed.
    C. Always position the wheelchair next to the toilet so that the person's strong side is near the toilet.
    D. Unlock the wheelchair wheels to allow movement during the transfer.

66. Before transferring a person from a wheelchair to the toilet, you need to check
    A. The physician's order
    B. To make sure the grab bars are secure
    C. Whether the person has soiled the bed
    D. The amount of urine voided the last time the person used the toilet

67. When moving the person to the stretcher, which of the following is *not* needed?
    A. A drawsheet or lift sheet
    B. A stretcher with safety straps and side rails
    C. A transfer belt
    D. At least three workers to move the person

68. When moving the person from the bed to the stretcher, you
    A. Should have two workers stand behind the stretcher
    B. Should have two workers stand beside the bed
    C. Grab the edges of the lift sheet and spread it across the stretcher
    D. Need to loosen the bed sheets before beginning

69. How often does a person need to be repositioned?
    A. Once a shift
    B. Every 2 hours
    C. Once a day
    D. Every 4 hours

70. When positioning a person, you may also be delegated to
    A. Ambulate the person.
    B. Assist the person to the bathroom.
    C. Perform skin care measures.
    D. All of the above are true.

71. Persons with heart and respiratory disorders can usually breathe more easily in the
    A. Fowler's position
    B. Semi-Fowler's position
    C. Supine position
    D. Prone position

72. Most older persons do not tolerate the

    _____ position.

    A. Lateral
    B. Sims'
    C. Fowler's
    D. Prone

73. When positioning a person in the supine position, the nurse may ask you to place a pillow under the person's lower leg to
    A. Improve the circulation.
    B. Assist the person to breathe easier.
    C. Lift the heels off of the bed to prevent them from rubbing on the sheets.
    D. To prevent swelling of the legs and feet.

74. You usually place a pillow against the person's back

    when the person is in the

    _____.

    A. Lateral position
    B. Prone position
    C. Supine position
    D. Semi-Fowler's position

75. In the chair position, a pillow is not used
    A. To position paralyzed arms
    B. To support the feet
    C. Under the upper arm and hand
    D. Behind the back if restraints are used

76. When moving a person up in the wheelchair who cannot help, which of these steps would be *incorrect*?
    A. Have the tallest worker stand behind the wheelchair.
    B. A worker stands in front of the person and places the hands and arms under the person's knees.
    C. The person uses his arms and legs to push up on the count of "3."
    D. Lock the wheelchair wheels.

Fill in the Blanks

77. Where are strong, large muscles located that are used to lift and move heavy objects?

    A. _____

    B. _____

    C. _____

    D. _____

78. Back injuries constitute a major risk when lifting. Good body mechanics involve:

    A. _____

    B. _____

79. What three quality-of-life actions should be taken before performing procedures?

    A. _____

    B. _____

    C. _____

80. Many procedures for lifting and moving include the same pre-procedure guidelines, which are:

    A. Follow _____ .

    B. Ask _____ .

    C. Practice _____ .

    D. Identify _____ .

    E. Explain _____ .

    F. Provide _____ .

    G. Lock _____ .

    H. Raise _____ .

81. Many procedures for lifting and moving include the same post-procedure guidelines, which are:

    A. Provide _____ .

    B. Place _____ .

    C. Raise _____ .

    D. Lower _____ .

    E. Unscreen _____ .

    F. Practice _____ .

    G. Report _____ .

82. After dangling a person, you should report and record:

    A. _____

    B. _____

    C. _____

    D. _____

    E. _____

    F. _____

    G. _____

83. What is the purpose of the paper or sheet you collect when getting ready to transfer a person to a chair or wheelchair?

    _____

    _____

84. If your center has a "no-lift" policy, you must use

    _____

    _____ .

85. When you screen the person properly and expose only the body part involved when you lift, move, transfer, and position a person, you protect the person's right to

    _____ .

86. The right to _____

    is protected when you let the person choose things such as bed positions, where the chair or wheelchair is positioned after transfers, and when to go back to bed.

87. _____

    are considered restraints under OBRA and are used only with the person's consent.

Labeling

88. Label the positions in each of the drawings.

A. _____

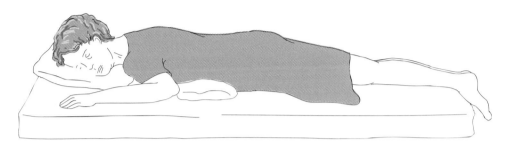

B. _____

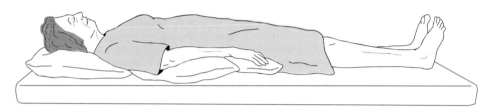

C. _____

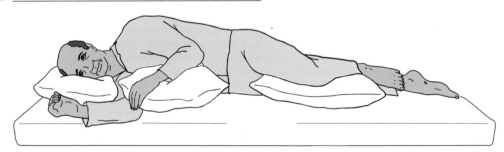

D. _____

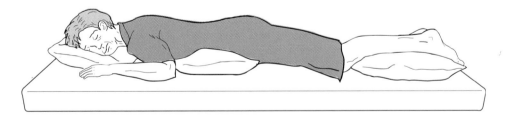

E. _____

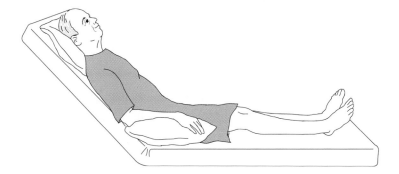

F. _____

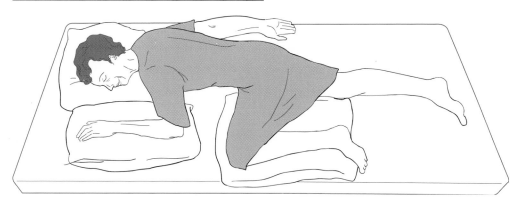

Nursing Assistant Skills Video Exercise

View the first part of the **Body Mechanics and Exercise** *video to answer these questions.*

89. What are the three principles of body mechanics that should be used when performing lifting and moving procedures?

   A. _____

   B. _____

   C. _____

90. When you are standing correctly, what body parts are bases of support?

   _____

   _____

91. When lifting and moving, when do you decide how to move the person and when to get help?

   _____

   _____

92. How do you provide privacy for the person?

   _____

   _____

93. What muscles do you use when moving a person up in bed?

    A. _____

    B. _____

    C. _____

    D. _____

94. When turning a person, after moving the person closer to your side the near leg is

    _____

    _____.

95. Where do you place your arms to position a person to dangle?

    _____

    _____

96. Place the wheelchair back even with the

    _____

    when preparing to transfer a person from the bed to

    a wheelchair.

97. As the person stands to transfer from the bed to the wheelchair, how do you brace and block the person's feet?

    _____

    _____

98. After the person is sitting in the wheelchair, where do you position the chair?

    _____

99. What observations are reported after transferring a person to the wheelchair?

    A. _____

    B. _____

    C. _____

    D. _____

Optional Learning Exercises

100. According to the Occupational Safety and Health Administration (OSHA), certain activities are associated with back injuries. Read the following examples and list the activity that can cause a back injury in each example.

    A. The nursing assistant does not raise the level of the bed when changing linens.

       _____

       _____

    B. While you are walking with Mr. Smith, he slips and starts to fall.

       _____

       _____

    C. Mrs. Tippett slides down in bed and looks uncomfortable.

       _____

       _____

    D. You are giving a complete bed bath to Mrs. Miller and she needs to be turned.

       _____

       _____

    E. You find Mrs. Watson lying on the floor.

       _____

       _____

    F. Mr. Brooks needs help to use the toilet. He is in a wheelchair.

       _____

       _____

101. When a person has been logrolled and is being positioned in good alignment, where would you place pillows?

   A. _____

   B. _____

   C. _____

   D. _____

102. Why is providing support important when a person is dangling on the side of the bed?

   _____

   _____

103. Regular position changes and good body alignment promotes:

   A. _____

   B. _____

   C. _____

   D. _____

These prevent:

   E. _____

   F. _____

104. Pressure ulcers occur when the person lays or sits

   _____;

   they may also occur when linens are

   _____.

105. Contractures can be prevented by

   _____

   _____.

Independent Learning Activities

1. After learning about using good body mechanics in this chapter, think about how well you practice body mechanics in your daily life and answer these questions.
   - How much do the books you carry with you each day weigh? How do you carry them? When carrying them, where is your base of support? Is your body in good alignment?
   - Do you have small children that you pick up? How do you lift them? What methods listed in this chapter do you use?
   - When carrying groceries into the house, do you carry them held close to the body? How well are you using good body mechanics?
   - At the end of the day, how do you feel? How might using good body mechanics help you avoid any discomfort?

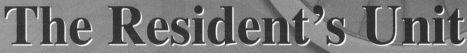

The Resident's Unit

Fowler's position	Reverse Trendelenburg's position
Full visual privacy	Semi-Fowler's position
Resident unit	Trendelenburg's position

Fill in the Blanks: Key Terms

Select your answers from the Key Terms listed above.

1. The personal space, furniture, and equipment provided for the individual by the nursing center make up the

   _____.

2. In _____,

   the head of the bed is raised 45 degrees, and the knee portion is raised 15 degrees; or the head of the bed is raised 30 degrees, and the knee portion is not raised.

3. _____

   is a semisitting position; the head of the bed is raised 45 to 90 degrees.

4. The head of the bed is raised, and the foot of the bed is lowered in

   _____.

5. In _____,

   the head of the bed is lowered, and the foot of the bed is raised.

6. The person has the means to be completely free from public view while in bed when they have

   _____.

Circle the BEST Answer

7. When residents share a room
   A. You may rearrange items and furniture in the room as needed.
   B. Each person has a private area.
   C. Residents may use each other's belongings.
   D. They generally share furniture such as a dresser.

8. OBRA requires that nursing centers maintain a temperature range of
   A. 68° to 74° Fahrenheit
   B. 61° to 71° Fahrenheit
   C. 71° to 81° Fahrenheit
   D. 78° to 85° Fahrenheit

9. Persons who are older and chronically ill
   A. Need cooler room temperatures
   B. Need warmer room temperatures
   C. Are insensitive to room temperature changes
   D. Need a warmer room at night

10. Which of these factors that affect comfort cannot be controlled by the nursing staff?
    A. Illness
    B. Temperature
    C. Noise
    D. Odors

11. If an older person complains of a draft
    A. Have the person go to bed.
    B. Give the person a hot shower.
    C. Offer a lap robe or a warm sweater to wear.
    D. Pull the privacy curtain around the person.

12. If unpleasant odors occur, do all of the following *except*
    A. Use spray deodorizers around residents with breathing problems.
    B. Provide good personal hygiene for residents.
    C. Change and dispose of soiled linens and clothing.
    D. Empty and clean bedpans, commodes, urinals, and kidney basins promptly.

13. Noises in a strange setting, such as a nursing center, may keep a resident from meeting the need for
    A. Love and belonging
    B. Self-esteem
    C. Rest
    D. Safety and security

14. Which of these measures will *not* reduce noises in a nursing center?
    A. Have drapes in rooms.
    B. Use only metal equipment.
    C. Answer the telephone promptly.
    D. Oil wheels on equipment.

15. Soft, nonglare lighting is helpful for all of the following *except*
    A. Helping residents to relax
    B. Decreasing agitation in residents with dementia
    C. Improving orientation in residents with dementia
    D. Helping residents rest

16. Cranks on manual beds are kept down when not in use to
    A. Prevent residents from operating the bed.
    B. Prevent anyone walking past the crank from bumping into it.
    C. Keep the bed in the correct position.
    D. Make sure they are ready to use at all times.

17. How can the staff prevent a person from adjusting an electric bed to unsafe positions?
    A. Lock the bed into a position.
    B. Unplug the bed.
    C. Assign the person to a bed that cannot be repositioned.
    D. Keep reminding the person not to change the position.

18. What bed position may adjust the head of the bed and the knee portion to prevent sliding down in bed?
    A. Fowler's
    B. Semi-Fowler's
    C. Trendelenburg's
    D. Reverse Trendelenburg's

19. What items should *not* be placed on the overbed table?
    A. Meals
    B. Personal care items
    C. Writing and reading materials
    D. Bedpans, urinals, and soiled linens

20. Where are the bedpan and urinal kept in the bedside table?
    A. Wherever the person wants
    B. On the top shelf
    C. On the bottom shelf
    D. In the top drawer

21. OBRA requires that the resident unit always has
    A. Two chairs
    B. A straight-back chair
    C. A reclining chair
    D. At least one chair for personal and visitor use

22. Privacy curtains
    A. Are sometimes used in rooms with more than one bed
    B. Are always pulled completely around the bed when care is given
    C. Can block sounds and conversations
    D. May be open when giving personal care

23. Personal care items
    A. Must be supplied by the nursing center
    B. May be brought by the residents
    C. Must be ordered by the physician
    D. Are required by OBRA

24. When the resident is weak on the left side, the signal light
    A. Is placed on the left side
    B. Is removed from the room
    C. Is placed on the right side
    D. Is replaced by an intercom

25. If a confused resident cannot use a signal light
    A. Explain often how to use the signal light.
    B. Use an intercom instead of the signal light.
    C. Remove the signal light.
    D. Check the resident often.

26. Elevated toilet seats
    A. Help residents with joint problems.
    B. Make wheelchair transfers easier.
    C. May be removable.
    D. All of the above are true.

27. When a person uses a bathroom signal light
    A. It flashes above the room door and at the nurse's station.
    B. It makes the same sound as the room signal light.
    C. It activates the intercom.
    D. All of the above are true.

28. Closet and drawer space
    A. Is shared by residents in a room with more than one person
    B. Can be cleaned out by a staff member
    C. Cannot be searched without the resident's permission
    D. Must have free access for the resident

29. What equipment may be in rehabilitation and subacute rooms that are not usually in long-term care centers?
    A. Televisions
    B. Commode chairs
    C. Piped-in wall oxygen and suctioning
    D. Electric beds

30. Residents can bring some furniture and personal items to use in the room as long as the choices
    A. Do not interfere with the rights of others
    B. Match the color and decoration in the room
    C. Can be cared for by the resident or the family
    D. Do not need to be attached to the wall

Labeling

31. In this figure:

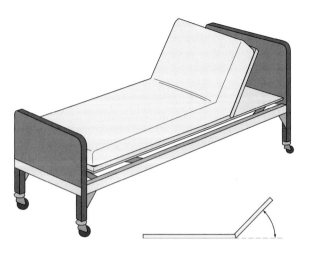

A. What is the bed position called?

_____

_____

B. What is the angle of the head of the bed?

_____

_____

C. Why is this position used?

_____

_____

32. In this figure:

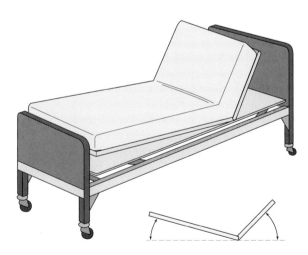

A. What is the bed position called?

_____

_____

B. What is the angle of the head of the bed?

_____

_____

C. Why is this position used?

_____

_____

34. In this figure:

A. What is the bed position called?

_____

_____

B. What is the position of the head of the bed and the foot of the bed?

_____

_____

C. Who decides this position is to be used?

_____

_____

33. In this figure:

A. What is the bed position called?

_____

B. What is the position of the head of the bed and the foot of the bed?

_____

_____

C. Who decides this position is to be used?

_____

_____

Optional Learning Exercises

35. Comfort is affected by three factors that cannot be controlled. These factors are:

A. _____

B. _____

C. _____

36. Four factors that can be controlled to increase comfort are:

    A. _____

    B. _____

    C. _____

    D. _____

37. In these situations, how would you help protect a resident from drafts?

    A. The person is dressing for the day.

    _____

    _____

    B. The person is sitting in a wheelchair.

    _____

    _____

    C. You are assisting a resident who is going to bed for the night.

    _____

    _____

    D. You are giving personal care to the resident.

    _____

    _____

38. How can you help eliminate odors in these situations?

    A. You are caring for a resident who is frequently incontinent.

    _____

    _____

B. The resident is vomiting and has wound drainage.

    _____

    _____

C. The resident changes his own ostomy drainage bag in his bathroom.

    _____

    _____

D. The resident keeps a urinal at his bedside and uses it himself during the day.

    _____

    _____

39. When the staff talks loudly and laughs in hallways, some residents may think that

    _____

    _____.

40. Why do persons with dementia react more to loud noises at night?

    _____

    _____

41. How can the staff reduce noises and increase resident comfort?

    A. Control

    _____

    B. Handle

    _____

    C. Answer

    _____

42. What are two situations in which bright lights are helpful for a resident with poor vision?

    A. _____

    B. _____

43. In dementia units, how does adjusting lighting help the residents?

    A. Soft, nonglare:

    _____

    _____

    B. Brighter:

    _____

    _____

44. The bed in the flat position is used for

    A. _____

    B. _____

45. Fowler's position is used for persons with

    _____.

46. Semi-Fowler's has two definitions:

    A. _____

    B. _____

47. How do you know which of the ways in #46 to position the bed when semi-Fowler's position is ordered?

    _____

    _____

48. To raise the foot of the bed with Trendelenburg's position, you may place

    _____

    _____.

49. When the nursing team uses the over-bed table as a work area, what are the only items that can be placed on it?

    _____

    _____

50. What are your responsibilities in these situations regarding the signal light?

    A. The resident is sitting in a chair next to the bed.

    _____

    _____

    B. The person is weak on the right side.

    _____

    _____

    C. The person calls out instead of using the signal light.

    _____

    _____

    D. The resident is embarrassed because she soiled the bed after signaling for assistance.

    _____

    _____

    E. The emergency light in a room signals while you are busy in another room.

    _____

    _____

51. The resident is allowed to bring personal items to make his space as homelike as possible. The health team must make sure the resident's choices

    A. _____

    B. _____

    C. _____

52. List the OBRA requirement that relates to each of these items in the resident unit.

    A. Number of residents in a room:

    _____

    _____

    B. Windows:

    _____

    _____

    C. Closets:

    _____

    _____

    D. Call system:

    _____

    _____

    E. Odors, noise, lighting:

    _____

    _____

    F. Hand rails, bedrails:

    _____

    _____

Independent Learning Activities

1. When you are in the health care center as a student, find an empty resident room and practice using the equipment. Answer these questions about the equipment.
   - Where are the controls for the bed?
     - How do you operate the head of the bed?
     - How do you operate the knee control of the bed?
     - How do you adjust the height of the bed?
   - Where is the signal light located?
   - Where are controls for the television and radio?
   - Does the center have an intercom system? How is it used?

2. Ask the staff these questions about the signal lights.
   - How does the staff know when a resident turns on the signal light?
   - When a resident uses a bathroom signal light, how does the staff know the difference?

3. Think about what temperature is comfortable for you and answer these questions. This exercise will help you understand the importance of individual preferences for residents in the health care center.
   - What is the usual temperature of your home?
   - Who decides what the temperature will be in your home? Partner, spouse, roommate, children?
   - Would the temperature you prefer be comfortable for an infant? An older person? Why or why not?

4. Think about the noises in your home and how they affect you. This exercise will help you understand why noise levels in the nursing center can affect the residents.
   - When you study, do you turn on the television or radio? Listen to music? Prefer complete silence?
   - What noises do you like when going to sleep? Television? Radio? Soft music?
   - Does everyone in your household agree on how loud or soft to play a radio or television? How are conflicts about noise levels resolved?
   - If the noise in your surroundings is unacceptable, how do you react? How does it affect your ability to think? To rest? To study? How does it affect your relationship with others?

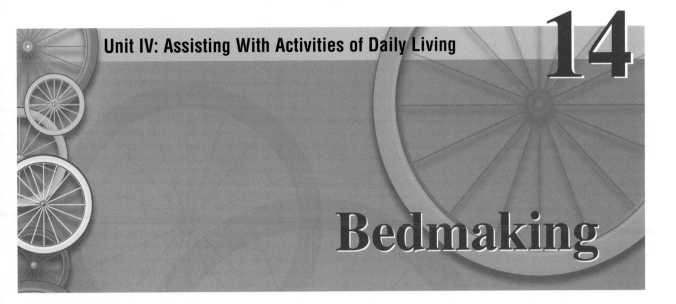

Bedmaking

Drawsheet
Plastic drawsheet

Fill in the Blanks: Key Terms

Select your answers from the Key Terms listed above.

1. A drawsheet that is placed between the bottom sheet

   and cotton drawsheet to keep the mattress and

   bottom linens clean and dry is a

   _____.

2. A _____ is a

   small sheet placed over the middle of the bottom

   sheet; it helps to keep the mattress and bottom

   linens dry and clean.

Circle the BEST Answer

3. In nursing centers, bed linens are changed
   A. Only when the linens are wet or soiled
   B. Every day after baths
   C. On the person's bath or shower day
   D. Once a week

4. You should follow Standard Precautions and
   Bloodborne Pathogen Standard when you
   A. Change any bed linens
   B. Make the bed every morning
   C. May have contact with wet, soiled, or damp
      linens soiled with the person's blood, body
      fluids, secretions, or excretions
   D. Place clean linens on the bed

5. Which of the following statements about a closed
   bed is *not* true?
   A. A closed bed is made after a person is
      discharged.
   B. The top linens are fan-folded back, which en-
      ables the person to get into bed with ease.
   C. Closed beds are made for people who are out of
      bed most of the day.
   D. If a bedspread is used, it covers the pillow and is
      tucked under the pillow.

6. When making a bed, good body mechanics are used by
   A. Bending from the waist when removing and replacing the linens
   B. Stretching across the bed to smooth the linens
   C. Raising the bed to a comfortable height to prevent injury to the nursing assistant
   D. Locking the wheels

7. If extra clean linens are brought to a person's room, you should
   A. Return the unused linens to the linen room.
   B. Store the extra linens in the person's closet.
   C. Place the unused linens in the dirty laundry.
   D. Use the linens for a person in the next room.

8. An open bed is
   A. Made with the person in it
   B. In use; top linens are folded back so that the person can get into bed
   C. Not in use until bedtime; top linens are not folded back
   D. Made to transfer a person from a stretcher to the bed

9. When handling linens and making beds, which of these actions *do not* follow the rules of medical asepsis?
   A. Place the dirty linens on the floor.
   B. Hold the linens away from your body and uniform.
   C. Never shake linens in the air.
   D. Place clean linens on a clean surface.

10. Which of these linens will be collected first?
    A. Bath towel
    B. Bath blanket
    C. Mattress pad
    D. Top sheet

11. When you remove dirty linens, which of these actions is *incorrect?*
    A. Gather all the linens in one large roll.
    B. Roll each piece away from you.
    C. Top and bottom sheets, drawsheets, and pillowcases are always changed.
    D. The blanket and bedspread may be reused for the same person.

12. A plastic drawsheet can
    A. Cause discomfort and skin breakdown
    B. Be hard to keep tight and wrinkle free
    C. Keep the mattress and bottom linens clean and dry
    D. All of the above

13. When you are delegated to make a bed, why do you need to know the person's schedule for treatments, therapies, and activities?
    A. You need to make sure the bed is flat.
    B. It is best to change linens after the treatment or when the person is out of the room.
    C. You need to unlock beds that have been locked in a certain position.
    D. You will know what type of bed to make.

14. When you are assigned to make a bed, which of the following is *not* information you need from the nurse or care plan?
    A. What type of bed to make
    B. If the person uses bed rails
    C. When the bed was changed last
    D. How to position the person and positioning devices needed

15. When a person is discharged from a hospital or nursing center, what is done in addition to changing the bed?
    A. New pillows are placed on the bed
    B. The bed frame and mattress are cleaned according to center policy
    C. The bed is sterilized
    D. The bedspread and blanket may be reused

16. When making a bed, position the bottom sheet with
    A. The lower edge even with the top of the mattress
    B. The hemstitching facing downward
    C. The large hem at the bottom and the small hem at the top
    D. All of the above

17. When the top sheet, blanket, and bedspread are in place on the bed
    A. Each one is tucked under the mattress separately.
    B. The sheet and blanket are tucked together, and the bedspread is allowed to hang loosely over them.
    C. All three are tucked together under the foot of the bed, and the corners are mitered.
    D. All three items are allowed to hang loosely over the foot of the bed.

18. The pillow is placed on the bed so that
    A. The open end is away from the door
    B. The seam of the pillowcase is toward the foot of the bed
    C. It is leaning against the head of the bed
    D. The open end is toward the door

19. If you are making a bed that is occupied by a person who is comatose, it is important to
    A. Keep the bed in the low position
    B. Unlock the wheels
    C. Use special linens
    D. Explain each step of the procedure to the person before it is done

20. When making an occupied bed, a bath blanket is used to
    A. Protect the person while he or she is being bathed
    B. Cover the person for warmth and privacy
    C. Protect the bed linens
    D. Protect the person from dirty linens

21. To provide safety when making a bed that is occupied by a person who does not use bed rails, you should
    A. Have a co-worker work on the opposite side of the bed.
    B. Push the bed against the wall.
    C. Always keep one hand on the person while you are making the bed.
    D. Change linens only when the person is out of the bed for tests or therapies.

22. When making an occupied bed, how is privacy provided?
    A. Close the door.
    B. Cover the person with a bath blanket when linens are removed.
    C. Pull the curtain around the bed in a semiprivate room.
    D. All of the above are true.

23. Which of these steps is *not* done when making a surgical bed?
    A. Tuck all top linens under the mattress together and make a mitered corner.
    B. Remove all linens from the bed.
    C. Place the mattress pad on the mattress.
    D. Place the bottom sheet with the lower edge even with the bottom of the mattress.

24. You allow the person the right of personal choice when you
    A. Allow the person to use bed linens from home.
    B. Decide which linens will look best in the room.
    C. Tell the person that you will make the bed at 9:00 AM.
    D. Choose the pillows and blanket the person needs for comfort.

Fill in the Blanks

25. Number the following list from 1 to 15 in the order you would collect the linens to make a bed.

    _____ Pillowcases

    _____ Top sheet

    _____ Hospital gown

    _____ Bottom sheet (flat or fitted)

    _____ Laundry bag

    _____ Mattress pad

    _____ Bedspread

    _____ Plastic drawsheet

    _____ Bath blanket

    _____ Hand towel

    _____ Cotton drawsheet

    _____ Gloves

    _____ Bath towels

    _____ Blanket

    _____ Washcloth

Nursing Assistant Skills Video Exercise

View the **Bedmaking** *video to answer these questions.*

26. The following are the basic principles of bedmaking. Two are missing. List the two missing basic principles.
    • Protect privacy and confidentiality.
    • Prevent infection.
    • Promote comfort and safety.
    • Select appropriate equipment.

    • _____

    • _____

27. As part of the procedural guidelines, you should use standard precautions and

    _____

    standards.

28. Gloves are worn when

    _____.

29. If the blanket and bedspread are to be reused, they

    should be _____.

30. Before removing the dirty top sheet, cover

    the person with a _____

    to provide warmth and privacy.

31. When you have removed all of the dirty linens, you

    should remove _____

    and wash _____.

32. After the person rolls over the fan-folded linens, what does the worker on the second side of the bed remove?

    _____

    _____

33. When you put the top sheet on the bed, the hemstitching should be

    _____

    _____

34. When do you remove the bath blanket that covers the person while the linens are changed?

    _____

    _____

Optional Learning Exercises

35. When is a complete linen change made in a nursing center?

    _____

    _____

    How does this policy differ from linen changes in a hospital?

    _____

    _____

    Why are linen changes done less often in a nursing center than they are in a hospital?

    _____

    _____

36. Beds are made every day to increase

    _____

    and to prevent _____

    and _____.

37. Even when a complete linen change is not scheduled, you should do the following to keep beds neat and clean:

    A. _____

    B. _____

    C. _____

    D. _____

    E. _____

38. When handling linens, practice medical asepsis. Explain why each of the following actions would be *poor* medical asepsis.

    A. Holding the linens close to your body and uniform:

    _____

    _____

    B. Shaking the linens to straighten them:

    _____

    _____

    C. Placing the dirty linens on the floor:

    _____

    _____

39. The mattress pad, plastic drawsheet, blanket, and bedspread are reused for the same person unless they are

    _____

    _____.

40. Family and visitors may question the quality

    _____

    and the quality _____

    if the bed is unmade, messy, or dirty.

Independent Learning Activities

1. When you make beds at home this week, practice the methods you learned in this chapter.
   - What linens did you collect? What was the order of the linens?
   - Did you remember to make as much of one side of the bed as possible before moving to the other side?
   - What step cannot be carried out at home that may have helped you use good body mechanics?
   - Think about the methods you used to change your bed before reading this chapter. How did you change your bedmaking practices now that you studied this chapter?

2. Practice with a classmate and take turns as a resident who must have an occupied bed made. Ask these questions about your feelings.
   - In what ways was your privacy protected?
   - Did the caregiver offer you any choices before making your bed? What were these choices?
   - Did you feel safe at all times? If not, what made you feel unsafe?
   - What was uncomfortable during the bed change?
   - How were you positioned after the bed was made?

Remembering the order that linens are collected is sometimes difficult for a new nursing assistant. If you have difficulty with the correct order, make a list in a pocket notebook or on a 3 × 5 index card so you can carry it with you when you are working.

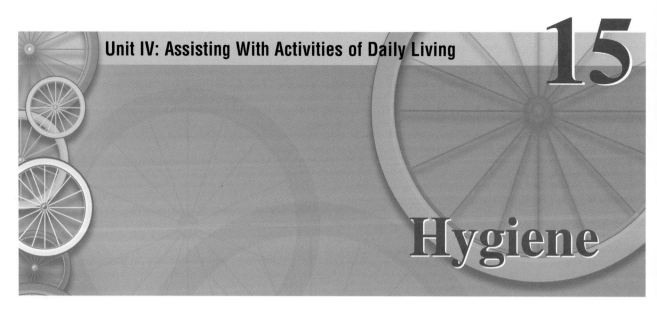

Hygiene

AM care	HS care	Perineal care
Aspiration	Morning care	Plaque
Early morning care	Oral hygiene	PM care
Evening care	Pericare	Tartar

Fill in the Blanks: Key Terms

Select your answers from the Key Terms listed above.

1. Another name for HS care or PM care is

   _____.

2. _____

   is cleansing the genital and anal areas.

3. Sometimes HS care or evening care is called

   _____.

4. Routine care before breakfast or early morning care

   is called

   _____.

5. _____

   is mouth care.

6. Hardened plaque on teeth is

   _____.

7. _____

   occurs when breathing fluid or an object into the

   lungs.

8. Care given after breakfast when cleanliness and skin

   care are more thorough is called

   _____.

9. Another name for perineal care is

   _____.

10. _____

    is a thin film that sticks to the teeth and contains

    saliva, microorganisms, and other substances.

11. Another name for AM care is

    _____.

12. Care given in the evening at bedtime is

    _____.

    Care given at this time is also called evening care or

    afternoon care.

Circle the BEST Answer

13. If a person needs help with personal hygiene, you
    can find out what needs he or she has by
    A. Looking at the care plan
    B. Asking the family
    C. Asking other staff members
    D. Making your own decisions

14. You should assist a person with personal hygiene
    A. Only when the person asks
    B. Only in the morning
    C. Whenever necessary
    D. Only when you are assigned to do so

15. When giving personal hygiene, you need to re-
    member to protect the person's right to
    A. Privacy and personal choice
    B. Care and security of personal possessions
    C. Activities
    D. Environment

16. Which of these hygiene measures is _not_ done before
    breakfast?
    A. Assisting with elimination
    B. Straightening resident units, including making
       beds
    C. Assisting with personal hygiene: face and hand
       washing, oral hygiene, bathing, back massage,
       and perineal care
    D. Assisting with oral hygiene

17. Which of these is done every time you offer hygiene
    measures throughout the day?
    A. Dressing and hair care assistance
    B. Face and hand washing
    C. Activity assistance
    D. Helping the person change into sleepwear

18. If good oral hygiene is not practiced regularly, the
    person may develop periodontal disease, which will
    lead to
    A. Dry mouth
    B. Tartar buildup
    C. Tooth loss
    D. Cavities

19. All of the following health team members may as-
    sess the person's need for mouth care _except_ the
    A. Speech-language pathologist
    B. Physical therapist
    C. Nurse
    D. Dietician

20. Sponge swabs are used for
    A. Persons with sore, tender mouths and for persons
       who are unconscious
    B. Cleaning dentures
    C. Oral care on children
    D. Oral care on all residents

21. You should follow Standard Precautions and
    Bloodborne Pathogen Standard when giving oral
    hygiene because
    A. You will prevent the spread of bacteria to the
       person.
    B. It will help you avoid bad breath odors from the
       person.
    C. It will prevent contact with bleeding gums and
       microbes in the mouth.
    D. You will avoid any loose teeth or rough dentures.

22. When the person is able to perform oral hygiene in
    bed, you arrange the items on
    A. Overbed table
    B. Bedside table
    C. Sink counter
    D. Bed

23. When you are brushing the person's teeth, which of
    these steps would be _incorrect?_
    A. Let the person rinse the mouth with water.
    B. Use a sponge swab to clean the teeth.
    C. Brush the person's tongue gently, if needed.
    D. Floss the person's teeth.

24. Teeth are flossed to
    A. Remove plaque from the teeth
    B. Remove tartar from the teeth
    C. Remove food from between the teeth
    D. All of the above

25. Which of these steps is *incorrect* when flossing the teeth?
    A. Start at the lower back tooth on the right side.
    B. Hold the floss between the middle fingers when flossing the upper teeth.
    C. Move the floss gently up and down between the teeth.
    D. Move to a new section of floss after every second tooth.

26. When providing mouth care for an unconscious person, position the person on one side with the head turned well to the side to
    A. Make it easier to brush the teeth.
    B. Make the person more comfortable.
    C. Prevent or reduce the risk of aspiration.
    D. Make it easier for the person to breathe.

27. Mouth care is given to an unconscious person
    A. After each meal
    B. When AM and PM care is given
    C. At least every 2 hours
    D. Once a day

28. A padded tongue blade is used when giving oral hygiene to an unconscious person to
    A. Separate the upper and lower teeth.
    B. Clean the teeth.
    C. Clean the tongue.
    D. Prevent aspiration.

29. When cleaning dentures at a sink, line the sink with a towel to
    A. Prevent infections.
    B. Prevent damage to the dentures if they are dropped.
    C. Dry the dentures.
    D. Clean the dentures.

30. If the person cannot remove the dentures, what can you can use to get a good grip on the slippery dentures?
    A. Gloves
    B. Washcloth
    C. Gauze squares
    D. Your bare hands

31. If dentures are not worn after cleaning, store them in
    A. Cool water
    B. Hot water
    C. Soft towel
    D. Soft tissues or a napkin

32. Older persons usually need a complete bath or shower once a week because
    A. They are less active.
    B. They are often ill.
    C. They have increased perspiration.
    D. Dry skin often occurs with aging.

33. If a person with dementia resists care, you should
    A. Hurry through the bath.
    B. Speak firmly in a loud voice to get the person's attention.
    C. Calm the person, and try the bath later.
    D. Use restraints so the person will not harm you.

34. When choosing skin care products for bathing, you should use
    A. Soap
    B. Products that the person chooses
    C. Bath oils
    D. Creams and lotions

35. The water temperature for a complete bed bath is usually between 110° and 115° Fahrenheit for adults. For older adults, the temperature
    A. Should be 110° and 115° Fahrenheit
    B. May need to be lower
    C. Should be whatever you believe is comfortable
    D. May need to be warmer

36. A complete bed bath is given to people who
    A. Cannot bathe themselves
    B. Are unconscious or paralyzed
    C. Are weak from illness or surgery
    D. All of the above

37. When you are giving a complete bed bath, the bed linens
    A. May be changed if needed
    B. Are changed before the bath begins
    C. Are changed after the bath is complete
    D. Are changed after the person gets out of bed

38. The bedpan or urinal is
    A. Offered before the bath begins
    B. Offered after the bath ends
    C. Is left in place during the bath
    D. Not offered at all during the bath procedure

39. During the bath, the bath blanket is placed
    A. Over the top linens
    B. Under the top linens
    C. Over the top linens, which are then removed
    D. Under the person

40. Soap is not used when washing
    A. The face, ears, and neck
    B. Around the eyes
    C. The abdomen
    D. The perineal area

41. How do you avoid exposing the person when washing the chest?
    A. Keep the bath blanket over the area.
    B. Keep the top linens over the chest.
    C. Place a bath towel over the chest crosswise.
    D. Make sure the curtains are closed.

42. Bath water is changed
    A. Every 5 minutes during the bath
    B. Only when it becomes cool and soapy
    C. After washing the legs, feet, and back
    D. After washing the face, ears, and neck

43. A towel bath may be used to give a bath to a resident
    A. With dementia
    B. Who has been incontinent
    C. With breaks in the skin
    D. Who needs a partial bath

44. A partial bath involves bathing
    A. Areas the person cannot reach
    B. The person's face, hands, axillae (underarms), back, buttocks, and perineal area
    C. Arms, legs, and feet
    D. Chest, abdomen, and underarms

45. A tub bath should not last longer than
    A. 10 minutes
    B. 15 minutes
    C. 20 minutes
    D. 30 minutes

46. If a person is weak or unsteady, which of the following should be used when the person showers?
    A. Shower chair
    B. Transfer belt
    C. Wheelchair
    D. Stretcher

47. When assisting with a tub bath or shower, which of these steps is performed first?
    A. Help the person undress and remove footwear.
    B. Assist or transport the person to the tub or shower room.
    C. Display the "occupied" sign on the door.
    D. Place a rubber bath mat in the tub or on the shower floor.

48. The best position for a back massage is
    A. Prone position
    B. Supine position
    C. Side-lying position
    D. Semi-Fowler's position

49. Back massages are dangerous for persons with all of these problems *except*
    A. Heart diseases
    B. Lung disorders
    C. Arthritis
    D. Reddened areas on bony areas

50. When giving a back massage, the strokes
    A. Should start at the shoulders and go down to the buttocks
    B. Should be light and gentle
    C. Should start at the buttocks and go up to the shoulders
    D. Are continued for at least 10 minutes

51. When cleaning the perineal area
    A. You do not need to wear gloves.
    B. Work from the anal area to the urethra.
    C. Work from the urethra to the anal area.
    D. Work from the dirtiest area to the cleanest.

52. When gathering equipment for perineal care, you will need
    A. One washcloth
    B. Two washcloths
    C. At least three washcloths
    D. At least four washcloths

53. When giving perineal care to a man, you
    A. Retract the foreskin if he is uncircumcised.
    B. Wash from the scrotum to the tip of the penis.
    C. Use one washcloth for the entire procedure.
    D. Leave the foreskin retracted after finishing the care.

54. If a family member or friend offers to help provide hygiene to a person
    A. You should check the center policy.
    B. Allow the person to decide if this is acceptable.
    C. Accept the offer and allow him or her to give the care.
    D. Tell the family or friend that this is not allowed.

Matching

Match the skin-care product with the benefits or the problem that may occur if you use the product.

55. _____ Absorbs moisture and prevents friction

56. _____ Makes showers and tubs slippery

57. _____ Protects skin from the drying effect of air and evaporation

58. _____ Too much can cause caking and crusts that irritate the skin

59. _____ Masks and controls body odors

60. _____ Tends to dry and irritate skin

61. _____ Keeps skin soft and prevents drying

62. _____ Removes dirt, dead skin, skin oil, some microbes, and perspiration

A. Soaps

B. Bath oils

C. Creams and lotions

D. Powders

E. Deodorants and antiperspirants

Fill in the Blanks

63. To prevent microbes from entering the body and causing an infection, the skin and

_____

must be kept clean and intact.

64. The religion of East Indian Hindus requires at least

_____ a day.

65. Some Hindus believe that bathing

_____

causes injury.

66. When would you give oral hygiene to a person?

_____

_____

67. When you are delegated to give oral hygiene, what observations should you report?

A. _____

B. _____

C. _____

D. _____

E. _____

F. _____

68. If flossing is done only once a day, the best time to

floss is _____.

69. When giving oral care to an unconscious person, explain what you are doing, because you always assume

_____

_____.

70. When following the rules for bathing in Box 15-1, you protect the skin by following these rules:

Rinse

_____

_____

Pat

_____

_____

Remember to dry

_____

_____

71. What two methods can be used to measure the water temperature used for a bed bath?

A. _____

B. _____

72. When you place a person's hand in the basin during

the bed bath, you may have the person

_____

the hands and fingers.

73. When a partial bath is needed, you assist as needed,

particularly in washing

_____.

74. A tub bath can cause a person to feel

_____,

especially if the person is on bedrest.

75. When the shower room has more than one stall or cabinet, you must protect the person's right

_____.

What are four things you can do to protect this right?

A. _____

B. _____

C. _____

D. _____

76. When giving a tub bath or shower, you use safety

measures to protect the person from

_____ and

_____.

77. After the back massage, apply lotion to the

_____

to keep the skin soft.

78. When you are delegated to give a back massage, what observations should you report and record?

A. _____

B. _____

C. _____

79. When you are assisting a person with perineal care, what terms may be used to explain where the care will be done?

_____

_____

80. When assisting residents with hygiene, you should

report _____

immediately.

Labeling

81. Using arrows, show in which direction the teeth should be brushed. Describe the position and motion used in each drawing.

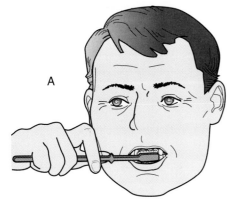

A

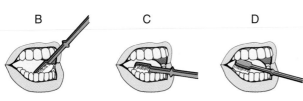

B   C   D

A. _____

B. _____

C. _____

D. _____

82. Look at this drawing to answer the following questions:

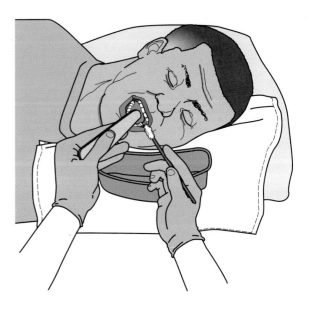

A. Why is the person positioned on his side?

_____

_____

B. What is the purpose of the padded tongue blade?

_____

_____

83. What is being used to remove the upper denture?

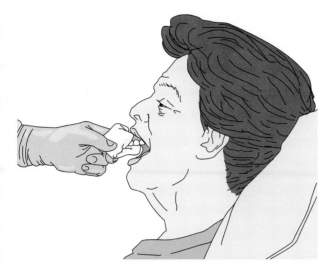

_____

_____

Why?

_____

_____

84. Using an arrow, show the direction to wash the eye when assisting with hygiene. Describe the direction.

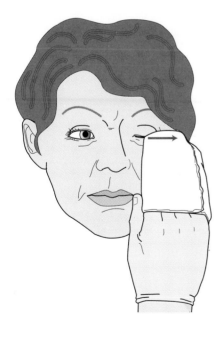

_____

_____

85. Explain what the staff member is doing.

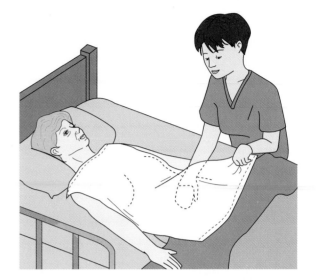

_____

_____

Why is the towel positioned vertically on the person?

_____

_____

86. Using an arrow, show the direction the back is washed. What rule of bathing is being followed by washing in this direction?

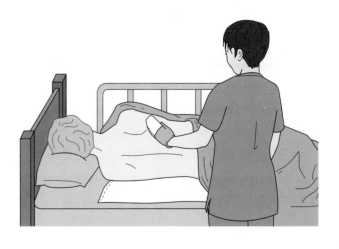

_____

_____

Nursing Assistant Skills Video Exercise

View the **Bathing** *video to answer these questions.*

87. When giving a bath, you should observe the person for:

    A. _____

    B. _____

    C. _____

    D. _____

    E. _____

88. If you observe any bleeding, discharge, drainage

    when bathing a person, you should

    _____.

89. When you are giving a back massage, what should you do if you find a reddened area?

    _____

    _____

90. When you clean the perineal area, you clean from

    clean to dirty areas. This technique means that you

    wash from the _____

    to the _____

    area.

91. The water temperature should be

    _____

    when you wash the perineal area.

Optional Learning Exercises

92. Hygiene promotes comfort, safety, and health. Answer these questions about hygiene:

    A. Intact skin prevents

    _____

    What other areas must be clean to maintain intact skin?

    _____

    B. Besides cleansing, what are the other benefits of good hygiene?

    _____

    _____

    C. Good hygiene also promotes

    _____

    _____.

93. Why is mouth care for the unconscious person especially important?

    _____

    A. What do these factors cause?

    _____

    B. Oral hygiene will help

    _____

    and prevent

    _____.

94. List all of the benefits of bathing.

   A. _____

   B. _____

   C. _____

   D. _____

   E. _____

   F. _____

   G. _____

   H. _____

95. When you are bathing a person with dementia, what measures are important to help the person understand you are trying to help them?

   A. _____

   B. _____

   C. _____

   D. _____

   E. _____

   F. _____

   G. _____

96. You are delegated to give Mrs. Johnson a bath. Before beginning, what information do you need?

   A. _____

   B. _____

   C. _____

   D. _____

   E. _____

   F. _____

   G. _____

97. As you are bathing Mrs. Johnson, what observation should you report and record?

   A. _____

   B. _____

   C. _____

   D. _____

   E. _____

   F. _____

   G. _____

   H. _____

   I. _____

   J. _____

98. When you are preparing to give perineal care to Mrs. Johnson. How many washcloths should you gather?

   _____

   Why?

   _____

   _____

Independent Learning Activities

1. Discuss the following questions with several classmates to understand personal preferences about personal hygiene.
   - Do you prefer a shower or tub bath?
   - What time of day do you usually bathe?
   - What skin-care products do you use to keep your skin healthy?
   - What special measures do you use when brushing your teeth? Special toothbrush? Toothpaste? Do you floss? How often?

2. As part of your preparation for caring for residents, you may give a classmate a back massage and receive a back massage. Answer these questions about how you felt when you were the "resident."
   - How did the lotion feel on your back? Was it warm or cold?
   - Which strokes were relaxing? Which were more stimulating?
   - How long do you think the back massage lasted? Did you look at the clock to see the actual time?
   - What would you like to tell the person who is giving the back massage that would improve the back massage?
   - How will this practice help you when you give a back massage to another person?

3. As part of your preparation for caring for residents, you may give a classmate oral hygiene. Answer these questions about how you felt when you were the "resident."
   - What did the "nursing assistant" tell you before beginning the oral hygiene?
   - What choices were offered? Position? Equipment? Products?
   - How did it feel to have someone else give you oral hygiene? Flossing your teeth?
   - How clean did your teeth feel when the oral hygiene was complete?
   - What would you like to tell the person who gave the oral hygiene that would help improve the procedure?
   - How will this experience help you when you give oral hygiene to a resident?

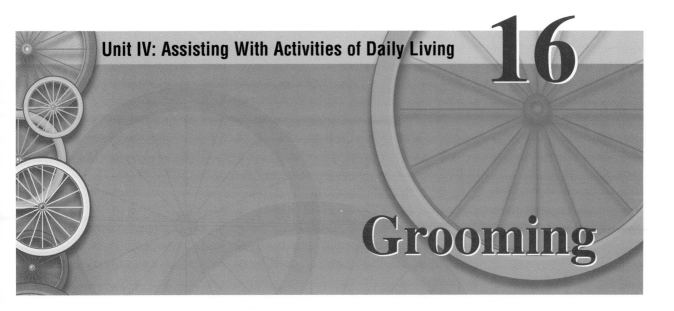

16

Grooming

Alopecia	Pediculosis
Anticoagulant	Pediculosis capitis
Dandruff	Pediculosis corporis
Hirsutism	Pediculosis pubis

Fill in the Blanks: Key Terms

Select your answers from the Key Terms listed above.

1. The infestation with lice is

   _____ .

2. _____

   is the excessive amount of dry, white flakes from the

   scalp.

3. The infestation of the body with lice is

   _____ .

4. Hair loss is

   _____ .

5. _____

   is the infestation of the pubic hair with lice.

6. Excessive body hair in women and children is

   _____ .

7. The infestation of the scalp with lice is

   _____ .

8. A drug that prevents or slows blood-clotting time is

   an _____ .

Circle the BEST Answer

9. If you see any signs of lice, you should report it to
   the nurse because
   A. Lice bites can cause severe infections.
   B. Lice are easily spread to other persons through
      clothing, furniture, bed linens, and sexual
      contact.
   C. Lice can cause the person's hair to fall out.
   D. The lice will cause the hair to mat and tangle.

10. When a person is taking an anticoagulant drug, you should
    A. Shave the person with an electric razor.
    B. Shave the person with a safety razor.
    C. Allow the beard to grow to prevent accidentally cutting the person.
    D. Allow only a professional barber to shave the person.

11. Hair care, shaving, and nail and foot care are important to residents because they affect
    A. Safety and security needs
    B. Love and belonging and self-esteem needs
    C. Physical needs
    D. Self-actualization needs

12. Who or what dictates how you will brush, comb, and style a person's hair?
    A. The person
    B. You
    C. The nurse
    D. The care plan

13. If long hair becomes matted or tangled, you should
    A. Braid the hair.
    B. Cut the hair to remove the tangles and matting.
    C. Talk to the nurse and ask for directions.
    D. Decide what is the easiest thing to do.

14. If hair is curly, coarse, and dry, which of the following would *not* be done?
    A. Braid or cut the hair.
    B. Use a wide-toothed comb.
    C. Work upward, lifting and fluffing hair outward.
    D. Apply a conditioner or petrolatum jelly to make combing easier.

15. If a person has the hair styled in small braids, when you are assisting with grooming,
    A. Undo the hair and rebraid each day.
    B. The braids are left intact for shampooing.
    C. Undo the braids to make lying in bed more comfortable.
    D. Ask the nurse to decide what should be done.

16. If the beautician styles woman's hair
    A. Wash her hair only once a week.
    B. Wash her hair on the day she goes to the beautician.
    C. Make sure she wears a shower cap during the tub bath or shower.
    D. Wash her hair each time she gets a shower or tub bath.

17. Shampooing at the sink or on a stretcher
    A. Is not tolerated by persons with limited range of motion in their necks and upper backs
    B. Can be used in place of shampooing in bed
    C. Is easier than is shampooing in the shower or tub
    D. Is used only for a person with limited range of motion in the neck and upper back

18. Which of the following is *not* an observation that is made when shampooing?
    A. Scalp sores
    B. The presence of lice
    C. The amount of hair on the head
    D. Hair falling out in patches

19. If safety razors (blade razors) are used, which of the following is *not* true?
    A. You may use the nursing center's razor if it is cleaned between residents.
    B. Use the resident's own razor.
    C. Use disposable razors.
    D. Safety razors are not used to shave persons who are receiving anticoagulants.

20. When shaving a person, you should wear gloves
    A. When you fill the basin with water
    B. To wipe off the overbed table with paper towels.
    C. To apply the shaving cream
    D. When you wash the person's face

21. When caring for a mustache and beard, which of the following is *not* done?
    A. Wash the mustache or beard daily.
    B. Combing daily is usually needed.
    C. Ask the person how to groom his beard or mustache.
    D. Trim or shave a beard or mustache when needed.

22. Nursing assistants do not cut or trim toenails if a person
    A. Has just taken a bath or shower
    B. Asks the nursing assistant to use nail clippers
    C. Has diabetes or poor circulation
    D. Has shoes that fit poorly

23. When caring for the fingernails or toenails, which of the following is *wrong?*
    A. Cut the nails with small scissors.
    B. Clean under the nails with an orange stick.
    C. Clip the nails straight across with nail clippers.
    D. Shape the nails with an emery board or nail file.

24. When changing clothing, remove the clothing from
    A. The weak side first
    B. The lower limbs first
    C. From the right side last
    D. From the strong or "good" side first

25. When you are delegated to undress a person, it is usually done
    A. In the bed
    B. With the person sitting in a chair
    C. By having the person stand at the bedside
    D. In the bathroom

26. When you are changing the person's clothes, you use good body mechanics by
    A. Having a good base of support
    B. Holding objects close to your body
    C. Raising the bed to a good working level
    D. Lifting with the large muscles

27. To provide warmth and privacy when changing clothes, you
    A. Keep the top sheets in place.
    B. Cover the person with a bath blanket.
    C. Close the curtains.
    D. Close the door.

28. When changing the gown of a person with an IV, you
    A. Turn off the IV.
    B. Lay the IV bag on the bed.
    C. Gather the sleeve of the arm with the IV and slide it over the IV.
    D. Slide the gown over the IV and down the pole.

29. When you have finished changing the gown of a person with an IV, you should
    A. Restart the pump.
    B. Reconnect the IV.
    C. Check the flow rate or ask the nurse to check it.
    D. Ask the person if it is running properly.

Fill in the Blanks

30. If long hair is matted and tangled, the nurse may

    have you brush by taking a small section of hair

    near _____.

31. If you give hair care to a person in bed after a linen change, collect falling hair by

    _____

    _____.

32. When you brush and comb the hair, you should report and record

    A. _____

    B. _____

    C. _____

    D. _____

    E. _____

33. If a person cannot tip the head back as you shampoo in the shower or tub, he or she can protect the eyes by holding a

    _____

    _____.

34. When rinsing the hair, you can keep soapy water from running down the person's forehead and into the eyes by

    _____

    _____.

35. What delegation guidelines do you need when shaving a person?

    A. _____

    B. _____

    C. _____

36. When you are shaving the face and underarms, which direction do you shave?

    _____

    _____

37. When shaving legs, which direction do you shave?

    _____

    _____

38. What two actions should you take if you nick someone while shaving?

    A. _____

    B. _____

39. When you give nail and foot care, report and record

    A. _____

    B. _____

    C. _____

    D. _____

    E. _____

40. When undressing the person, if you cannot raise the person's head and shoulders, you should

    A. _____

    B. _____

    C. _____

    D. _____

    E. _____

41. Before changing a person's hospital gown, what information do you need from the nurse or the care plan about the IV?

    A. _____

    B. _____

    C. _____

Nursing Assistant Skills Video

View the **Personal Hygiene and Grooming** *video to answer these questions.*

42. What observations should be made when giving hair care?

    A. _____

    B. _____

    C. _____

    D. _____

43. When washing the hair in bed, how is the head supported in the trough?

    _____

    _____

44. When washing hair in bed, the water temperature

    should be _____.

45. When shaving the face, keep the skin

    _____

    and shave at a _____-degree angle.

46. Razors are discarded in the

    _____.

47. Because injury is a risk, many centers only allow a

    _____

    or _____

    to trim toenails.

48. Feet and hands should be soaked for

_____

before cleaning under the nails and trimming or

shaping the nails.

49. When dressing a person in bed, cover the person

with a

_____.

50. To pull up the resident's pants, have the person

_____

_____.

Optional Learning Exercises

51. You are caring for a person who is receiving cancer
treatments. What effect might this treatment have on
the person's hair?

_____

_____

52. Dandruff occurs not only on the scalp, but it also

may involve the

_____.

53. You should report any signs of lice to the nurse im-

mediately because it easily

_____.

54. When brushing and combing the hair, you need to

inspect the comb and brush because

_____.

55. Many older or disabled persons cannot tolerate

having the hair shampooed at the sink because

_____

_____.

56. Electric shavers are used when shaving a person

who is taking anticoagulants because a

_____.

57. Injuries to the feet of a person with poor circulation

is serious because

_____.

58. Why are grooming measures important? What
needs does this care meet?

A. _____

B. _____

C. _____

D. _____

Independent Learning Activities

1. Ask another person if you may shave him or her with a safety razor. (**WARNING:** SOME INSTRUCTORS MAY BE CONCERNED ABOUT THE LIABILITY OF THIS EXERCISE. MAKE SURE THAT THE INSTRUCTOR APPROVES THIS EXERCISE, ESPECIALLY IF YOU USE A CLASSMATE AS A PARTNER.) Ask the person you shaved to help you answer these questions.
   - What did you use for lubricating the skin? Shaving cream? Soap? Water only? How did it feel to the person? What worked best?
   - Which technique worked best? When you applied more pressure? Less pressure?
   - Shave one side of face *with* hair growth and one side *against* the hair growth. Which way was more effective? Why?
   - In what way can the person help you shave the face better?
   - What area was the most difficult to shave? How did you deal with this area?
   - Ask the person you shaved for any tips on how to improve your shaving skills.

2. Role-play this situation with a classmate. Take turns being the resident and the nursing assistant. Remember to keep your left arm and leg limp when you are the resident.

   SITUATION: Mr. Olsen is a 58-year-old resident who has weakness on the left side. You are assigned to take off his sleepwear and dress him for the day. You need to remove his pajamas and dress him in a shirt, a pullover sweater, slacks, socks, and shoes.

   - How did you provide privacy?
   - How was Mr. Olsen positioned for the clothing change?
   - What difficulties did you have when you removed his pajamas?
   - Which arm did you redress first? What difficulty did you have getting his arms into the shirt?
   - How did you put on the sweater? What was most difficult about this?
   - What was the most difficult part of putting on the slacks?
   - How did you put on the socks and shoes?
   - What did you learn from this role-play situation? Did you follow the procedure in the chapter to assist you?
   - Discuss with each other how it felt to have someone dress you when you were "Mr. Olsen."

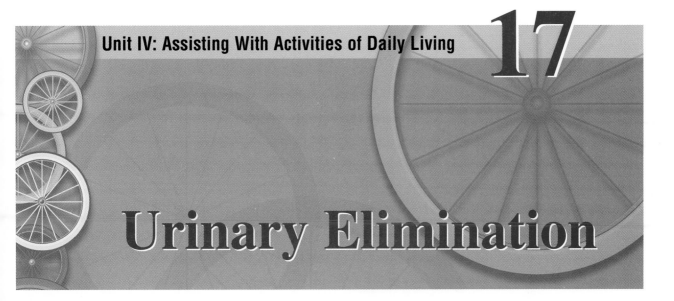

Urinary Elimination

Acetone	Ketone body	Stoma
Catheter	Micturition	Stress incontinence
Catheterization	Nocturia	Ureterostomy
Dialysis	Oliguria	Urge incontinence
Dysuria	Ostomy	Urinary frequency
Functional incontinence	Overflow incontinence	Urinary incontinence
Glucosuria	Peritoneal dialysis	Urinary urgency
Glycosuria	Polyuria	Urination
Hematuria	Reflex incontinence	Voiding
Hemodialysis		

Fill in the Blanks: Key Terms

Select your answers from the Key Terms listed above.

1. Abnormally large amounts of urine is

    _____.

2. _____

    removes waste and fluid from the body by filtering

    the blood through an artificial kidney.

3. Sugar in the urine is

    _____

    or glycosuria.

4. Inserting a catheter is

    _____.

5. _____ is the

    loss of bladder control.

6. Frequent urination at night is

    _____.

7. Ketone bodies that appear in the urine because of

    the rapid breakdown of fat for energy is

    _____.

8. A _____

is an artificial opening between the ureter and

abdomen.

9. The loss of urine when the bladder is too full is

_____.

10. The process of emptying the bladder is called urina-

tion, voiding, or

_____.

11. _____

is the involuntary, unpredicted loss of urine from the

bladder.

12. An artificial opening to the outside of the body is a

_____.

13. Another name for micturition, or voiding, which is

the process of emptying urine from the bladder, is

_____.

14. A _____

is a tube used to drain or inject fluid through a body

opening.

15. Blood in the urine is

_____.

16. Acetone, the production of which occurs because of

the rapid breakdown of fat for energy, is also called

_____.

17. A process that uses the lining of the abdominal

cavity to remove waste from the body is

_____.

18. Voiding at frequent intervals is

_____.

19. Sugar in the urine is called glucosuria, or

_____.

20. _____

is a process to remove waste and excess fluid from

the body.

21. The loss of small amounts of urine with exercise

and certain movements is

_____.

22. Another word for urination or micturition is

_____.

23. The need to void immediately is

_____.

24. Surgical creation of an artificial opening is an

_____.

25. The involuntary loss of urine after feeling a strong

need to void is

_____.

26. Painful or difficult urination is

_____.

27. The loss of urine at certain intervals is unconscious

incontinence, or

_____.

28. A scant amount of urine, usually less than 500 ml in

24 hours, is

_____.

Circle the BEST Answer

29. Solid wastes are removed from the body by the
    A. Digestive system
    B. Urinary system
    C. Blood
    D. Integumentary system

30. A healthy adult excretes approximately how much urine a day?
    A. 500 ml
    B. 1000 ml
    C. 1500 ml
    D. 2000 ml

31. You can provide privacy when the person is voiding by doing all of the following *except*
    A. Pulling drapes or window shades
    B. Staying in room to give assistance if needed
    C. Pulling the curtain around the bed
    D. Closing room and bathroom doors

32. If the person has difficulty starting the urine stream, you can
    A. Play music on the radio.
    B. Provide perineal care.
    C. Use a stainless steel bedpan.
    D. Run water in a nearby sink.

33. The urine may be bright yellow if the person eats
    A. Asparagus
    B. Carrots and sweet potatoes
    C. Beets and blackberries
    D. Rhubarb

34. When using a steel bedpan, you should
    A. Keep the pan in the utility room.
    B. Warm the pan with water and dry it before use.
    C. Sterilize the pan after each use.
    D. Cool the pan with water and dry before use.

35. When you are getting ready to give a person the bedpan, you should
    A. Raise the head of the bed slightly.
    B. Position the person in the Fowler's position.
    C. Wash the person's hands.
    D. Place the bed in a flat position.

36. Urinals are usually placed at the bedside on
    A. Bed rails
    B. Overbed tables
    C. Bedside stands
    D. Floor

37. A commode chair is used when the person
    A. Is unable to walk to the bathroom
    B. Cannot sit up unsupported on the toilet
    C. Needs to be in the normal position for elimination
    D. All of the above

38. When you place a commode over the toilet
    A. Restrain the person.
    B. Stay in the room with the person.
    C. Lock the wheels.
    D. Make sure the container is in place.

39. Dribbling of urine that occurs with laughing, sneezing, coughing, lifting, or other activities mean the person has
    A. Urge incontinence
    B. Stress incontinence
    C. Overflow incontinence
    D. Functional incontinence

40. Which of the following will *not* help prevent urinary tract infections?
    A. Encourage adequate fluid intake as directed by the nurse.
    B. Decrease fluid intake before bedtime.
    C. Encourage the person to wear cotton underpants.
    D. Keep perineal area clean.

41. When providing perineal care, which of the following steps would be *incorrect?*
    A. Provide perineal care once a day.
    B. Wash, rinse, and dry the perineal area and buttocks.
    C. Remove wet incontinent products, garments, and linens.
    D. Provide dry garments and linens.

42. A catheter that is inserted to collect a sterile urine specimen and is then removed is
    A. An indwelling catheter
    B. A straight catheter
    C. A condom catheter
    D. A Foley catheter

43. An indwelling catheter is used for all of the following *except*
    A. To keep the bladder empty before, during, and after surgery
    B. When a person is dying
    C. To measure urine left in the bladder after voiding (residual urine)
    D. To protect wounds and pressure ulcers from contact with urine

44. A last resort for incontinence is
    A. Bladder training
    B. Answering signal lights promptly
    C. An indwelling catheter
    D. Adequate fluid intake

45. When cleaning a catheter, you should
    A. Wipe 4 inches up the catheter to the meatus.
    B. Disconnect the tubing from the drainage bag.
    C. Hold the catheter near the meatus.
    D. Wash and rinse the catheter by washing up and down the tubing.

46. The drainage bag from a catheter should *not* be attached to the
    A. Bed frame
    B. Back of a chair
    C. Lower part of an IV pole
    D. Bed rail

47. If a catheter is accidentally disconnected from the drainage bag, you should
    A. Cover the tip of the catheter with tape.
    B. Clamp the catheter to prevent leakage.
    C. Wipe the end of the tube and the end of the catheter with antiseptic wipes.
    D. Discard the drainage bag and get a new bag.

48. If a person uses a leg drainage bag, it
    A. Is switched to a drainage bag when the person is in bed
    B. Is attached to the clothing with tape or safety pins
    C. Is attached to the bed rail when the person is in bed
    D. Can be worn 24 hours a day

49. A leg bag needs to be emptied more often than does a drainage bag because
    A. It holds 1000 ml, and the drainage bag holds about 2000 ml.
    B. It is more likely to leak than is the drainage bag.
    C. It holds about 250 ml, and the drainage bag holds 1000 ml.
    D. It interferes with walking if it is full.

50. When you empty a drainage bag, you should
    A. Disconnect the bag from the tubing.
    B. Clamp the catheter to prevent leakage.
    C. Open the clamp and drain into a measuring container.
    D. Take the bag into the bathroom to empty it.

51. When applying a condom catheter
    A. Apply elastic tape in a spiral around the penis.
    B. Make sure the catheter tip is touching the head of the penis.
    C. Apply tape securely in a circle entirely around the penis.
    D. Remove and reapply every shift.

52. The goal of bladder training is
    A. To keep the person dry and clean
    B. Voluntary control of urination
    C. To prevent skin breakdown
    D. To prevent infection

53. When you are assisting the person with bladder training to have normal elimination, you should
    A. Help the person to the bathroom every 15 or 20 minutes.
    B. Give the person 15 to 20 minutes to start voiding.
    C. Make sure the person drinks at least 1000 ml each shift.
    D. Tell the person he or she can void only once a shift.

54. When you assist with bladder training for a person with an indwelling catheter, you should
    A. Empty the drainage bag every hour.
    B. At first, clamp the catheter for 1 hour.
    C. At first, clamp the catheter for 3 to 4 hours.
    D. Give the person 15 to 20 minutes to start voiding.

55. When you collect a urine specimen, you label the
    A. Container
    B. Container lid
    C. The plastic bag
    D. Only the requisition slip

56. When you collect a specimen, you ask the person
    A. Not to have a bowel movement during the specimen collection
    B. To put toilet tissue in the toilet or the wastebasket
    C. Not to touch the inside of the container
    D. All of the above

57. When collecting a random urine specimen, which of the following is *not* true?
    A. It is collected at any time.
    B. You may collect the specimen in a bedpan, urinal, or specimen pan.
    C. The specimen container is sterile.
    D. Pour about 120 ml (4 oz) of urine into the specimen container.

58. When collecting a midstream specimen, you should
    A. Collect the first urine that is voided.
    B. Clean the perineal area with soap and water.
    C. Use sterile technique when you open the specimen container.
    D. Collect about 180 ml (3 oz) of urine.

59. When collecting a 24-hour urine specimen, you should
    A. Save the first specimen voided.
    B. Save the last specimen voided.
    C. Keep the urine at room temperature.
    D. Save each voiding in a separate container.

60. Fresh-fractional or double-voided specimens test for
    A. Blood in the urine
    B. Glucose and ketones in the urine
    C. Bacteria in the urine
    D. Particles in the urine

61. When you collect a double-voided specimen, you should
    A. Test both the first and second voidings.
    B. Send the specimen to the laboratory immediately.
    C. Test only the first voiding.
    D. Test only the second voiding.

62. If you are testing urine for occult blood, you
    A. Will notice a strong odor from the urine
    B. Know the blood is unseen in the urine
    C. Will see blood in the urine
    D. Will check the urine to see if it is acidic or alkaline

63. When you use reagent strips to test urine, which of the following is *not* true?
    A. Remove the strip from the urine after the correct amount of time.
    B. Compare the strip with the color chart on the bottle.
    C. You use sterile technique when you collect the specimen.
    D. Follow the manufacturer's instructions to carry out the test.

64. When you strain urine, you should
    A. Strain urine only when the person complains of pain.
    B. Send urine to the laboratory and discard the strainer.
    C. Place the strainer in the specimen container if any crystals, stones, or particles appear.
    D. Examine the strainer or gauze, and discard any crystals, stones, or particles.

65. A person with a ureterostomy
    A. Has an indwelling catheter from the bladder to a drainage bag
    B. Will be able to void normally
    C. Has had the bladder removed and has a urinary diversion
    D. Has no urine output

66. When changing a ureterostomy pouch, you should
    A. Clean around the stoma with adhesive remover.
    B. Use soap or other cleansing agent to clean around the stoma.
    C. Apply a skin barrier to area around the stoma if it is a separate device.
    D. All of the above are true.

67. When a person needs dialysis, it means that the
    A. Person has urinary incontinence
    B. Urine contains sugar or blood
    C. Person has nocturia
    D. Kidneys are producing little or no urine

68. When you care for a person who has dialysis done, you know the person
    A. Is transported to the hospital or dialysis centers two to three times a week
    B. Will void large amounts of urine
    C. Will drink a large amount of fluids
    D. Eats a regular diet

Fill in the Blanks

69. What substances increase urine production?

    A. _____

    B. _____

    C. _____

    D. _____

70. A normal position for voiding for women is

    _____.

    For men, a normal position is

    _____.

71. What can you do to mask urination sounds?

    _____

    _____

72. Fracture pans are used for persons with

    _____

    and those in

    _____.

    Persons with limited

    _____

    may also use fracture pans.

73. When a person voids in a bedpan or urinal, what observations are important?

    A. _____

    B. _____

    C. _____

    D. _____

74. When you are handling bedpans, urinals, and commodes and their contents, you should practice

    _____

    and follow

    _____.

75. When you transfer a person to a commode from bed, you must practice safe transfer practices and use a

    _____.

76. Name five causes of urge incontinence.

    A. _____

    B. _____

    C. _____

    D. _____

    E. _____

77. Stress incontinence is common in women because the pelvic muscles weaken after

    _____

    and with

    _____.

78. Overflow incontinence may occur in men because of a

    _____

    _____.

79. _____

    incontinence occurs with nervous system disorders and injuries.

80. A catheter that is inserted after a person voids is measuring how

    _____

    _____.

81. When you provide perineal care after a person is incontinent, you should remember to

    A. _____

    B. _____

    C. _____

    D. _____

    E. _____

    F. _____

82. A catheter is secured to the inner thigh or the man's abdomen to prevent

    _____

    _____.

83. When a person has a catheter, what observations should you report and record?

    A. _____

    B. _____

    C. _____

    D. _____

    E. _____

84. When you give catheter care, clean the catheter

    about _____ inches. Clean

    _____

    from the meatus with

    _____ stroke.

85. Is the urinary system sterile or nonsterile?

    _____

86. What happens if a drainage bag is higher than is the bladder?

    _____

    _____

87. When you are changing a leg bag to a drainage bag, what should you do if you accidentally contaminate the end of the catheter?

    _____

    _____

88. Before applying a condom catheter, you should

    provide _____

    and observe the penis for

    _____.

89. The catheter is clamped for 1 hour at first and eventually for 3 to 4 hours when

    _____

    is being done.

90. What information is written on the label for a specimen that has been collected?

    _____

    _____

91. When collecting a midstream urine specimen, the

    perineal area is cleaned with

    _____

    _____.

92. When you start a 24-hour specimen collection,

    place one label in the

    _____

    and the other label

    _____.

93. The first time the bladder is emptied when collecting a double-voided specimen, the urine is

    "_____."

    The person voids the second time in _____

    minutes.

94. A routine urine specimen is collected when testing

    the urine for

    _____

    and _____.

95. When testing urine you should report and record

A. _____

B. _____

C. _____

D. _____

E. _____

Labeling

96. Mark the places you would secure the catheter. Explain why the catheter is secured this way.

_____

_____

97. Mark the places you would secure the catheter. Explain why the catheter is secured this way.

_____

_____

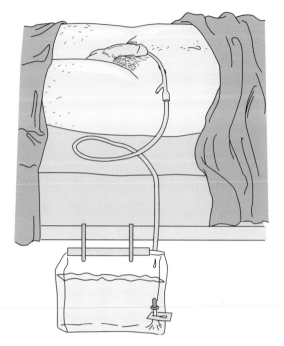

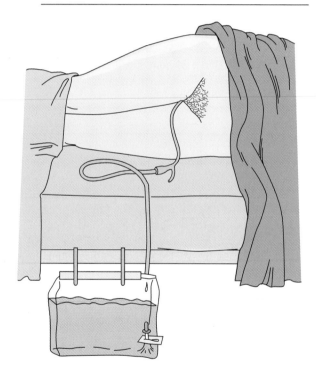

Crossword

Fill in the crossword puzzle.

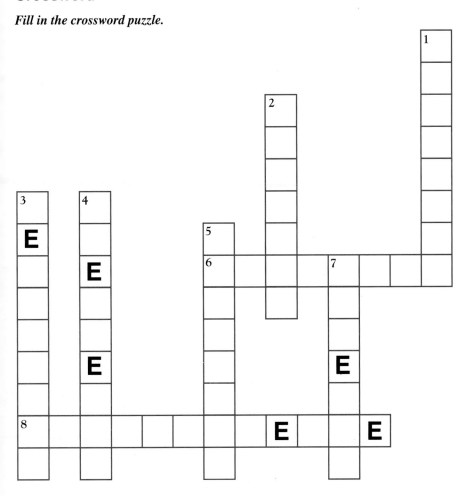

Across

6. Scant amount of urine, usually less than 500 ml in 24 hours.
8. Inability to control loss of urine from bladder.

Down

1. Production of abnormally large amount of urine.
2. Painful or difficult urination.
3. Blood in the urine.
4. Voiding at frequent intervals.
5. Frequent urination at night.
7. Need to void immediately.

Nursing Assistant Skills Video Exercise

View the **Normal Elimination** *video to answer these questions.*

98. A healthy adult normally produces how much urine each day?

    _____

99. What is the normal color of urine?

    _____

100. After a person has used the bedpan or urinal, you

    should offer _____

    and _____.

101. Before handling a bedpan or urinal, you should put

    on _____.

Optional Learning Exercises

102. When a person eats a diet that is high in salt, it

    causes the body _____.

    When this event happens, how does it affect urine output?

    _____

    _____

103. When a person does not have nervous system or urinary system injuries but has involuntary, unpredictable loss of urine, the condition is called what?

    _____.

104. What can you do to make sure the person can use the bathroom, bedpan, urinal, or commode in time?

    A. _____

    B. _____

    C. _____

    D. _____

105. If you caring for an incontinent person and you become short-tempered and impatient,

    _____.

    What right are you protecting when you take this action?

    _____

106. You know that catheters are a last resort for incontinent persons. If a person is weak, disabled, and dying, a catheter may be used for what?

    _____

    _____.

107. In addition to the reasons in #106, list two other reasons why a catheter may be used.

    A. _____

    B. _____

108. What can happen if microbes enter a closed drainage system?

    _____

    _____

109. What type of tape is used to apply a condom catheter?

    _____

    Why?

    _____

    _____

    What can happen if you use the wrong tape?

    _____

    _____

110. What kind of specimen can many persons collect by themselves?

_____

_____

Why?

_____

_____

111. Why is it important to clean the perineal area before collecting a midstream specimen?

_____

_____

112. Signs are placed in the room when a 24-hour urine collection is being done. What information is written on these signs?

_____

_____

113. Why is a ureterostomy pouch replaced any time it leaks?

_____

_____

Independent Learning Activities

1. Role-play the following situation with a classmate. Take turns playing the person using the bedpan and the nursing assistant. Answer the questions about the activity.

   SITUATION: Mrs. Donnelly is a 70-year-old woman who must use the bedpan. She finds it difficult to move easily and usually does not have enough strength to raise her hips to get on the bedpan. She tells you that she will try to help as much as she can.

   As Mrs. Donnelly:
   - When you tried to assist, how easy was it to raise your hips? How did the nursing assistant help you get on the pan?
   - When you were rolled onto the bedpan, how did it feel? How well was the pan positioned under you?
   - How did you feel about sitting on the pan in bed? Did you feel as if this would be an easy or difficult way to void? Explain your feelings.
   - How might the nursing assistant make this procedure better?

   As the nursing assistant:
   - How did you position the bedpan to get ready to slide it under Mrs. Donnelly? Did this method work? How can you improve this?
   - When you rolled Mrs. Donnelly onto the pan, how well positioned was she? What adjustments were necessary?
   - When you rolled her off the pan, what happened? If urine had been in the pan, what would have occurred?
   - How might you change some of your steps to make this procedure better?

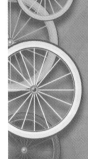

Bowel Elimination

Anal incontinence	Enema	Ileostomy
Colostomy	Fecal impaction	Melena
Constipation	Fecal incontinence	Peristalsis
Defecation	Feces	Stool
Dehydration	Flatulence	Suppository
Diarrhea	Flatus	

Fill in the Blanks: Key Terms

Select your answers from the Key Terms listed above.

1. The process of excreting feces from the rectum through the anus is a bowel movement, or

   _____.

2. The excessive formation of gas or air in the stomach and intestines is

   _____.

3. A _____ is a cone-shaped solid medication that is inserted into a body opening.

4. The frequent passage of liquid stools is

   _____.

5. _____, or anal incontinence, is the inability to control the passage of feces and gas through the anus.

6. _____ is the excessive loss of water from tissues.

7. Gas or air passed through the anus is

   _____.

8. The introduction of fluid into the rectum and lower colon is an _____.

9. Excreted fecal matter is

   _____.

10. An artificial opening between the colon and abdominal wall is a

    _____.

11. The prolonged retention and accumulation of feces in the rectum is

    _____.

12. _____

    is the alternating contraction and relaxation of intestinal muscles.

13. The passage of a hard, dry stool is

    _____.

14. Another name for fecal incontinence is

    _____.

15. _____

    is a black, tarry stool.

16. The semi-solid mass of waste products in the colon

    is _____.

17. An opening between the ileum and the abdominal wall is an

    _____.

Circle the BEST Answer

18. People normally have a bowel movement
    A. Every day
    B. Every 2 to 3 days
    C. 2 or 3 times a day
    D. Any of the above

19. Bleeding in the stomach and small intestines causes stool to be
    A. Brown
    B. Black
    C. Red
    D. Clay colored

20. The characteristic odor of stool is caused by
    A. Poor personal hygiene
    B. Poor nutrition
    C. Bacterial action in the intestines
    D. Adequate fluid intake

21. If you are caring for a person and observe that the stool is abnormal, you should
    A. Ask the nurse to observe the abnormal stool.
    B. Report your observation and discard the stool.
    C. Ask the person if the stool is normal for him or her.
    D. Record your observation when you finish his or her care.

22. Which of the following might interfere with defecation?
    A. Being able to relax by reading a book or newspaper
    B. Eating a diet with high-fiber foods
    C. Using a bedpan or commode in a semiprivate room
    D. Drinking six to eight glasses of water daily

23. A person who must stay in bed most of the time may have irregular elimination and constipation because of
    A. Poor diet
    B. Poor fluid intake
    C. Lack of activity
    D. Lack of privacy

24. Which of the following would provide safety for the person during bowel elimination?
    A. Make sure the bedpan is warm.
    B. Place the signal light and toilet tissue within the person's reach.
    C. Provide perineal care.
    D. Allow enough time for defecation.

25. Constipation can be relieved by
    A. Giving the person a low-fiber diet
    B. Increasing activity
    C. Decreasing fluids
    D. Ignoring the urge to defecate

26. A person tries several times to have a bowel movement and cannot. Liquid feces seeps from the anus. This event probably means that the person has
    A. Diarrhea
    B. Constipation
    C. Fecal impaction
    D. Fecal incontinence

27. If the nurse finds that a fecal impaction is present, he or she will first try to relieve it by
    A. Changing the person's diet
    B. Telling the nursing assistant to give more fluids
    C. Removing the fecal mass with a gloved finger
    D. Increasing the activity of the person

28. Good skin care is important when a person has diarrhea because
    A. It prevents odors.
    B. Skin breakdown and pressure ulcers are risks of diarrhea.
    C. It prevents the spread of microbes.
    D. It prevents fluid loss.

29. Why is diarrhea very serious in older persons?
    A. It causes skin breakdown.
    B. It causes odors.
    C. It can cause dehydration.
    D. It increases activity.

30. When fecal incontinence occurs, the nurse may plan all of the following *except*
    A. Increased fluid intake
    B. Bowel training
    C. Assisting with elimination after meals
    D. Incontinent products to keep garments and linens clean

31. If flatus is not expelled, the person may complain of
    A. Abdominal cramping or pain
    B. Diarrhea
    C. Fecal incontinence
    D. Nausea

32. Which of the following is *not* a goal of bowel training?
    A. Giving laxatives daily to maintain regular bowel movements
    B. Gaining control of bowel movements
    C. Developing a regular pattern of elimination
    D. Preventing fecal impaction, constipation, and fecal incontinence

33. When bowel training is planned, which of the following is included in the care plan?
    A. The amount of stool the person expels
    B. How many bowel movements the person has each day
    C. The time of day the person usually has a bowel movement
    D. The foods that cause flatus

34. When the nurse gives a suppository to a person, you would expect the person to have a bowel movement
    A. Immediately
    B. Within about 10 minutes
    C. In about 30 minutes
    D. 3 to 4 hours later

35. When the nurse delegates you to prepare a soapsuds enema, you will mix
    A. 2 teaspoons of salt in 1000 ml of tap water
    B. 5 ml of castile soap in 1000 ml of tap water
    C. 5 ml of castile soap in 500 ml of tap water
    D. Mineral oil with sterile water

36. When you give a cleansing enema, it should be given to the person
    A. Within 5 minutes
    B. Over about 30 minutes
    C. In about 10 to 15 minutes
    D. Within about 15 to 20 minutes

37. The person receiving an enema is usually placed in a
    A. Supine position
    B. Prone position
    C. Semi-Fowler's position
    D. Side-lying or Sims' position

38. When you prepare and give an enema, you will do all of the following *except*
    A. Preparing the solution at 110° Fahrenheit
    B. Inserting the tubing 3 to 4 inches into the rectum
    C. Holding the solution container about 12 inches above the bed
    D. Lubricating the enema tip before inserting it into the rectum

39. When the physician orders enemas until clear, you should
    A. Give one enema.
    B. Give as many enemas as is necessary to return a clear fluid.
    C. Ask the nurse how many enemas to give.
    D. Give only tap-water enemas.

40. If you are giving an enema and the person complains of cramping, you should
    A. Tell the person that cramping is normal and continue to give the enema.
    B. Clamp the tube until the cramping subsides.
    C. Discontinue the enema immediately and tell the nurse.
    D. Lower the bag below the level of the bed.

41. When giving a commercial enema, do not release pressure on the bottle because
    A. It will cause cramping if pressure is released.
    B. The fluid will leak from the rectum.
    C. Solution will be drawn back into the bottle.
    D. It will cause flatulence.

42. When giving a commercial enema, you should
    A. Place the person in the prone position.
    B. Insert the enema tip 2 inches into the rectum.
    C. Heat the solution to 105° Fahrenheit.
    D. Clamp the tubing if cramping occurs.

43. An oil-retention enema is given to
    A. Cleanse the bowel to prepare for surgery
    B. Regulate the person who is receiving bowel training
    C. Relieve flatulence
    D. Soften the feces and lubricate the rectum

44. The physician may order a rectal tube
    A. To relieve flatulence and intestinal distention
    B. After rectal surgery
    C. To give cleansing enemas
    D. When the person has an impaction

45. If you feel resistance when you are giving an enema or inserting a rectal tube, you should
    A. Lubricate the tube more thoroughly.
    B. Push more firmly to insert the tube.
    C. Stop and call the nurse.
    D. Ask the person to take a deep breath and relax.

46. After inserting a rectal tube, you should
    A. Hold it in place until it can be removed.
    B. Have the person lie on his or her back to hold it in place.
    C. Tape the rectal tube to the buttocks.
    D. Cover the person with a bath blanket and tell him or her to lie still to keep the tube in place.

47. When you are caring for a person with an ostomy, you know that
    A. All of the stools are solid and formed.
    B. Stomas do not have nerve endings and are not painful.
    C. An ostomy is always temporary and is reconnected after healing.
    D. A pouch is worn to protect the stoma.

48. Which of these statements is *true* about an ileostomy?
    A. The stool is solid and formed.
    B. The stoma is an opening into the colon.
    C. The pouch is changed daily.
    D. Digestive juices in the stool can irritate the skin around the ileostomy.

49. When caring for a person with a stoma, the pouch is
    A. Changed daily
    B. Changed every 3 to 7 days and when it leaks
    C. Worn only when the person thinks he or she will have a bowel movement
    D. Changed every time the person has a bowel movement

50. The best time to change the ostomy bag is before breakfast because
    A. The stoma is less likely to expel stool at this time.
    B. The person has more time in the morning.
    C. It should be changed before morning care.
    D. The person tolerates the procedure better before eating.

51. When cleaning the skin around the stoma, you use
    A. Sterile water and sterile gauze squares
    B. Alcohol and sterile cotton
    C. Gauze squares or washcloths, water or soap, and other cleansing agent as directed by the nurse
    D. Adhesive remover and sterile cotton balls

52. When you collect a stool specimen that needs to be kept warm, you should
    A. Place the specimen in a warm place, such as the kitchen.
    B. Wrap the specimen thoroughly in several layers of paper towels.
    C. Take the specimen to the laboratory immediately.
    D. Place the specimen in a special sterile, insulated container to keep it warm.

53. A stool specimen is collected by
    A. Taking the bedpan with stool to the laboratory
    B. Using a tongue blade to take about 2 tablespoons of feces to the specimen container
    C. Telling the person to hold the specimen container in place to catch the stool specimen
    D. Using your gloved hand to put a small amount of stool into the container

54. If you are delegated to collect a stool specimen for occult blood, which of the following should you report to the nurse?
    A. The person has soft, formed stool.
    B. The person tells you that he or she did not have a bowel movement yesterday.
    C. The person tells you that he or she had red meat for dinner last evening.
    D. The specimen is collected from a bedpan.

55. You give the person with an ostomy the right of personal choice when you
    A. Allow the person to manage the ostomy care
    B. Allow the person to follow special routines in care
    C. Choose the care measures and equipment used
    D. All of the above

Fill in the Blanks

56. Name six foods that may cause gas in the bowel.

    A. _____

    B. _____

    C. _____

    D. _____

    E. _____

    F. _____

57. Drinking warm fluids such as coffee, tea, cider, and

    warm water will increase

    _____.

58. Three serious signs of dehydration are

    A. _____

    B. _____

    C. _____

59. Flatulence may be caused when the person

    _____

    while eating and drinking.

60. A commercial enema contains

    _____ of solution.

61. Because you will likely contact stool while giving

    an enema, you should follow

    _____

    and _____.

62. When you start to insert the rectal tube to give an

    enema, ask the person to

    _____.

63. What can you place in the ostomy pouch to prevent
    odors?

    _____

64. Showers and baths are delayed 1 or 2 hours after

    applying a new pouch to allow

    _____.

Labeling

Answer Questions 65 through 68 using the following illustrations.

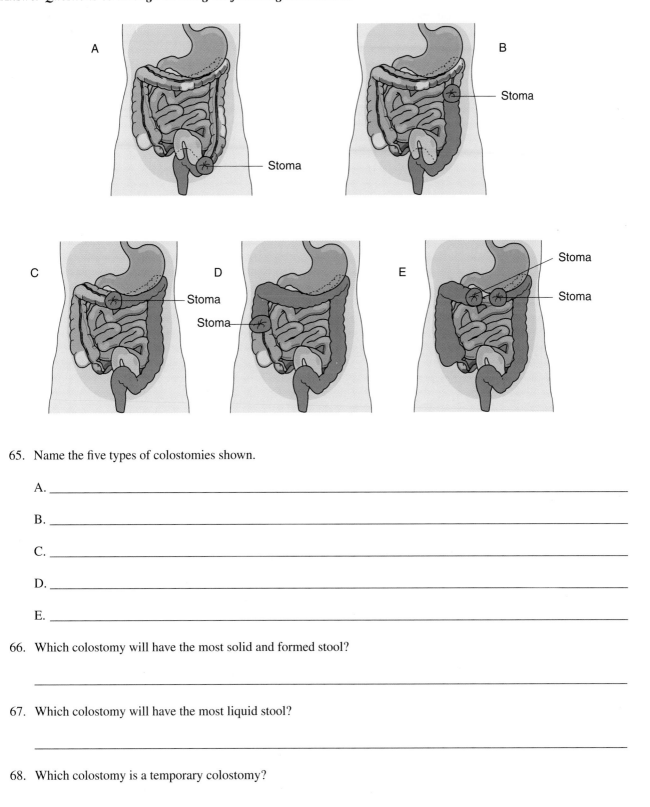

65. Name the five types of colostomies shown.

A. _____

B. _____

C. _____

D. _____

E. _____

66. Which colostomy will have the most solid and formed stool?

_____

67. Which colostomy will have the most liquid stool?

_____

68. Which colostomy is a temporary colostomy?

_____

Answer Questions 69 through 71 using the following illustration.

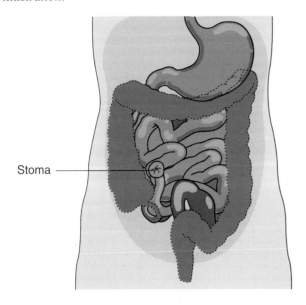

Stoma

69. Name the type of ostomy shown?

_____

70. What part of the bowel has been removed?

_____

71. Will the stool from the ostomy be liquid or formed?

_____

Nursing Assistant Skills Video Exercise

View the **Normal Elimination** *video (the section on administering an enema) to answer these questions.*

72. The enema tube should be

_____

in place during the enema.

73. The water temperature of an enema should luke-warm or _____ for an adult.

74. What is added to 1000 ml of water to prepare these enemas?

A. Saline: _____

B. Soapsuds: _____

C. Tap water: _____

75. After you have filled the bag and hung it from the IV, you must unclamp the tubing to

_____.

76. To relax the anal sphincter, ask the person to

_____

before inserting the tube.

77. Unless the nurse instructs you otherwise, you should lubricate the enema tube _____ inches.

78. The enema tube is *never* inserted more than _____ inches.

79. Stop the enema if

A. _____

B. _____

C. _____

80. To prevent air from entering the rectum, you should clamp the tube and remove it before

_____.

Optional Learning Exercises

81. You are caring for Mr. Evans who is in a semiprivate room. He has not had a bowel movement in 3 days, even though he is eating well and taking medications to assist elimination. What might be a reason that he has not had a bowel movement?

_____

_____

82. Mrs. Weller usually has a bowel movement after breakfast. What are some activities that may assist her to defecate more easily?

_____

_____

83. The nurse tells you to make sure Mr. Johnson eats the high-fiber foods in his diet to assist in his elimination. What foods are high in fiber?

_____

_____

84. Mrs. Shaffer tells you that she cannot digest fruits and vegetables, and she refuses to eat them. What may be added to her cereal and prune juice to provide fiber?

_____

_____

85. You offer Mr. Murphy

_____

of water each day to promote normal bowel

elimination.

86. Mr. Hernandez has been taking an antibiotic to treat

his pneumonia, and he has developed diarrhea. You

know he has diarrhea because

_____

_____.

87. You are caring for 83-year-old Mrs. Chen, and you helped her to the bathroom where she had a bowel movement 30 minutes ago. When you enter her room to make her bed, she tells you she needs to use the bathroom for a bowel movement. You know that older people do what?

_____.

_____.

88. The two goals of bowel training are

_____

and

_____.

89. Why are tap-water enemas dangerous?

_____

_____

How many tap-water enemas can be given? _____

Why?

_____

_____

90. Compare commercial enemas and oil-retention enemas.

A. Commercial enemas are given to

_____.

Oil-retention enemas are given to

_____.

B. Commercial enemas take effect in about _____

minutes. Oil-retention enemas should be retained

for at least _____ minutes.

C. The nurse may want an oil-retention enema re-

tained for _____ hours.

Independent Learning Activities

1. Think about the times when you have had a problem with bowel irregularity. Answer these questions about how you handled the problems.
   - What causes you to have irregularity? Foods? Illness? Stress? Inactivity?
   - What methods have you used to treat irregularity? Diet? Medication?
   - How does irregularity affect you physically? Your appetite? Energy level? Sleep and rest?
   - How does irregularity affect your mood? Your daily activities?

2. Interview a person who has a colostomy or an ileostomy. You may know someone who has an ostomy, or you may care for someone who has one. Your community may have an ostomy support group that you can contact. Talk to the person and ask these questions.
   - How long has the person had the ostomy? Is it permanent or temporary?
   - What was the hardest part of learning to live with an ostomy? What was the easiest part?
   - How has living with an ostomy affected the person's life? Has the person's work been affected? Were leisure activities affected?
   - How has the ostomy affected the person's family? What changes have occurred?
   - What equipment works best for the person? How expensive is the equipment? How much time is required each day to care for the ostomy?

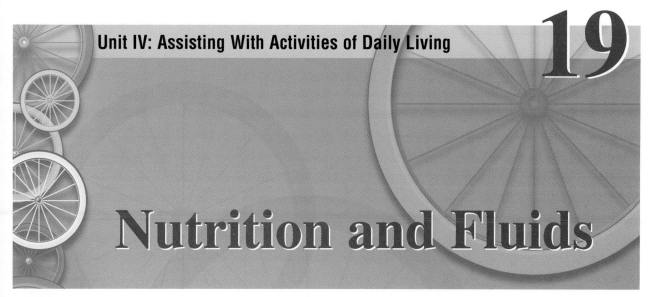

Nutrition and Fluids

19

Anorexia	Edema	Nasogastric (NG) tube
Aspiration	Enteral nutrition	Nasointestinal tube
Calorie	Gastrostomy	Nutrient
Daily reference values (DRVs)	Gavage	Nutrition
Daily value (DV)	Graduate	Percutaneous endoscopic
Dehydration	Intravenous (IV) therapy	gastrostomy (PEG) tube
Dysphagia	Jejunostomy	Regurgitation

Fill in the Blanks: Key Terms

Select your answers from the Key Terms listed above.

1. A _____

    is a tube that is inserted through the nose into the

    duodenum or jejunum of the small intestine.

2. Giving nutrition through the gastrointestinal (GI)

    tract is _____.

3. _____

    is the backward flow of food from the stomach into

    the esophagus.

4. The _____

    is how a serving fits into the daily diet and is ex-

    pressed in a percentage based on a daily diet of

    2000 calories.

5. A tube inserted into the stomach through a stab or

    puncture wound made through the skin is a

    _____.

6. The loss of appetite is

    _____.

7. _____ is fluid

given through a needle that is inserted into a vein.

8. A substance that is ingested, digested, absorbed,

and used by the body is a

_____.

9. _____ is difficulty

in swallowing.

10. The breathing of fluid or an object into the lungs is

_____.

11. The many processes involved in the ingestion, di-

gestion, absorption, and use of food and fluids by

the body is _____.

12. A tube feeding is called

_____.

13. The amount of energy produced from the burning of

food by the body is a

_____.

14. A _____

is an opening into the middle part of the small

intestine.

15. A decrease in the amount of water in body tissues is

_____.

16. A surgically created opening in the stomach is a

_____.

17. The maximum daily intake values for total fat,

saturated fat, cholesterol, sodium, carbohydrate, and

dietary fiber are the

_____.

18. A tube inserted through the nose into the stomach is a

_____.

19. A _____

is a container used to measure fluid.

20. _____

is the swelling of body tissues with water.

Circle the BEST Answer

21. Which of the following does *not* occur when the
person has a poor diet and poor eating habits?
A. Increased risk for infection and chronic diseases
B. Healing problems
C. Improved physical and mental well-being
D. Increased risk for accidents and injuries

22. Body fuel for energy is found in
A. Vitamins
B. Minerals
C. Fats, proteins, and carbohydrates
D. All of the above

23. Which of these foods are found in level 3 of the
Food Guide Pyramid?
A. Rice and pasta
B. Milk, meat, and beans
C. Fats and sweets
D. Vegetables and fruits

24. Which of these food groups in the Food Guide
Pyramid are low in sugar and fat?
A. Bread, cereal, rice, and pasta
B. Milk, yogurt, and cheese
C. Meat, poultry, fish, and nuts
D. Fats, oils, and sweets

25. How many servings are allowed each day from the
breads, cereals, rice, and pasta group?
A. 6 to 11 servings a day
B. 3 to 5 servings a day
C. 2 to 4 servings a day
D. 2 to 3 servings a day

26. Which group in the Food Guide Pyramid should be
used sparingly?
A. Bread, cereal, rice, and pasta
B. Meat, poultry, fish, dry beans, eggs, and nuts
C. Milk, yogurt, and cheese
D. Fats, oils, and sweets

27. Which nutrient is needed for tissue growth and repair?
    A. Carbohydrates
    B. Fats
    C. Vitamins
    D. Protein

28. Food labels have all of the following information *except*
    A. Serving size
    B. All vitamins and minerals in the food
    C. Total amount of fat and amount of saturated fats
    D. Amount of cholesterol and sodium

29. What percentage of calories should come from fat?
    A. 30%
    B. 10%
    C. 50%
    D. 18%

30. A culture that eats a diet that is low in fat and high in sodium is in
    A. The Philippines
    B. China
    C. Poland
    D. Mexico

31. All pork and pork products are forbidden by which religion?
    A. Seventh Day Adventists
    B. Muslim or Islam
    C. Church of Jesus Christ of Latter Day Saints
    D. Roman Catholic

32. People with limited incomes often buy
    A. More protein foods
    B. Carbohydrate foods
    C. Food high in vitamins and minerals
    D. Fatty foods

33. When people buy cheaper foods, the diet may lack
    A. Fats
    B. Starchy foods
    C. Protein and certain vitamins and minerals
    D. Sugars

34. Appetite can be stimulated by
    A. Illness and medications
    B. Decreased senses of taste and smell
    C. Aromas and thoughts of food
    D. Anxiety, pain, and depression

35. Personal choice of foods is influenced by
    A. Foods served at home
    B. Age and social experience
    C. Allergies
    D. All of the above

36. During illness,
    A. Appetite increases.
    B. Fewer nutrients are needed.
    C. Nutritional needs increase to fight infection and heal tissue.
    D. The person will prefer protein foods.

37. All of the following may occur with aging *except*
    A. Increases in taste and smell
    B. Secretion of digestive juices decreases
    C. Difficulty in swallowing
    D. A need for fewer calories compared with younger people

38. What foods should be avoided to help a person with swallowing and digestion problems?
    A. High-fiber foods
    B. Whole-grain cereals
    C. Dry, fried, and fatty foods
    D. Protein foods

39. Requirements for food served in long-term care centers are made by
    A. The Food Guide Pyramid
    B. OBRA
    C. The nursing center
    D. The public health department

40. Which of the following is *not* a requirement for food that is served in long-term care centers?
    A. Food is prepared to meet the person's individual needs.
    B. The person's diet is well balanced, nourishing, and tastes good.
    C. All food is served at room temperature.
    D. Each person must receive at least three meals a day and be offered a bedtime snack.

41. A general diet
    A. Is ordered for a person with difficulty swallowing
    B. Has no dietary limits and is also called a regular or house diet
    C. May have restricted amounts of sodium
    D. Increases the amount of sugar in the diet

42. The body needs no more than _____ of sodium each day.
    A. 2400 mg
    B. 3000 mg
    C. 5000 mg
    D. 1000 mg

43. When the body tissues swell with water, what organ has to work harder?
   A. Kidneys
   B. Liver
   C. Heart
   D. Lungs

44. When you are caring for a person with diabetes, which of the following should you *not* do?
   A. Serve the person's meals and snacks on time.
   B. Report to the nurse what the person did and did not eat.
   C. Give the person extra food and snacks whenever it is requested.
   D. Provide a between-meal nourishment if all the food was not eaten.

45. A person may be given a mechanical soft diet because
   A. Nausea and vomiting have occurred.
   B. The person has chewing difficulties.
   C. The person has been advanced from a clear-liquid diet.
   D. The person has constipation.

46. If you were serving a meal to a person on a fiber- and residue-restricted diet, the meal would not include
   A. Raw fruits and vegetables
   B. Strained fruit juices
   C. Canned or cooked fruit without skin or seeds
   D. Plain pasta

47. A person who has serious burns would receive a
   A. Sodium-controlled diet
   B. Fat-controlled diet
   C. High-calorie diet
   D. High-protein diet

48. When a person has dysphagia, the thickness of the food served is chosen by the
   A. Person
   B. Nursing assistant
   C. Family
   D. Speech-language pathologist, dietician, and physician or nurse

49. Food on a dysphagia diet that is a thickened liquid is served
   A. From a cup
   B. In a bowl
   C. By stirring right before serving
   D. With a spoon

50. Which of the following may be a sign of a swallowing problem (dysphagia)?
   A. The person complains that food will not go down or that food is stuck.
   B. Foods that need chewing are avoided.
   C. There is excessive drooling of saliva.
   D. All of the above are true.

51. When assisting a person with meals, you can help prevent aspiration while the person is eating by placing the person in
   A. A semi-Fowler's position
   B. A Fowler's position
   C. The side-lying position
   D. The supine position

52. If fluid intake exceeds fluid output, the person will
   A. Have edema in the tissues
   B. Be dehydrated
   C. Have vomiting and diarrhea
   D. Have increased urinary output

53. How much fluid is needed every day for normal fluid balance?
   A. 500 ml
   B. 1000 to 1500 ml
   C. 2000 to 2500 ml
   D. 3000 to 4000 ml

54. If the person for whom you are caring has an order for restricted fluids, which of the following should you do?
   A. Offer a variety of liquids.
   B. Thicken all fluids.
   C. Keep the water pitcher out of sight.
   D. Do not allow the person to swallow any liquids during oral hygiene.

55. When you are keeping intake and output (I&O) records, you should measure all of the following *except*
   A. Milk, water, coffee, and tea
   B. Mashed potatoes and creamed vegetables
   C. Creamed cereals and gelatin
   D. Ice cream, custard, and pudding

56. When you are measuring I&O, you need to know that one ounce equals
   A. 10 ml
   B. 500 ml
   C. 100 ml
   D. 30 ml

57. When you are using the graduate to measure output, you read the amount by
    A. Holding the graduate at waist level and reading the amount
    B. Looking at the graduate while it is held above eye level
    C. Keeping the container at eye level
    D. Setting the graduate on the floor and reading it

58. What is the advantage for residents when they receive their meals in assistive dining?
    A. The person is with others at mealtime.
    B. The food is served in bowls and on platters.
    C. Assistive dining prevents distractions during meals.
    D. Food is served as it is in a restaurant.

59. Which of the following needs to be done before the person is served a meal?
    A. Give complete personal care.
    B. Change all linens.
    C. Make sure the person is clean and dry.
    D. Make sure the person has been shaved or has makeup applied.

60. You can provide comfort during meals by
    A. Making sure unpleasant sights and sounds are removed
    B. Making sure dentures, eyeglasses, or hearing aids are in place
    C. Giving the person good oral care before and after meals
    D. All of the above

61. What should you do if a food tray has not been served within 15 minutes?
    A. Recheck the food temperatures.
    B. Serve the tray immediately.
    C. Throw the food away.
    D. Serve only the cold items on the tray.

62. How can you make sure that the food tray is complete?
    A. Ask the person being served.
    B. Ask the nurse.
    C. Call the dietary department.
    D. Check items on the tray with the dietary card.

63. If you become impatient while feeding a resident with dementia, you should
    A. Refuse to continue caring for the person.
    B. Return the person to his or her room.
    C. Talk to the nurse.
    D. Make the person eat his or her food.

64. When you are feeding a person, you should
    A. Not allow the person to assist.
    B. Give the person a fork and knife to assist with cutting the food.
    C. Feed the person in a private area to maintain confidentiality.
    D. Use a spoon because it is less likely to cause injury.

65. When feeding a person, liquids are given
    A. Only at the start of feeding
    B. Alternating with solid foods
    C. At the end of the meal when all solids have been eaten.
    D. Only if the person has difficulty swallowing

66. When providing fresh water to residents, you would *not*
    A. Give fresh water when the pitcher is empty.
    B. Put ice in all pitchers.
    C. Practice the rules of medical sepsis.
    D. Ask the nurse about any special orders.

67. When you keep track of calorie intake, you include
    A. When the person ate
    B. Only the liquids that the person drinks
    C. All of the food that was served to the person
    D. What the person ate and how much

68. Enteral nutrition is used to feed a person when
    A. The person has cancer of the head, neck, or esophagus.
    B. The person has trauma or surgery to the face, mouth, head, or neck.
    C. The person has dementia and no longer knows how to eat.
    D. Any of the above situations are true.

69. Which of the following is *not* a type of enteral nutrition feeding?
    A. An NG tube
    B. IV therapy
    C. A PEG tube
    D. Jejunostomy

70. A major risk with NG and nasointestinal tubes is
    A. Nausea
    B. Complaints of flatulence
    C. Aspiration
    D. Elevated temperature

71. When a person has a feeding tube, it is especially important to provide
    A. Frequent sips of water
    B. Frequent oral hygiene and lubricant for the lips
    C. Linen changes every shift
    D. Snacks between meals

72. When a person has an NG tube, it is important to
    A. Give the person sips of water frequently.
    B. Clean the nose and nostrils every 4 to 8 hours.
    C. Provide oral care once a day.
    D. Remove the tape securing the tubing every 2 hours.

73. If you hear an IV pump alarm, you should
    A. Tell the nurse immediately.
    B. Reset the pump to see if it stops.
    C. Turn off the pump.
    D. Reposition the person to see if the alarm stops.

74. When a person is seriously ill or injured, the person may need to receive hyperalimentation, which is a highly concentrated nutritional solution given
    A. As an oral feeding
    B. Through an NG tube
    C. As an IV administration
    D. Through a PEG tube

75. When residents are included in deciding what foods they eat, which one of the following rights is being met?
    A. Personal choice
    B. Privacy
    C. Confidentiality
    D. Good nutrition

Fill in the Blanks

76. List seven countries in which the main meal is eaten generally at midday.

    A. _____

    B. _____

    C. _____

    D. _____

    E. _____

    F. _____

    G. _____

77. How many calories are in each of the following?

    A. 1 g of fat: _____

    B. 1 g of protein: _____

    C. 1 g of carbohydrate: _____

78. Eating more foods from levels 1 and 2 of the Food Guide Pyramid will help a person eat a

    _____ diet.

79. As you move up the Food Guide Pyramid, the

    amounts of _____ increase.

80. List the food groups in the levels of the Food Guide Pyramid.

    A. Level 1: _____

    B. Level 2: _____ and

    _____

    C. Level 3: _____ and

    _____

    D. Level 4: _____

81. What is the size of the serving in the Food Guide Pyramid for each of these foods?

    A. Milk or yogurt: _____

    B. Butter or margarine: _____

    C. Chopped, cooked, or canned fruit: _____

    D. Cooked cereal, rice, or pasta: _____

    E. Cooked lean meat, poultry, or fish: _____

    F. Vegetable juice: _____

82. How many servings are recommended for each level of the Food Guide Pyramid?

    A. Breads: _____

    B. Vegetables: _____

    C. Fruits: _____

    D. Milk: _____

    E. Meats: _____

    F. Fats, oils, sweets: _____

83. How many calories are in 1 cup of whole milk?

    _____

    How many of these calories come from fat?

    _____

84. When a person eats a 12-ounce steak, how many servings of meat are used?

    _____

85. A well-balanced diet ensures an adequate intake of the essential nutrients. These nutrients are

    A. _____

    B. _____

    C. _____

    D. _____

    E. _____

86. Which vitamins can the body store?

    _____

87. Which vitamins must be ingested daily?

    _____

88. Vitamin _____ is important for these functions:
    A. Formation of substances that hold tissues together
    B. Healthy blood vessels, skin, gums, bones, and teeth
    C. Wound healing; prevention of bleeding
    D. Resistance to infection

89. Milk and milk products, liver, green leafy vegetables, eggs, breads, and cereals are good sources of which vitamin?

    _____

90. What mineral allows red blood cells to carry oxygen?

    _____

91. A diet that does not have enough

    _____,

    may affect nerve function, muscle contraction, and

    heart function.

92. Calcium is needed for _____

    _____.

93. What information is found on food labels?

    A. _____

    B. _____

    C. _____

    D. _____

    E. _____

    F. _____

    G. _____

94. What religious group may forbid the eating of meat?

    _____

95. People who practice _____

    as their religion cannot eat shellfish.

96. The following religious groups do not allow the consumption of alcohol and coffee:

    A. _____

    B. _____

    C. _____

    D. _____

97. What religious group may have members that fast from meats on Fridays?

_____

_____

98. Nutritional needs increase during illness when the body must _____

_____ .

99. Older persons need _____

than do younger people.

100. Why do the diets of some older people lack protein?

_____

_____

101. What two OBRA requirements are related to the temperature of foods that are served in long-term care centers?

A. _____

B. _____

102. Describe the food that is served when the person is receiving a clear-liquid diet.

_____

_____

103. When the person receives a full-liquid diet, it will include all of the foods on the clear-liquid diet, as well as these foods:

_____

_____

104. If a person has poorly fitted dentures and has

chewing difficulties, the physician may order a

_____ diet.

105. A person who is constipated and has other GI disor-

ders may receive a _____

diet. The foods in this diet increase the

_____ to

stimulate _____ .

106. If a person is receiving a high-calorie diet, the

calorie intake is

_____ .

107. If there is too much sodium in the body, the body

retains _____ .

108. When a person is receiving a diabetic diet, the same

amount of _____

is eaten each day. _____

109. If you are feeding a person a dysphagia diet, what observations should be reported to the nurse immediately?

_____

_____

110. Why is it important to offer water often to older persons?

_____

_____

111. When you give oral hygiene to a person who is re-

ceiving nothing by mouth, the person must not

_____ .

112. List the four special dining programs found at care centers.

    A. _____

    B. _____

    C. _____

    D. _____

113. What are four things you need to do for a person when you are preparing to feed the person?

    A. _____

    B. _____

    C. _____

    D. _____

114. When you are serving meal trays, you make sure the right person gets the right tray by checking

    _____.

115. When you are feeding a person, the spoon should be filled _____.

116. Give three reasons why it is important to sit facing the person when you feed him or her.

    A. _____

    B. _____

    C. _____

117. What should be reported after you have fed a person?

    A. _____

    B. _____

    C. _____

118. If a person receives scheduled feedings through a feeding tube, it is done _____ times a day. Usually, about 400 ml is given over

    _____.

119. Why is feeding-tube formula given at room temperature?

    _____

    _____

120. To prevent regurgitation with tube feedings, the person sits or is in

    _____.

    The person remains in this position for

    _____.

Labeling

121. Label each level of the Food Guide Pyramid, and list how many daily servings of each one should be eaten daily.

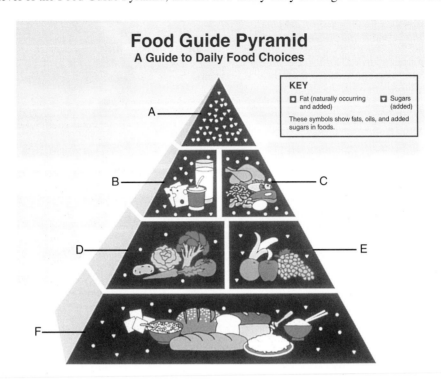

A. _____ _____

B. _____ _____

C. _____ _____

D. _____ _____

E. _____ _____

F. _____ _____

122. Enter this information on the I&O record. Total amounts for the 8-hour and 24-hour periods. Amounts in parentheses indicate how much the person ate or drank. (USC 0700-1500, 1500-2300, 2300-0700 as 8-hour periods)

0200	Voided	300 ml		1430	Water pitcher	500 ml (refilled)
0600	Voided	500 ml		1530	Vomited	50 ml
0730	Breakfast			1545	1 can of soda (whole can)	
	Orange juice (whole glass)			1730	Dinner	
	Milk (½ carton)				Soup (whole bowl)	
	Coffee (1 cup)				Tea (1 cup)	
0700	Voided	300 ml			Juice (whole glass)	
1000	Water pitcher filled				Ice cream (all)	
1130	Lunch			1730	Voided	250 ml
	Soup (whole bowl)			1830	Vomited	100 ml
	Milk (½ carton)			1915	Voided	500 ml
	Tea (1 cup)			2000	Milk (1 carton)	
	Jell-O (1 serving)			2015	Voided	300 ml
1330	Voided	450 ml		2330	Voided	200 ml

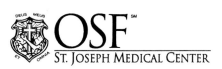

FLUID BALANCE CHART

ST. JOSEPH MEDICAL CENTER

Bloomington, Illinois

Water Glass	250cc
Styrofoam Cup	180cc
Cup (coffee)	250cc
Milk Carton	240cc
Pop (1 can)	360cc
Broth-Soup	175cc
Juice Carton	120cc
Juice Glass	120cc
Jello	120cc

Ice Cream	120cc
Ice Chips	1/2 amt. of cc's in cup
Pitcher (Yellow)	1000cc

DATE _____

TIME	ORAL	Parenteral	Amt. cc Absbd.	URINE Method Collected	Amt. (cc)	OTHER Method Collected	Amt. (cc)	CONT. IRRIGATION In	Out
		INTAKE				**OUTPUT**			
2400-0100		cc from previous shift							
0100-0200									
0200-0300									
0300-0400									
0400-0500									
0500-0600									
0600-0700									
0700-0800									
		8 - hour Sub-total		8-hr T		8-hr T			
0800-0900		cc from previous shift							
0900-1000									
1000-1100									
1100-1200									
1200-1300									
1300-1400									
1400-1500									
1500-1600									
		8 - hour Sub-total		8-hr T		8-hr T			
1600-1700		cc from previous shift							
1700-1800									
1800-1900									
1900-2000									
2000-2100									
2100-2200									
2200-2300									
2300-2400									
		8 - hour Sub-total		8-hr T		8-hr T			
		24 - hour Sub-total		24-hr T		24-hr T			

310' Marie Mills

Source Key:

URINE

V	- Voided
C	- Catheter
INC	- Incontinent
U.C.	- Ureteral Catheter

Source Key:

OTHER

G.I.T.	- Gastric Intestinal Tube
T.T.	- T. Tube
Vom.	- Vomitus
Liq S.	- Liquid Stool
H.V.	- Hemovac

Form No. MF36722 (Rev. 5/97)   **MFI**

123. Label the plate with numbers so that you can describe the location of food to a blind person. How would you tell that person where to find the following food items on the plate?

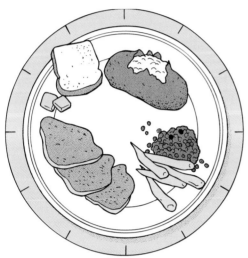

A. Bread: _____

B. Baked potato: _____

C. Vegetables: _____

D. Meat: _____

Nursing Assistant Skills Video Exercise

View the **Nutrition and Fluids** *video to answer these questions.*

124. What are signs and symptoms of dysphagia?

A. _____

B. _____

C. _____

D. _____

125. When you help a person eat, when should you assist them in washing the hands?

_____

and _____

126. When you help a person eat, when should you assist the person with oral hygiene?

_____

and _____

127. When you serve meal trays, what procedural guidelines should be followed?

A. _____

B. _____

C. _____

D. _____

Optional Learning Exercises

128. The following is a person's food intake for 1 day. List the foods and the servings eaten under the correct level in the Food Group Pyramid.

Breakfast
$3/4$ cup orange juice
1 cup oatmeal
2 slices toast
$1/4$ cup milk
2 cups black coffee
Lunch
1 cup tomato soup
Grilled cheese sandwich
$1/2$ cup applesauce
Can of regular soda
Candy bar
Dinner
2- to 4-ounce pork chops
Baked potato with butter
$1/4$ cup green beans
2 brownies
2 cups black coffee
Snacks
1 apple
1- to 4-ounce bag potato chips
$1/3$ cup nuts
1 can regular soda
$1/2$ cup ice cream

A. Breads: _____

_____;

servings _____

B. Vegetables: _____

_____;

servings _____

C. Fruits: _____

_____;

servings _____

D. Milk: _____

_____;

servings _____

E. Meat: _____

_____;

servings _____

F. Fats: _____

_____;

servings _____

129. Which group or groups meet the needs for daily servings?

_____

_____

130. Which group or groups do not meet the needs for daily servings?

_____

_____

Independent Learning Activities

1. Now that you have learned about good nutrition, use this exercise to find out whether you eat a nutritious diet. List your intake for 1 day. Be sure to include the amount of each item. Remember, the portion size is important. Group the foods and liquids you eat according to the parts of the Food Guide Pyramid. Either draw a Food Guide Pyramid and place your food items in the Pyramid, or make a list of the groups of foods. Answer the following questions:
   - How many servings did you eat of breads, cereals, rice, and pasta? How many of these servings were whole grain?
   - How many servings of fruit did you eat? How many were fresh fruit? Canned fruit? Fruit juice? Had added sugars?
   - How many vegetable servings did you eat? How many were raw? Cooked?
   - How many servings of milk, yogurt, and cheese did you eat? How many were low in fat or fat-free?
   - How many servings of meat, poultry, fish, dry beans, eggs, and nuts did you eat? How many were high in fat? Low in fat? High in sodium?
   - How many foods did you eat that count as fats, oils, and sweets?
   - In which food groups are you meeting your daily needs?
   - In which groups do you need to increase your intake? Decrease your intake?
   - After completing this exercise, what changes in your diet will you consider?

2. Role-play with a classmate and take turns feeding each other as you would a resident. You may choose any spoon-fed foods you wish. (Pudding, gelatin, and soup are suggestions.) You should also give a beverage to the person.

3. After you have fed each other, answer these questions:
    *   How were your physical needs (toileting, hand washing, oral hygiene) met before you were fed?
    *   Where were you fed? Bed, chair, at a table? Who made the decision about your location?
    *   Which food was offered first? Who made the choice of how food was offered? Were you offered a variety of foods?
    *   When was a beverage offered? Between food items? Only at the end of feeding? How did the person feeding you decide the order of foods and beverages? The temperature of these items?
    *   When you were being fed, how was the nursing assistant positioned? Sitting? Standing? How did the person's position make you feel?
    *   What kind of conversation was carried on while you were eating? What chances were offered to rest while you were eating? Did you feel relaxed or rushed?
    *   After this exercise, what will you do differently when you feed a resident?

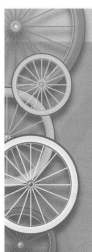

Exercise and Activity

Abduction	Extension	Plantar flexion
Adduction	External rotation	Postural hypotension
Ambulation	Flexion	Pronation
Atrophy	Footdrop	Range of motion (ROM)
Contracture	Hyperextension	Rotation
Deconditioning	Internal rotation	Supination
Dorsiflexion	Orthostatic hypotension	Syncope

Fill in the Blanks: Key Terms

Select your answers from the Key Terms listed above.

1. If _____

   is present, the foot is bent down at the ankle.

2. A brief loss of consciousness or fainting is

   _____.

3. Bending a body part is

   _____.

4. Moving a body part away from the midline of the

   body is _____.

5. _____

   is the movement of a joint to the greatest extent pos-

   sible without causing pain.

6. Turning the joint outward is

   _____.

7. A drop in blood pressure when the person stands is

   postural hypotension or

   _____.

8. _____

   occurs when moving a body part toward the midline

   of the body.

9. Turning upward is called

   _____.

10. Bending the toes and foot up at the ankle is

    _____.

11. Excessive straightening of a body part is

    _____.

12. A decrease in size or a wasting away of tissue is

    _____.

13. Turning the joint is

    _____.

14. _____

    is the straightening of a body part.

15. _____

    is another name for orthostatic hypotension.

16. _____

    is permanent plantar flexion; the foot falls down at

    the ankle.

17. The act of walking is

    _____.

18. _____

    is turning downward.

19. The loss of muscle strength from inactivity is

    _____.

20. _____

    is turning the joint inward.

21. The lack of joint mobility caused by abnormal

    shortening of a muscle is a

    _____.

Circle the BEST Answer

22. If a person is on bedrest, he or she
    A. May be allowed to perform some activities of daily living (ADL)
    B. Can use the bedside commode for elimination needs
    C. May not perform any ADL
    D. Can use the bathroom for elimination needs

23. Complications of bedrest include all of the following *except*
    A. Contractures in fingers, wrists, knees, and hips
    B. Urinary tract infections and renal calculi
    C. Increased appetite and improved muscle strength
    D. Orthostatic hypotension and syncope

24. If a contracture develops,
    A. It will require extra ROM exercises to correct it.
    B. You need to position the person in good body alignment.
    C. The person is permanently deformed and disabled.
    D. It will be relieved as soon as the person is able to walk and exercise.

25. When you are caring for a person who has orthostatic hypotension, you should
    A. Raise the head of the bed to Fowler's position before getting the person out of bed.
    B. Have the person get out of bed quickly to prevent weakness.
    C. Keep the bed flat when getting the person out of bed.
    D. Have the person walk around to decrease weakness and dizziness.

26. Good nursing care that prevents complications from bedrest includes
    A. Positioning in good body alignment
    B. ROM exercises
    C. Frequent position changes
    D. All of the above

27. If a person sitting on the edge of the bed complains of weakness, dizziness, or spots before the eyes, you should
    A. Assist the person to stand.
    B. Help the person to sit in a chair or walk around.
    C. Assist the person to Fowler's position.
    D. Tell the person that this is a normal response and continue to get the person up.

28. Bed boards are used to
    A. Keep the person in alignment by preventing the mattress from sagging.
    B. Prevent plantar flexion that can lead to foot drop.
    C. Keep the hips abducted.
    D. Keep the weight to top linens off the feet.

29. Plantar flexion must be prevented to
    A. Keep the feet from bending down at the ankle.
    B. Keep the hips from rotating outward.
    C. Keep the wrist, thumb, and fingers in normal position.
    D. Maintain good body alignment.

30. To prevent the hips and legs from turning outward, you can use
    A. Bed cradles
    B. Hip abduction wedges
    C. Trochanter rolls
    D. Splints

31. Exercise occurs when
    A. ADLs are done.
    B. The person turns and moves in bed without help.
    C. The person uses a trapeze to lift the trunk off the bed.
    D. All of the above are true.

32. When another person moves the joints through their ROM, it is called
    A. Active ROM
    B. ADL
    C. Active-assistive ROM
    D. Passive ROM

33. ROM exercises are performed on the

    _____

    only if allowed by center policy.
    A. Shoulder
    B. Neck
    C. Hip
    D. Knee

34. The goal in rehabilitation and subacute care is to
    A. Send the person home.
    B. Improve the person's independence so he or she can go home.
    C. Give complete care and meet all of the person's needs.
    D. Perform only passive ROM activities.

35. When exercising the wrist, you will perform all of these motions *except*
    A. Abduction
    B. Supination
    C. Flexion
    D. Extension

36. Which joint is adducted and abducted?
    A. Neck
    B. Hip
    C. Forearm
    D. Knee

37. When you help a person who is too weak and unsteady to walk, you should
    A. Use a gait belt.
    B. Help the person use the hand rails along the wall.
    C. Check the person for orthostatic hypotension.
    D. All of the above are true.

38. If you are walking a person and he or she starts to fall, you should
    A. Support the person and prevent the fall.
    B. Call for help while you hold the person upright.
    C. Ease the person to the floor.
    D. Let the person fall so you do not injure him or her by stopping the fall.

39. When the person is walking with crutches, the person should wear
    A. Soft slippers on the feet
    B. Clothes that fit well
    C. Clothes that are loose
    D. A gait belt

40. When walking with a cane, it is held
    A. On the strong side of the body
    B. On the weak side of the body
    C. In the right hand
    D. On the left side of the body

41. When a person is using a walker, it is
    A. Picked up and moved 3 to 4 inches in front of the person
    B. Moved forward with a rocking motion
    C. Moved first on the left side and then on the right
    D. Picked up and moved 6 to 8 inches in front of the person

42. When you are caring for a person who wears a brace, it is important to report immediately
    A. How far the person walks
    B. What care measures the person can do alone
    C. The amount of mobility in joints when doing ROM exercises
    D. Any redness or signs of skin breakdown when you remove a brace

43. Recreational activity is important for all of these reasons *except*
    A. It forces the person to take part in activities to find new interests.
    B. Joints and muscles are exercised.
    C. Circulation is stimulated.
    D. Activities are mentally stimulating.

Fill in the Blanks

44. To prevent deconditioning, is it important to encourage each resident to be as

    _____.

45. Bedrest is ordered to

    A. _____

    B. _____

    C. _____

    D. _____

    E. _____

46. The nurse tells you that the resident is on bedrest but can use the bathroom for elimination, which means that the resident is ordered

    _____

    _____.

47. When a person has a contracture, the joint is deformed and disabled

    _____

    _____.

48. When a person is moved from lying or sitting to a standing position, the blood pressure may

    _____.

    This condition is called

    _____.

49. Bed boards keep the person in

    _____

    by preventing the mattress from sagging.

50. When you use a footboard, the soles of the feet

    are _____

    against it to prevent _____.

51. A trochanter roll is placed along the body to prevent the hips and legs from

    _____.

52. Handrolls or grips prevent

    _____

    of the thumb, fingers, and wrists. A device used to keep the wrist, thumb, and fingers in normal position is a _____.

53. Bed cradles are used because the weight of top

    linens can cause _____

    and _____ .

54. A trapeze bar allows the person to lift the

    _____

    off the bed; it also allows the person to

    _____

    and _____ in bed.

55. When ROM exercises are done, what should be re-
    ported or recorded?

    A. _____

    B. _____

    C. _____

    D. _____

    E. _____

56. When performing ROM exercises, each movement

    should be repeated _____ times or the

    _____ .

57. List the rules to follow when performing ROM
    exercises.

    A. _____

    B. _____

    C. _____

    D. _____

    E. _____

    F. _____

    G. _____

58. When you help a person walk, you should walk to

    the _____

    and _____

    the person. Provide support with the

    _____ ,

    or have _____

    _____ .

59. If a person falls, do not allow him or her to move or

    get up before the _____

    _____ .

60. If a person falls, what is reported to the nurse?

    A. _____

    B. _____

    C. _____

    D. _____

    E. _____

Labeling

61. ROM exercises for the

_____

joint are shown in these drawings. Name the movements shown in each drawing.

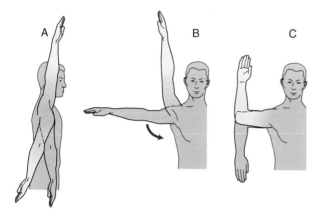

A. _____

B. _____

C. _____

62. ROM exercises for the

_____

joint are shown in these drawings. Name the movements shown in each drawing.

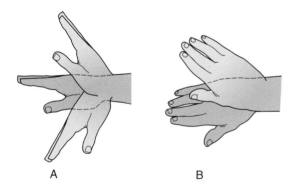

A. _____

B. _____

63. ROM exercises for the

_____

joint are shown in these drawings. Name the movements shown in each drawing.

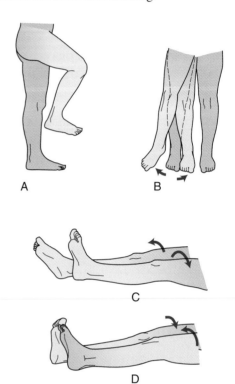

A. _____

B. _____

C. _____

D. _____

Crossword

Fill in the crossword puzzle by answering the clues with words from this list.

Abduction   Extension   Hyperextension   Pronation
Adduction   External rotation   Internal rotation   Rotation
Dorsiflexion   Flexion   Plantar flexion   Supination

Across

5. Turning upward
7. Turning the joint inward
10. Straightening a body part
11. Bending the toes and foot up at the ankle
12. Turning downward

Down

1. Bending a body part
2. Bending the foot down at the ankle
3. Turning the joint outward
4. Excessive straightening of a body part
6. Turning the joint
8. Moving a body part from the midline of the body
9. Moving a body part toward the midline of the body

Nursing Assistant Skills Video

View the related portions of the **Body Mechanics and Exercise** *video to answer these questions.*

64. When doing ROM exercises, you should support the

_____.

65. When exercising the knee, your hands should be

under the _____

and _____.

66. The person should wear

_____

footwear when being ambulated.

67. When using a gait belt, you should grasp the belt

_____

when helping the person stand.

68. When ambulating the person, grasp the gait belt at

the _____

and _____.

69. What observations should be reported after ambu-lating a person?

A. _____

B. _____

Optional Learning Exercises

70. What kind of ROM exercises would be used with each of these residents?
    A. The resident needs complete care for bathing, grooming, and feeding.

    _____

    B. The resident takes part in many activities in the center. She walks to most activities independently.

    _____

    C. The resident has weakness on his left side. He is able to feed himself but needs help with bathing and dressing.

    _____

71. As you plan to help a person out of bed, you are concerned about orthostatic hypotension. To make sure the person is able to stand and get up safely, you plan to take the blood pressure, pulse, and res-pirations several times. When would you take the blood pressure?

    A. _____

    B. _____

    C. _____

    D. _____

    E. _____

72. If you are caring for a confused person and he or she falls, you may need to let the person move. Why?

    _____

    _____

Independent Learning Activities

1. Role-play with a classmate and take turns acting as the nursing assistant and a person with left-sided weakness. Perform ROM exercises on the person. Answer these questions about how you felt after this activity.
   - What did the nursing assistant explain to you before performing the exercises?
   - How were you positioned for exercising? What did the nursing assistant ask about your comfort and personal wishes in the position used?
   - How was your privacy maintained? Was there anything that made you feel exposed or embarrassed?
   - How were your joints supported during the exercises? Did you feel any discomfort or pain during the exercises?
   - What exercises were you encouraged to carry out independently? With some assistance?
   - Which exercises were done first? Were the exercises carried out in an organized pattern? How did you know what exercise would be done next?
   - After this activity, what will you do differently when giving ROM exercises to a person?

2. With a classmate, role-play assisting a weak, older person to ambulate. Take turns acting as the person and the nursing assistant. Answer these questions about how you felt and what you learned.
   - What did the nursing assistant tell you before preparing to walk with you? What choices were offered about the time you were to ambulate, what clothing to wear, and where you were going to walk?
   - What safety devices were used? What did the nursing assistant tell you about the devices or equipment used?
   - What assessments were made before you sat up? When you dangled? After walking?
   - Did the nursing assistant make you feel secure during ambulation? How did the nursing assistant hold you?
   - What did you learn from this activity that will help you when you ambulate a person?

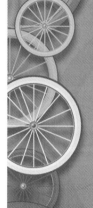

Comfort, Rest, and Sleep

Acute pain	Guided imagery	Radiating pain
Chronic pain	Insomnia	Relaxation
Circadian rhythm	Non–rapid-eye-movement	REM sleep
Comfort	(NREM) sleep	Rest
Discomfort	NREM sleep	Sleep
Distraction	Pain	
Enuresis	Phantom pain	

Fill in the Blanks: Key Terms

Select your answers from the Key Terms listed above.

1. Another name for discomfort is

   _____.

2. _____

   is pain that is felt suddenly from injury, disease,

   trauma, or surgery; it generally lasts less than 6

   months.

3. _____

   is a way to change a person's center of attention.

4. A state of unconsciousness, reduced voluntary

   muscle activity, and lowered metabolism is

   _____.

5. Pain lasting longer than 6 months is

   _____;

   it may be constant or occur off and on.

6. _____

   is to be free from mental or physical stress.

7. _____

   is a state of well-being. The person has no physical

   or emotional pain and is calm and at peace.

8. NREM sleep is also called

   _____.

9. To be calm, at ease, and relaxed is to

_____.

The person is free of anxiety and stress.

10. Creating and focusing on an image is

_____.

11. The phase of sleep when there is rapid eye

movement is

_____.

12. _____ is a

chronic condition in which the person cannot sleep

or stay asleep throughout the night.

13. The day-night cycle or body rhythm is also called

_____.

This daily rhythm is based on a 24-hour cycle.

14. _____

is pain felt at the site of tissue damage and in nearby

areas.

15. The stage of sleep when there is no rapid eye move-

ment is _____.

16. To ache, hurt, or be sore is

_____;

it is also called pain.

17. Pain felt in a body part that is no longer there is

_____.

18. Urinary incontinence in bed at night is

_____.

Circle the BEST Answer

19. Comfort, rest, and sleep are needed for
    A. Well-being and energy
    B. Decreasing function and quality of life
    C. Increasing muscle strength
    D. All of the above

20. OBRA requirements related to comfort, rest, and
    sleep include
    A. Only two people in a room
    B. Bright lighting in all areas
    C. Room temperature between 65° and 71° F
    D. Adequate ventilation and room humidity

21. When a person complains of pain,
    A. The person has pain.
    B. It must be carefully measured to see if the person
       really has pain.
    C. You can easily measure to find out how much
       pain is present.
    D. You can tell if the person really has pain by the
       way he or she acts.

22. When a person complains of pain that is located
    near an area of tissue damage, this is what kind of
    pain?
    A. Acute
    B. Chronic
    C. Radiating
    D. Phantom

23. If pain is ignored or denied, it may be because the
    person thinks pain is a sign of weakness. Which
    factor that affects pain would this thought be?
    A. Attention
    B. Past experience
    C. Value or meaning of pain
    D. Support from others

24. A person from which of the following countries may
    refuse pain relief the first time it is offered?
    A. Vietnam
    B. China
    C. Mexico
    D. Philippines

25. When a person has anxiety, the person
    A. Will usually feel increased pain
    B. Will usually feel less pain
    C. May deny having pain
    D. May be stoic and show no reaction to pain

26. When you ask a person, "Where is the pain?" you are asking the person to
    A. Describe the pain.
    B. Explain the intensity of the pain.
    C. Tell you the onset and duration of the pain.
    D. Tell you the location of the pain.

27. When a person tells you that he or she has pain when coughing or deep breathing, this is
    A. A factor causing pain
    B. A measurement of the onset of pain
    C. Words used to describe the pain
    D. The location of the pain

28. A distraction measure to promote comfort and relieve pain may be
    A. Asking the person to focus on an image
    B. Teaching the person to breathe deeply and slowly
    C. Having the person listen to music or playing games
    D. Instructing the person to contract and relax muscle groups

29. If the nurse has given a person pain medication, you should
    A. Give the person a bath.
    B. Walk the person according to the care plan.
    C. Wait $1/2$ hour before giving care.
    D. Give care before the medication makes the person sleepy.

30. You may help promote comfort and relieve pain by doing all of the following *except*
    A. Allowing family members and friends at the bedside as requested by the person
    B. Keeping the room brightly lit and playing loud music
    C. Providing blankets for warmth and to prevent chilling
    D. Handling the person gently

31. You can help promote rest by
    A. Meeting physical needs such as thirst, hunger, and elimination needs
    B. Making sure the person feels safe
    C. Allowing the person to practice rituals or routines before resting
    D. All of the above

32. When caring for an ill or injured person, you know that the person may need more rest. You can help the person get rest by making sure that you
    A. Provide plenty of exercise to prevent weakness.
    B. Provide rest periods during or after a procedure.
    C. Give complete hygiene and grooming measures quickly.
    D. Spend time talking with the person to distract him or her.

33. Which of the following does *not* occur during sleep?
    A. The person is unaware of the environment.
    B. Metabolism is reduced during sleep.
    C. Blood pressure, temperature, pulse, and respirations are higher during sleep.
    D. There are no voluntary arm or leg movements.

34. Some people function better in the morning because of
    A. Circadian rhythm
    B. Getting enough sleep
    C. Interference with the body rhythm
    D. Changes in the work schedule

35. During REM sleep, the person
    A. Is hard to arouse
    B. Has a gradual fall in vital signs
    C. Is easily aroused
    D. Will relax muscles completely

36. Which stage of sleep is usually not repeated during the cycles of sleep?
    A. REM
    B. Stage 1: NREM
    C. Stage 2: NREM
    D. Stage 3: NREM

37. Which age-group requires the least amount of sleep?
    A. Toddlers
    B. Young adults
    C. Adolescents
    D. Older adults

38. Which of these factors increases the need for sleep?
    A. Illness
    B. Weight loss
    C. Emotional problems
    D. Drugs and other substances

39. When a person takes sleeping pills, sleep may not restore the person mentally because
    A. Caffeine prevents sleep.
    B. Some people have difficulty falling asleep.
    C. The length of REM sleep is reduced.
    D. It upsets the usual sleep routines.

40. Exercise should be avoided for 2 hours before sleep because
    A. It requires energy.
    B. People usually feel good after exercise.
    C. It causes the release of substances in the bloodstream that stimulate the body.
    D. The person tires after exercise.

41. Persons who are ill or in intensive care units are at great risk for
    A. Sleep deprivation
    B. Sleepwalking
    C. Insomnia
    D. Increased sleep times

42. If a person has decreased reasoning, red, puffy eyes, and coordination problems, report these signs and symptoms to the nurse because the person
    A. Is having a reaction to sleeping medications
    B. Is experiencing sleep disorders
    C. Needs more exercise before bedtime
    D. May need an increase in sleeping pills

43. Which of these measures would *not* help promote sleep?
    A. Provide blankets or socks for persons who tend to be cold.
    B. Have the person void, or make sure incontinent persons are clean and dry.
    C. Follow bedtime rituals.
    D. Offer the person a cup of coffee or tea at bedtime.

Fill in the Blanks

44. OBRA has requirements about the person's room. List the requirements that relate to each of the following.

    A. Suspended curtain: _____

    B. Linens: _____

    C. Bed: _____

    D. Room temperature: _____

    E. Persons in room: _____

45. Name the type of pain described.
    A. A person with an amputated leg may still sense leg pain.

    _____

    B. There is tissue damage. The pain decreases with healing.

    _____

    C. Pain from a heart attack is often felt in the left chest, left jaw, left shoulder, and left arm.

    _____

    D. The pain remains long after healing. Common causes are arthritis and cancer.

    _____

46. What is the reason that persons from the Phillipines may appear stoic in reaction to pain?

    _____

    _____

47. Older persons may ignore or deny pain because

    A. _____.

    B. _____.

48. Persons with dementia may signal pain by changes

    _____.

49. When gathering information about a person in pain, you can use a scale from 1 to 10. Which end of the scale is the most severe pain?

    _____

50. What happens to vital signs when the person has pain?

    _____

51. When the person uses words such as aching, knife-like, or sore to describe pain, what do you report to the nurse?

    _____

52. What body responses may be signs that the person has pain?

    A. _____

    B. _____

    C. _____

    D. _____

    E. _____

53. What changes in these behaviors may be symptoms of pain?

    A. Speech: _____

    B. Affected body part: _____

    C. Body position: _____

54. List nursing measures to promote comfort and relieve pain related to these clues.

    A. Position of the person: _____

    B. Linens: _____

    B. Blankets: _____

    C. Pain medications: _____

    D. Family members: _____

55. If a person is receiving strong pain medication or sedatives, what safety measures are important?

    A. _____

    B. _____

    C. _____

    D. _____

    E. _____

    F. _____

56. When you explain the procedure before performing it, you may help a person rest better because you met the need for _____.

57. A clean, neat, and uncluttered room can promote rest by meeting _____ needs.

58. The mind and body rest, the body saves energy, and body functions slow during

    _____.

59. Mental restoration occurs during a phase of sleep called _____.

60. The deepest stage of sleep occurs during

    _____.

61. If work hours change, it can affect the normal

    _____ cycle

    and the _____ rhythm.

62. Alcohol tends to cause drowsiness and sleep, but it interferes with _____.

63. Insomnia may be caused by

    A. Fear of _____.

    B. Afraid of not _____.

    C. Fear of not being able _____.

    D. Physical and emotional _____.

64. When a person has dementia and wanders at night, the best approach for some persons is to allow

    _____.

Optional Learning Exercises

65. You are caring for two residents who both have arthritis. Mr. Forman tells you that this is the first time he has had any health problems. Mrs. Wegman tells you that she has had several surgeries and has had three children. Which of these two persons is likely to be more anxious than is the other about the pain and to be unable to handle the pain well?

_____

_____

Why? _____

_____

66. Mr. Forman tells you that his pain seems much worse at night. What might be the reason for this reaction?

_____

_____

67. You are caring for Mrs. Reynolds. She tells you that she misses her children who have moved to another state. Today, Mrs. Reynolds is complaining of pain in her abdomen. In spite of providing nursing comfort measures, she still rates her pain at a 7. What is a possible reason Mrs. Reynolds is not getting relief of her pain?

_____

_____

68. When a person is ill, how do the following circumstances affect sleep?

A. Treatments and medications:

_____

B. Traction or a cast:

_____

C. Emotions that affect sleep include

_____.

69. Certain foods affect sleep. Indicate how these foods affect sleep, and list foods that contain the substances.

A. Caffeine _____

sleep and is found in _____

_____

B. L-tryptophan _____

sleep and is found in _____

_____

Independent Learning Activities

1. Form a group with several classmates and share your personal experiences with pain. Discuss these questions to understand the different ways you respond to and treat the pain.
   - What experiences have you had with pain? Accidents? Illnesses? Childbirth? Surgery?
   - What type of pain have you had? Acute? Chronic? Other types?
   - How would you rate your pain on a scale from 1 to 10? How long did it last?
   - How did your family and friends respond to your pain? How much support did you receive from them? How did the support (or lack of it) affect the pain?
   - What measures were used to treat the pain? Which measure was the most effective? The least effective?
   - What did you learn from this discussion with other classmates about their pain? How will this help you as you care for people with pain?

2. Form a group with several classmates to talk about differences in sleep habits. Answer these questions to understand differences in personal practices concerning rest and sleep.
    *   How many hours do you sleep each day? How many hours of sleep do you think you *should* get each day?
    *   If you did not have to follow a schedule (work, school, etc.), when would you go to bed and wake up?
    *   What rituals do you perform before going to bed? How is your sleep affected if you cannot perform these rituals?
    *   What factors interfere with your sleep? What do you do to avoid these factors?
    *   When do you feel most alert? Morning? Afternoon? Night?
    *   How do you feel when you wake up? Alert? Pleasant? Grouchy? Tired?
    *   How often do you take naps? What time of day do you like to nap? How do you feel when you wake from a nap?
    *   How will this discussion help you understand differences in sleep patterns when you are caring for others? How will it affect how you help the persons in your care get the rest and sleep they need?

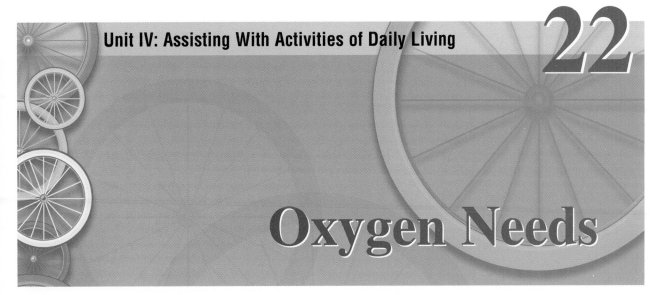

Oxygen Needs

Allergy	Hemothorax	Mechanical ventilation	Respiratory arrest
Apnea	Hyperventilation	Orthopnea	Respiratory depression
Biot's respirations	Hypoventilation	Orthopneic position	Sputum
Bradypnea	Hypoxemia	Oxygen concentration	Suction
Cheyne-Stokes	Hypoxia	Pleural effusion	Tachypnea
Dyspnea	Intubation	Pneumothorax	
Hemoptysis	Kussmaul's respirations	Pollutant	

Fill in the Blanks: Key Terms

Select your answers from the Key Terms listed above.

1. _____

   are rapid and deep respirations followed by 10 to 30

   seconds of apnea.

2. Bloody sputum is called

   _____.

3. _____

   is inserting an artificial airway.

4. Air in the pleural space is

   _____.

5. Rapid breathing in which respirations are more than

   24 per minute is called

   _____.

6. An _____

   is a sensitivity to a substance that causes the body to

   react with signs and symptoms.

7. Difficult, labored, or painful breathing is

   _____.

8. _____

   is blood in the pleural space.

9. Being able to breathe deeply and comfortably only while sitting or standing is

   _____.

10. Mucus from the respiratory system that is expectorated through the mouth is

    _____.

11. Respirations that are less than 12 per minute is slow breathing or

    _____.

12. A reduced amount of oxygen in the blood is

    _____.

13. _____ describes slow, weak respirations at a rate of less than 12 per minute.

14. The lack or absence of breathing is

    _____.

15. _____ is a pattern of respirations that are rapid and deeper than normal.

16. Using a machine to move air into and out of the lungs is _____.

17. A harmful chemical or substance in the air or water is a _____.

18. The process of withdrawing or sucking up fluid is

    _____.

19. _____ are respirations that gradually increase in rate and depth and then become shallow and slow. Breathing may stop for 10 to 20 seconds.

20. The _____ is sitting up and leaning over a table.

21. The escape and collection of fluid in the pleural space is _____.

22. _____ occurs when breathing stops.

23. Very deep and rapid respirations that occur in diabetic coma is called

    _____.

24. _____ is the amount of hemoglobin that contains oxygen.

25. Cells that do not have enough oxygen have

    _____.

26. _____ occurs when respirations are slow, shallow, and sometimes irregular.

Circle the BEST Answer

27. Capillaries and cells must exchange oxygen (O_2) and carbon dioxide (CO_2) in the
    A. Respiratory system
    B. Cardiovascular system
    C. Nervous system
    D. Red blood cells

28. O_2 needs increase when
    A. The person is aging.
    B. Drugs are taken.
    C. The person has fever or pain.
    D. The person is well nourished.

29. Respiratory depression can occur when
    A. The person exercises.
    B. Allergies are present.
    C. Narcotic drugs are taken in large doses.
    D. The person smokes.

30. Restlessness is an early sign of
    A. Hypoxia
    B. Apnea
    C. Hyperventilation
    D. Bradypnea

31. When you prepare a person for a chest x-ray, you should
    A. Make sure the person does not eat for several hours before the test.
    B. Help the person remove all clothing and jewelry from the waist to the neck.
    C. Tell the person not to drink any fluids before the x-ray test.
    D. All of the above are true.

32. You are caring for a person who just had a pulmonary function test done. You would expect the person to
    A. Tell you he has chest pain
    B. Be very tired
    C. Have hemoptysis
    D. Complain of nausea and vomiting

33. If a pulse oximeter were being used, which of these sites would be best?
    A. Toe in a foot that is swollen
    B. Finger with a fake fingernail
    C. Toe with an open wound
    D. Earlobe

34. When you are delegated to place a pulse oximeter on a person, you should report to the nurse if
    A. The person is sleeping.
    B. The person's pulse does not equal the pulse on the display.
    C. You remove nail polish from the nail on the site used.
    D. You tape the oximeter in place.

35. When collecting a sputum specimen, you should do all of the following *except*
    A. Having the person rinse the mouth with mouthwash
    B. Collecting the specimen in the morning
    C. Providing privacy
    D. Covering the specimen container

36. Which of these specimens collected would *not* be sputum? The specimen is
    A. Clear, thick, and frothy
    B. Thick and streaked with blood
    C. Thin, clear liquid
    D. Thick, green, and has a foul odor

37. For a person who has breathing difficulties, breathing is usually easier when the person is
    A. In the supine position
    B. Lying on one side for long periods
    C. In the semi-Fowler's or Fowler's position
    D. In the prone position

38. Coughing and deep-breathing exercises
    A. Help prevent pneumonia and atelectasis
    B. Decrease pain after surgery or injury
    C. Are done once a day
    D. Causes mucus to form in the lungs

39. When assisting with coughing and deep breathing, you tell the person to
    A. Take deep breaths through the mouth.
    B. Hold the breath for 30 seconds.
    C. Exhale slowly through pursed lips.
    D. Repeat the exercise 1 or 2 times.

40. When a person uses an incentive spirometer, it allows the person to
    A. Take shallow breaths.
    B. See air movement when inhaling.
    C. See air movement when exhaling.
    D. Exhale quickly.

41. If a person is receiving O_2, you may
    A. Set the flow rate.
    B. Start and maintain the therapy.
    C. Set up the system.
    D. All of the above are true.

42. If you are caring for a person with O_2 therapy, you may *not*
    A. Start and maintain oxygen therapy.
    B. Remove the mask for meals.
    C. Tell the nurse if the rate is too high or too low.
    D. Check for irritation from the device.

43. If a person receives O_2 through a nasal cannula, it is important to look for irritation
    A. On the nose, ears, and cheekbones
    B. Under the mask
    C. In the throat
    D. All of the above

44. If you are delegated to set up for O_2 administration, you will do all of the following *except*
    A. Collect the device with connecting tubing.
    B. Attach the flow meter to the wall outlet or tank.
    C. Apply the O_2 administration device to the person.
    D. Fill the humidifier with distilled water.

45. When you care for a person receiving O_2, you should know the O_2 flow rate. You should get this information from the
    A. Physician
    B. Nurse and care plan
    C. Respiratory therapist
    D. Chart

46. If the O_2 administration setup has a humidifier, you should report
    A. If the container is one half full of water
    B. If the humidifier is bubbling
    C. If the humidifier is not bubbling
    D. If moisture collects under the mask

47. Which of the following would *not* be a sign of hypoxia?
    A. Disorientation and confusion
    B. Decrease in pulse rate and respirations
    C. Apprehension and anxiety
    D. Cyanosis of the skin, mucous membranes, and nail beds

48. If you are caring for a person with an artificial airway, your care should always include
    A. Removing the device to clean it
    B. Comforting and reassuring the person that the airway helps breathing
    C. Suctioning to maintain the airway
    D. Making sure the person never takes a tub bath

49. When oropharyngeal and nasopharyngeal suctioning is done, the nurse
    A. Uses sterile technique
    B. Follows Standard Precautions and Bloodborne Pathogen Standard
    C. Applies suction for 20 to 30 seconds each time
    D. Uses suction as many times as is necessary to clear the airway

50. When you are caring for a person who has an artificial airway, tell the nurse at once if
    A. The person needs frequent oral hygiene.
    B. The person feels as if he or she is gagging or choking.
    C. The person cannot speak.
    D. The airway comes out or is dislodged.

51. When a person has a tracheostomy, the stoma is
    A. Uncovered when the person is outdoors
    B. Covered with plastic when outdoors to prevent dust from entering
    C. Covered when shaving
    D. Covered with a loose gauze dressing

52. If you are caring for a person with a mechanical ventilator and the alarm sounds, you should first
    A. Get the nurse.
    B. Reset the alarms.
    C. Reassure the person.
    D. Check to see if the person's tube is attached to ventilator.

53. If a person has chest tubes, petrolatum gauze is kept at the bedside to
    A. Cover the insertion site if a chest tube comes out.
    B. Lubricate the site of the chest tube.
    C. Cleanse the skin around the chest tube.
    D. Apply to any open areas that occur.

54. To avoid upsetting the person or family when a mechanical ventilator is being used,
    A. Avoid eye contact.
    B. Work quietly and do not talk to the person.
    C. Watch what you say and do.
    D. Stay out of the room as much as possible.

55. To provide safe care to a resident with O_2 needs, you should do all of the following *except*
    A. Make sure a nurse supervises you if you are doing complex tasks.
    B. Have the necessary training to perform or assist in care.
    C. Give O_2 when you understand O_2 therapy and its safety rules.
    D. Refuse to perform any procedure that you do not understand.

Fill in the Blanks

56. As a person ages, the risk of pneumonia increases

    because _____

    weaken and lung tissue is

    _____.

57. Smoking affects O_2 needs because it causes

    _____

    and _____.

58. If a person has hypoxia, you may find that the

    person prefers a position in which he or she is

    _____.

59. Adults normally have _____ respirations per

    minute. If the person has tachypnea, the respirations

    are _____ per minute.

60. After a thoracentesis is done, the person is checked
    often for these respiratory signs and symptoms.

    A. _____

    B. _____

    C. _____

    D. _____

    E. _____

    F. _____

    G. _____

61. A pulse oximeter measures

    _____.

    The normal range is

    _____.

62. When recording the results of a pulse oximeter, you
    use SpO_2, where:

    S = _____

    p = _____

    O_2 = _____

63. When you have been delegated to collect a sputum
    specimen, what observations are reported and
    recorded?

    A. _____

    B. _____

    C. _____

    D. _____

    E. _____

64. Coughing and deep breathing help prevent atelec-

    tasis, which is the

    _____.

65. If you are assisting a person with coughing and
    deep-breathing exercises, how can you help the
    person support the incision?

    A. _____

    B. _____

66. What is the goal of using an incentive spirometer?

    _____

    This goal is met because

    A. Air moves _____.

    B. Secretions _____.

    C. O_2 and CO_2 _____.

67. O_2 needs to be humidified because it is a

    _____

    and dries the airway's

    _____.

68. If you are delegated setting up for O_2 administration, what information do you need from the nurse?

   A. _____

   B. _____

   C. _____

69. If you assist the nurse with suctioning, you check

   the person's pulse, respirations, and pulse oximeter

   _____

   _____.

70. When you are caring for a person who is suctioned, tell the nurse immediately if the following events occur:

   A. _____

   B. _____

   C. _____

   D. _____

   E. _____

71. If a person has mechanical ventilation, where do you find a plan for communication?

   _____

   Why is it important for everyone to use the same signals for communication?

   _____

Optional Learning Exercises

Situation: You are caring for Mr. Reynolds, age 84, who has chronic obstructive pulmonary disease. Answer Questions #72 and #73 about caring for Mr. Reynolds.

72. What position would make it easier for Mr. Reynolds to breathe when he is in bed?

   _____

73. How can you increase his comfort when he is sitting up?

   _____

   What is this position called?

   _____

Situation: Mrs. Fagan is receiving O_2 through a nasal cannula at 2 L/min. Her respirations are unlabored at 16 per minute unless she is walking around or doing personal care. Then, her respirations are 28 and dyspneic. Answer Questions #74 to #77 about her care.

74. Why is there no humidifier with the O_2 setup for Mrs. Fagan?

   _____

   _____

75. Where should you check for signs of irritation from the cannula?

   _____

   _____

76. You should make sure there are

   _____

   in the tubing and that Mrs. Fagan does not

   _____ of the tubing.

77. What are the abnormal respirations that Mrs. Fagan has with activity called?

   _____

Independent Learning Activities

1. Work with a classmate and carry out these exercises, which will help you understand how it feels to be a person with breathing problems.
   - Have your partner count your respirations while you are at rest. Then, exercise by running or jogging in place for at least 2 minutes. Now, have your partner check your respirations again. How have they changed? Rate? Rhythm or pattern? Easy or labored?
   - While you exercise, first, try to breathe only through your nose. Then, try breathing through your mouth. Which way makes you feel you are getting enough air?
   - Place a drinking straw in your mouth and close your lips tightly around it. Now, breathe only through the straw while at rest and during exercise. When you are at rest, how comfortable does this feel? Are you getting enough air? How is your air supply during exercise?
   - Take a drinking straw and place small pieces of paper in one end so that it is fairly tight. Now, try breathing through the straw at rest and exercise. What is the difference between the open and the blocked straw? Imagine if every breath you take feels like it does with the blocked straw. This is how many people with breathing problems feel all the time.

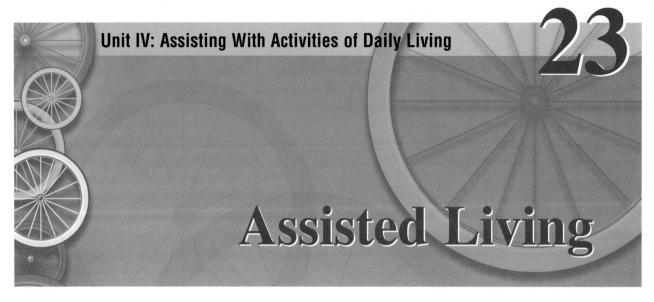

Assisted Living

Assisted living residence
Medication reminder
Service plan

Fill in the Blanks: Key Terms

Select your answers from the Key Terms listed above.

1. A _____

   is reminding the person to take drugs, observing

   that they were taken as prescribed, and charting that

   they were taken.

2. A written plan that lists the services that the person

   needs and who provides them is a

   _____.

3. An _____

   provides housing, support services, and health care

   to persons needing help with activities of daily

   living (ADL).

Circle the BEST Answer

4. Which of these persons would *not* be living in assisted living?
   A. Someone who needs help taking drugs
   B. A person who has problems with thinking, reasoning, and judgment
   C. A person who must stay in bed all the time because of failing health
   D. Someone who is lonely and wants to live with people

5. When a person lives in an assisted living unit, one requirement is
   A. At least two rooms and a bath
   B. Both a bathtub and a shower
   C. A door that locks and the person keeping the key
   D. A double or queen-sized bed

6. Environmental requirements in assisted living units include
   A. Common bathrooms that have toilet paper, soap, and cloth towels or a dryer
   B. Pets or animals that must be kept in kennels
   C. Hot water temperatures that are between 110° and 130° F
   D. Garbage that is stored in covered containers lined with plastic bags that are removed at least once a day

7. An Alzheimer's special care unit provides
   A. Programs that rehabilitate the person to normal function
   B. Activities that provide stimulation and promote the highest level of function
   C. Each person with a private room that locks
   D. A private apartment with cooking facilities

8. A staff member in an assisted living facility would be expected to have training in all of these areas *except*
   A. Assisting with medications
   B. Early signs of illness and the need for health care
   C. Food preparation, service, and storage
   D. Measuring and giving medications

9. Which of the following is *not* required of a resident in assisted living?
   A. The person must be able to leave the building in an emergency.
   B. The person must have stable health.
   C. The person may need some help with ADL.
   D. The person must not be paralyzed or be chronically ill.

10. A service plan for a person in assisted living
    A. Is reviewed every 90 days
    B. Lists the services that the person needs and who provides them
    C. States the medications that the person takes each day
    D. Is reviewed and revised only when needs change

11. Meals in an assisted living facility
    A. Are served in the person's room
    B. Include the noon meal only
    C. Are posted in a weekly menu
    D. Cannot meet special dietary needs

12. When you assist with housekeeping, you will be expected to
    A. Clean the tub or shower after each use.
    B. Put out clean towels and washcloths every week.
    C. Use a disinfectant or water and detergent to clean bathroom surfaces once a week.
    D. Dust furniture every day.

13. A measure that you should follow when handling, preparing, or storing foods is
    A. Use leftover food within 4 or 5 days.
    B. Wash all pots and pans in a dishwasher.
    C. Date and refrigerate containers of leftovers, and refrigerate as soon as possible.
    D. Clean kitchen appliances, counters, tables, and other surfaces once a day.

14. When assisting with laundry, a guideline to follow is
    A. Sort items according to the amount of soil on the items.
    B. Wear gloves when handling soiled laundry.
    C. Use hot water to wash all items.
    D. Use the highest setting on the dryer to sanitize the items.

15. When you assist a person with medication, it may involve
    A. Opening containers for the person who cannot do so
    B. Measuring the medications for the person
    C. Explaining to a person the action of the medication
    D. Preparing a pill organizer for the person each week

16. If a drug error occurs, you should
    A. Tell the person not to do it again.
    B. Make sure the person takes the correct medication at the next scheduled time.
    C. Report the error to the RN.
    D. Take all medications away from the person immediately.

17. An attendant is needed in an assisted living unit 24 hours a day to
    A. Give care to persons who need it.
    B. Make sure medications are dispensed when ordered.
    C. Assist persons who need assistance if an emergency occurs.
    D. Provide activities for the residents.

18. A resident can be transferred, discharge, or evicted from the facility if
    A. The facility closes.
    B. The person is a threat to the health and safety of self or others.
    C. The person fails to pay for services as agreed on.
    D. All of the above are true.

19. Which of the following is *not* a right of a resident in assisted living?
    A. The right to confidentiality of the medical record
    B. The right to have overnight guests whenever the resident wishes
    C. The right to refuse to work for the facility
    D. The right to request to relocate or refuse to relocate within the facility

Fill in the Blanks

20. When working in an assisted living setting, you

    should follow _____

    _____ when

    contact with blood, body fluids, secretions, excre-

    tions, or potentially contaminated items is likely.

21. According to the American Association of Retired
    Persons (AARP), most persons in assisted living
    settings need help with

    A. _____

    B. _____

    C. _____

    D. _____

    E. _____

    Almost one half of these persons are

    _____.

22. What are the requirements and features of a bath-
    room in an assisted living unit?

    A. _____

    B. _____

    C. _____

    D. _____

    E. _____

    F. _____

23. If you are assigned to work on an Alzheimer's unit,

    you know the staff must have training about

    _____.

    Many states require

    _____.

24. The assisted living facility cannot employ a person

    with a _____

    _____.

25. The service plan relates to these services that the
    person needs:

    A. _____

    B. _____

    C. _____

    D. _____

    E. _____

    F. _____

    G. _____

26. A 24-hour emergency communication system is

    provided so the person can communicate

    _____.

27. The time between the evening meal and breakfast

    is usually no more than

    _____.

    It can be longer if

    _____.

28. When you wash eating and cooking items by hand,
    what is the order in which they are washed?

    _____

    _____

    These items are placed in a drainer to dry because

    _____

    _____.

29. If you are assisting the person with taking medications, you should know the five rights of drug administration, which are

    A. _____

    B. _____

    C. _____

    D. _____

    E. _____

30. If a person is taking his or her drugs and states that a pill looks different, what should you do?

    _____

    _____

31. If a person needs a medication reminder, it means

    reminding _____ ,

    observing _____ ,

    and charting _____ .

32. If you are assisting in drug administration, you should report any drug error to the RN. Errors would include:

    A. _____

    B. _____

    C. _____

    D. _____

    E. _____

    F. _____

Optional Learning Exercises

You are working in an assisting living facility. What would you do in these situations?

33. You are providing housekeeping assistance to Mrs. Miller who lives alone. The stove is on, and a pan has burning food in it. Mrs. Miller tells you she did not put the pan on the stove. What should you do?

    _____

    _____

    What is a likely reason for her behavior?

    _____

    _____

34. A resident in the facility has lived there for 2 years and has needed little assistance. He recently had a stroke and now needs care for all of his ADL. Why is he being moved to a nursing facility?

    _____

    _____

35. Mrs. Jenkins tells you that she is expecting an important telephone call and wants to eat her lunch in her room. What should you do?

    _____

    _____

36. Mr. Shante asks you to get his medicines ready for him to take. What assistance are you allowed to give when the nurse has trained you?

    A. _____

    B. _____

    C. _____

    D. _____

    E. _____

    F. _____

    G. _____

    H. _____

37. When you are assisting Mrs. Clyde with her medicines, you notice two of the labels have an expired date. What should you do?

_____

_____

38. Mrs. Johnson asks you when the next meeting of the quilting group will be? She also asks what days the community crafts fair is planned. Where would you direct her to find this information?

_____

_____

Independent Learning Activities

1. Find out if your community has any assisted living facilities. These units may be part of another facility or may be an independent facility. Visit the facility to answer these questions.
   - What services are offered in the facility? Who provides the services? Nursing assistants? Other assistants? What training is required?
   - What kinds of living quarters are provided? What belongings can the person bring from home?
   - What activities are scheduled? How are residents given information about these activities?
   - How do the residents act? Happy? Withdrawn? Sad? How do the staff members act?

2. Find out laws in your state that apply to assisted living facilities. Answer these questions about the laws.
   - What type of license is required for an assisted living facility? Do the laws apply to independent facilities, as well as those attached to other facilities?
   - What laws apply to staff training for these facilities? Does the state require workers to be nursing assistants with special training?
   - What does the state law state about assisting with medications? What nonlicensed persons can assist with medications? What training is required?

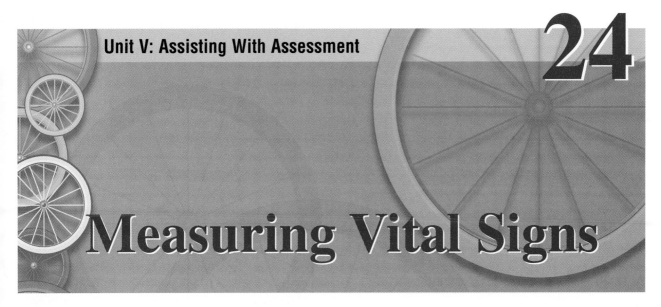

Unit V: Assisting With Assessment

24

Measuring Vital Signs

Apical-radial pulse	Hypertension	Sphygmomanometer
Blood pressure	Hypotension	Stethoscope
Body temperature	Pulse	Systole
Bradycardia	Pulse deficit	Systolic pressure
Diastole	Pulse rate	Tachycardia
Diastolic pressure	Respiration	Vital signs

Fill in the Blanks: Key Terms

Select your answers from the Key Terms listed above.

1. A rapid heart rate is

   _____.

   The heart rate is over 100 beats per minute.

2. The _____

   is taking the apical and radial pulse at the same

   time.

3. An instrument used to listen to the sounds that the

   heart, lungs, and other body organs produce is a

   _____.

4. When the systolic blood pressure is below 90 mm Hg

   and the diastolic pressure is below 60 mm Hg it is

   called _____.

5. The _____

   is the number of heartbeats or pulses felt in

   1 minute.

6. The amount of heat in the body that is a balance be-

   tween the amount of heat produced and amount lost

   by the body is the

   _____.

7. _____

   is the period of heart muscle contraction.

8. _____ is the persistent blood pressure measurements above the normal systolic (140 mm Hg) or diastolic (90 mm Hg) pressures.

9. A cuff measuring device used to measure blood pressure is a _____.

10. The beat of the heart felt at an artery as a wave of blood passes through the artery is the _____.

11. Temperature, pulse, respirations, and blood pressure are _____.

12. _____ is a slow heart rate; the rate is less than 60 beats per minute.

13. The amount of force required to pump blood out of the heart into the arterial circulation is the _____.

14. The period of heart muscle relaxation is _____.

15. The difference between the apical and radial pulse rate is the _____.

16. _____ is the amount of force exerted against the walls of an artery by the blood.

17. The act of breathing air into and out of the lungs is _____.

18. _____ is the pressure in the arteries when the heart is at rest.

Circle the BEST Answer

19. Residents usually have vital signs measured
    A. Once a shift
    B. Every 4 hours
    C. Once a month
    D. Daily or weekly

20. Unless otherwise ordered, take vital signs when the person
    A. Is lying or sitting
    B. Has been walking or exercising
    C. Has just finished eating
    D. Is getting ready to take a shower or tub bath

21. Body temperature is lower in the
    A. Afternoon
    B. Morning
    C. Evening
    D. Night

22. If you take a rectal temperature, the normal range of the temperature would be
    A. 96.6° to 98.6° F (35.9° to 37.0° C)
    B. 97.6° to 99.6° F (36.5° to 37.5° C)
    C. 98.6° to 100.6° F (37.0° to 38.1° C)
    D. 98.6° F (37° C)

23. If you are taking the temperature of an older person, you would expect the temperature to be
    A. At the lower end of the normal range
    B. At the upper end of the normal range
    C. About in the middle of the normal range
    D. The same as that of a younger adult

24. A glass rectal thermometer has
    A. A stubby tip color coded in red
    B. A long or slender tip
    C. A pear-shaped tip
    D. All of the above

25. To read a glass thermometer, you should hold it at the
    A. Stem above eye level and look up to read it
    B. Bulb end and bring it to eye level
    C. Stem and bring it to eye level to read it
    D. Bulb at waist level and look down to read it

26. An oral temperature may be taken with a glass thermometer for a person who
    A. Is receiving oxygen
    B. Has a history of convulsive disorders
    C. Breathes through the mouth
    D. Is alert and needs a routine temperature taken

27. If you are preparing to take an oral temperature, ask the person not to
    A. Eat, drink, or smoke for at least 15 to 20 minutes.
    B. Shower or bathe right before the temperature is taken.
    C. Exercise for 30 minutes before.
    D. Eat, drink, or smoke for at least 5 to 10 minutes.

28. A glass thermometer is inserted into the rectum
    A. 1 inch
    B. 2 inches
    C. $\frac{1}{2}$ inch
    D. 3 inches

29. When recording an axillary temperature of 97.6° F, it is written
    A. 97.6°
    B. 97.6° R
    C. 97.6° A
    D. 97.6° axillary

30. When using an electronic thermometer, you can prevent the spread of infection by
    A. Discarding the thermometer after each use
    B. Discarding the probe cover after each use
    C. Keeping a thermometer for each person at the bedside
    D. Sterilizing the thermometer after each use

31. Which pulse is most commonly used?
    A. Carotid
    B. Brachial
    C. Radial
    D. Popliteal

32. Which pulse is taken during cardiopulmonary resuscitation (CPR)?
    A. Carotid
    B. Temporal
    C. Femoral
    D. Radial

33. When using a stethoscope, you can help prevent infection by
    A. Warming the diaphragm in your hand
    B. Wiping the earpieces and diaphragm with alcohol before and after use
    C. Placing the diaphragm over the artery
    D. Placing the earpieces in your ears so the bend of the tips point forward

34. The pulse rate is the number of heartbeats or pulses felt in
    A. 30 seconds
    B. 15 seconds
    C. 1 minute
    D. 5 minutes

35. Which of the following pulse information cannot be determined with electronic blood pressure equipment?
    A. Rhythm and force
    B. Rate
    C. Tachycardia
    D. Bradycardia

36. When taking the radial pulse, place
    A. The thumb over the pulse site
    B. Two or three fingers on the middle of the wrist
    C. Two or three fingers on the thumb side of the wrist
    D. All of the above

37. The apical pulse is counted for 1 minute if
    A. It is irregular.
    B. It is required by the center policy.
    C. It is directed by the nurse.
    D. All of the above are true.

38. An apical pulse of 72 is recorded as
    A. Pulse 72
    B. 72—Apical pulse
    C. 72Ap
    D. P 72

39. An apical-radial pulse is taken by
    A. Taking the radial pulse for 1 minute and then taking the apical pulse for 1 minute
    B. Subtracting the apical pulse from the radial pulse
    C. Having two staff members take the pulses at the same time
    D. Having two persons take the apical pulse at the same time

40. When counting respirations, the best way is to
    A. Stand quietly next to the person and watch the chest rise and fall.
    B. Keep your fingers or stethoscope over the pulse site so the person thinks you are still counting the pulse.
    C. Tell the person to breathe normally so you can count the respirations.
    D. Use the stethoscope to hear the respirations clearly and count for 1 full minute.

41. The blood pressure may be higher in older persons because
    A. They have orthostatic hypotension.
    B. The diet is higher in sodium.
    C. Arteries narrow and are less elastic.
    D. They are usually overweight.

42. The blood pressure should not be taken on an arm
    A. If the person has had breast surgery on that side
    B. With a cast
    C. That has a dialysis access site
    D. All of the above

43. You will find out the size of blood pressure cuff needed
    A. In the care plan
    B. By measuring the person's arm
    C. In the physician's orders
    D. By asking the person

44. When taking the blood pressure, you place the stethoscope diaphragm
    A. Over the radial artery on the thumb side of the wrist
    B. Over the brachial artery at the inner aspect of the elbow
    C. Lightly against the skin
    D. Over the apical pulse site

45. When getting ready to take the blood pressure, position the person's arm
    A. Above the level of the heart
    B. Level with the heart
    C. Below the level of the heart
    D. Abducted from the body

46. The blood pressure is inflated _____ beyond the point at which you last felt the radial pulse.
    A. 10 mm Hg
    B. 20 mm Hg
    C. 30 mm Hg
    D. 40 mm Hg

Fill in the Blanks

47. Vital signs are taken when drugs are taken that

    affect _____.

48. When vital signs are taken, immediately report to the nurse if:

    A. _____

    B. _____

    C. _____

49. Sites for measuring temperature are:

    A. _____

    B. _____

    C. _____

    D. _____

50. Which site has the highest baseline temperature?

    _____

51. Which site has the lowest baseline temperature?

    _____

52. If a mercury-glass thermometer breaks,

    _____

    immediately because mercury

    _____.

53. When you read a Fahrenheit thermometer, the short

    lines mean _____.

54. List how long the glass thermometer remains in place for these sites:

    A. Oral: _____

       or as required by center policy

    B. Rectal: _____

       or as required by center policy

    C. Axillary: _____

       or as required by center policy

55. When taking an oral temperature, place the bulb end of the thermometer

_____.

56. When taking an axillary temperature, the axilla

must be _____.

57. A tympanic membrane thermometer is useful for confused persons because the temperature is measured in _____.

58. When using an electronic thermometer, what does the color of the probe mean?

A. Blue: _____

B. Red: _____

59. When you take a rectal temperature,

_____ the tip

of the thermometer, or the end of the covered probe.

60. When taking a tympanic membrane temperature,

pull back on the ear to

_____.

61. The adult pulse rate is between

_____

per minute.

62. List words used to describe the following:

A. Forceful pulse: _____

B. Hard-to-feel pulse: _____

63. If a pulse is irregular, count the pulse for

_____.

64. When you take a pulse, what observations should be reported and recorded?

A. _____

B. _____

C. _____

D. _____

65. Do not use your thumb to take a pulse because

_____

_____.

66. When taking an apical pulse each *lub-dub* sound is

counted as _____.

67. The apical pulse rate is never less than the

_____.

68. A healthy adult has _____ respirations per

minute.

69. What observations should be reported and recorded when counting respirations?

A. _____

B. _____

C. _____

D. _____

E. _____

F. _____

70. One respiration is counted for each

_____.

71. Respirations are counted for

_____

if they are abnormal or irregular.

72. Blood pressure is controlled by:

    A. _____

    B. _____

    C. _____

73. Normal ranges for blood pressures are as follows.

    A. Systolic: _____

    B. Diastolic: _____

74. If a person has been exercising, let the person rest

    for _____

    before taking the blood pressure.

75. In what position is the person placed to take the

    blood pressure?

    _____.

    Sometimes the physician orders blood pressure in the

    _____

    position.

76. When listening to the blood pressure, the first sound

    you hear is the

    _____

    pressure, and the point where the sound disappears

    is the _____

    pressure.

Labeling

77. Name the types of thermometers.

    A. _____

    B. _____

    C. _____

    D. Which thermometers are used for oral or axillary
       temperatures?

       _____

       _____

    E. A rectal temperature is taken with the

       _____

       thermometer.

78. Name the pulse sites.

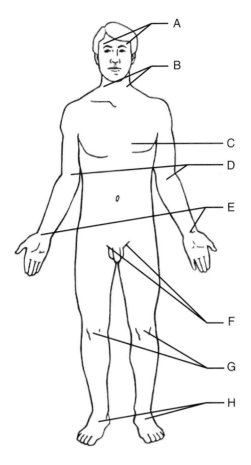

A. _____

B. _____

C. _____

D. _____

E. _____

F. _____

G. _____

H. _____

I. Which pulse is used during CPR?

_____

J. Which pulse is most commonly taken?

_____

K. Which pulse is used when taking the blood pressure?

_____

L. Which pulse is found with a stethoscope?

_____

79. Fill in the drawings below so that the thermometers read correctly.

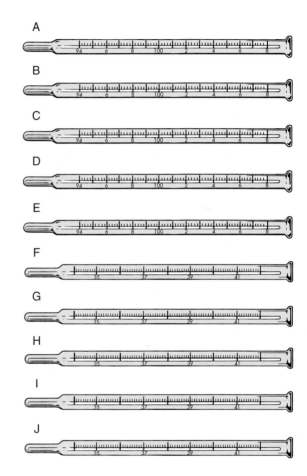

A. 95.8° F
B. 98.4° F
C. 100.2° F
D. 101° F
E. 102.6° F
F. 35.5° C
G. 36.5° C
H. 37° C
I. 38.5° C
J. 39.5° C

80. Fill in the drawings below so that the dials show the correct blood pressures.

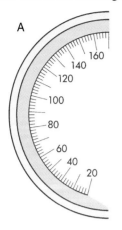 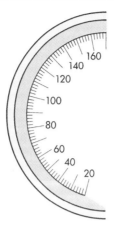 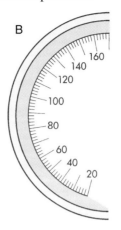 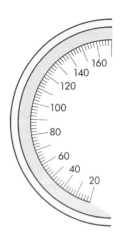

A

B

A. 168/102

B. 104/68

81. Fill in the drawings below so that the mercury columns show the correct blood pressures.

A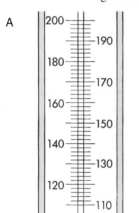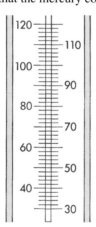

B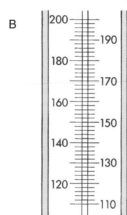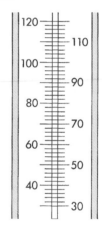

A. 152/86

B. 198/110

82. Record the temperatures shown.

A

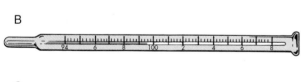

B

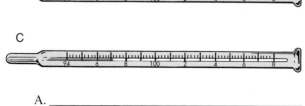

C

A. _____

B. _____

C. _____

Nursing Assistant Skills Video Exercise

View the parts of the Measurements *video that apply to this chapter to answer these questions.*

83. What information is needed before taking vital signs?

A. _____

B. _____

C. _____

D. _____

84. What procedure guidelines are important when taking vital signs?

    A. Temperature: _____

    B. Pulse: _____

    C. Respiration: _____

    D. Blood pressure: _____

85. Insert the rectal glass thermometer

    _____.

    If you meet resistance,

    _____.

86. When taking respirations in addition to counting, observe for

    A. _____

    B. _____

    C. _____

87. If you use the one-step method to take the blood pressure, what do you do after inflating the blood pressure cuff until the pulse disappears?

    _____

    _____

Optional Learning Exercises

Taking Temperatures

88. You prepare to take Mr. Harrison's temperature with a glass thermometer. When you take the thermometer from the container, it reads 97.8° F. What should you do?

    _____

89. If the thermometer registers between two short lines, record the temperature to the

    _____.

90. How would you record these temperature readings?

    A. An oral temperature of 97.4° F:

    _____

    36.5° C: _____

    B. A rectal temperature of 99.8° F:

    _____

    38.1° C: _____

    C. An axillary temperature of 96.2° F:

    _____

    36.1° C: _____

Taking Pulses and Respirations

91. You are assigned to take Mrs. Sanchez' pulse and respirations. You note that the pulse rate and respirations are regular, so you take each one

    for _____.

    When you complete counting the pulse, you keep

    your _____

    and count _____.

    This procedure is done so that Mrs. Sanchez will

    _____.

92. When you finish counting Mrs. Sanchez' pulse and respirations, your numbers are pulse 36 and respirations 9. What numbers should be recorded?

    Pulse: _____

    Respirations: _____

    Why? _____

    _____

93. The nurse tells you to take an apical-radial pulse on Mrs. Hellman. Why do you ask a co-worker to help you?

    _____

94. How long is an apical-radial pulse counted?

    _____

    After you have taken the apical-radial pulse, how do you find the pulse deficit?

    _____

Taking Blood Pressures

95. You are assigned to take Mr. Hardaway's blood pressure. You know that he goes for dialysis three times a week. What do you need to know before you take his blood pressure?

    _____

    Why? _____

96. When you inflate the cuff, you cannot feel the pulse after you pump the cuff to 130 mm Hg. How high will you inflate the cuff to take his blood pressure?

    _____

    _____

97. You should deflate the cuff at an even rate of

    _____

    per seconds.

Independent Learning Activities

1. Take turns measuring vital signs on three or four classmates. If possible, use glass, electronic, and tympanic thermometers for each person to see if they give similar results. Use this table to record the results.

Person	Temperature	Pulse	Respiration	Blood Pressure
#1	Glass Electronic Tympanic	Radial Apical	Rate Rhythm Depth	
#2	Glass Electronic Tympanic	Radial Apical	Rate Rhythm Depth	
#3	Glass Electronic Tympanic	Radial Apical	Rate Rhythm Depth	
#4	Glass Electronic Tympanic	Radial Apical	Rate Rhythm Depth	

2. Answer these questions about this exercise.
   - If you used different thermometers, how did the results compare?
   - What differences did you find in finding the radial pulses among your classmates?
   - What differences did you find in the rates and rhythms?
   - How were you able to measure respirations so that the person did not know you were watching?
   - What differences in rhythm and depth of respirations did you find among your classmates?
   - What differences did you find in locating the brachial artery in different people?
   - How did the sounds of the blood pressure differ among your classmates?
   - What difficulties did you have with any of the measurements taken?
   - What will you change about measuring vital signs on a resident after this practice?

3. Practice taking an apical-radial pulse with classmates. Take turns acting as the staff members and the person having the pulses taken. Answer these questions after the exercise has been completed.
   - How was privacy maintained for the person having the pulse measured?
   - How did the "staff members" decide who would begin and end the count?
   - What problems did you have in counting for a minute?
   - How did the apical and radial counts compare?
   - What will you change about measuring the apical-radial pulses on a resident after this experience?

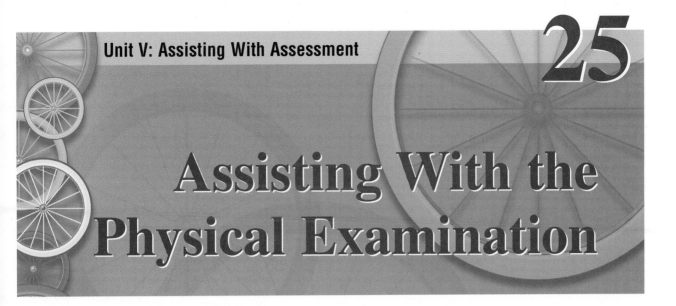

Assisting With the Physical Examination

Dorsal recumbent position	Lithotomy position	Percussion hammer
Horizontal recumbent position	Nasal speculum	Tuning fork
Knee-chest position	Ophthalmoscope	Vaginal speculum
Laryngeal mirror	Otoscope	

Fill in the Blanks: Key Terms

Select your answers from the Key Terms listed above.

1. An instrument used to test hearing is a

   _____.

2. When a person is in the

   _____,

   the hips are brought to the edge of the examination

   table, the knees are flexed, the hips are externally

   rotated, and the feet are supported in stirrups.

3. The supine position in which the legs are together is

   called the

   _____.

4. An _____

   is a lighted instrument used to examine the external

   ear and the eardrum (tympanic membrane).

5. A _____ is an

   instrument used to open the vagina so it and the

   cervix can be examined.

6. When a person kneels and rests the body on the

   knees and chest and the head is turned to one side,

   the arms are above the head or flexed at the elbows,

   the back is straight, and the body is flexed about

   90 degrees at the hip, the person is in the

   _____.

7. A _____ is an instrument used to tap body parts to test reflexes.

8. An instrument used to examine the mouth, teeth, and throat is called a

   _____.

9. An instrument used to examine the inside of the nose is a _____.

10. The dorsal recumbent position is also called the

    _____.

11. An _____ is a lighted instrument used to examine the internal structures of the eye.

Circle the BEST Answer

12. In nursing centers, residents have a physical examination
    A. Only when the person is admitted
    B. Once a month
    C. At least once a year
    D. Only when the person is ill

13. If a resident is having a physical examination, you may be asked to do all of the following *except*
    A. Measure vital signs, height, and weight.
    B. Assist the physician or nurse with an examination.
    C. Explain why the examination is being done and what to expect.
    D. Position and drape the person.

14. When the physician is examining the person's mouth, teeth, and throat, you may be asked to hand him or her the
    A. Ophthalmoscope
    B. Percussion hammer
    C. Tuning fork
    D. Laryngeal mirror

15. Which of the following would *not* protect the right to personal choice for a person having a physical examination?
    A. Having the person urinate before the examination begins
    B. Telling the person who will do the examination and when it will be done
    C. Explaining the procedure
    D. Allowing a family member to be present if the person requests

16. The right to privacy is protected by
    A. Removing all clothes for a complete examination
    B. Explaining the reasons for the examination
    C. Exposing only the body part being examined
    D. Explaining the examination results with a family member present

17. It is important to have a person empty the bladder before an examination because
    A. An empty bladder allows the examiner to feel the abdominal organs.
    B. A full bladder can change the normal position and shape of organs.
    C. A full bladder can cause discomfort when the abdominal organs are felt.
    D. All of the above are true.

18. Which of these steps would *not* be important in providing safety during an examination?
    A. Expose only the body part being examined.
    B. Have an extra bath blanket nearby.
    C. Prevent drafts to protect the person from chilling.
    D. Do not leave the person unattended.

19. After you have taken the person to the examination room and have placed the person in position, you should
   A. Put the signal light on for the nurse or examiner.
   B. Leave the room.
   C. Go to the nurse or examiner to report that the person is ready.
   D. Open the door so the nurse or examiner knows you are ready.

20. When the abdomen, chest, and breasts are to be examined, you will place the person in the
   A. Lithotomy position
   B. Sims' position
   C. Dorsal recumbent (horizontal recumbent) position
   D. Knee-chest position

21. If a person is asked to stand on the floor during an examination, you should
   A. Assist the person with putting on shoes or slippers.
   B. Place paper or paper towels on the floor.
   C. Place a sheet on the floor.
   D. Wipe the floor carefully with an antiseptic cleaner before the person stands on it.

Fill in the Blanks

22. List the equipment you need to collect when the ears are being examined.

   A. _____

   B. _____

23. What equipment is needed to examine the eyes?

   A. _____

   B. _____

24. When the nose, mouth, and throat are being examined, you should collect:

   A. _____

   B. _____

   C. _____

   D. _____

25. What are common fears the person may have when a physical examination is done?

   A. _____

   B. _____

26. To maintain the person's right to privacy, who are the only persons who have a right to see the person's body during the examination?

   _____

   _____

27. Who are the only people who need to know the reason for the examination and its results?

   _____

   _____

Labeling

Answer Questions 28 through 32 using the following illustration.

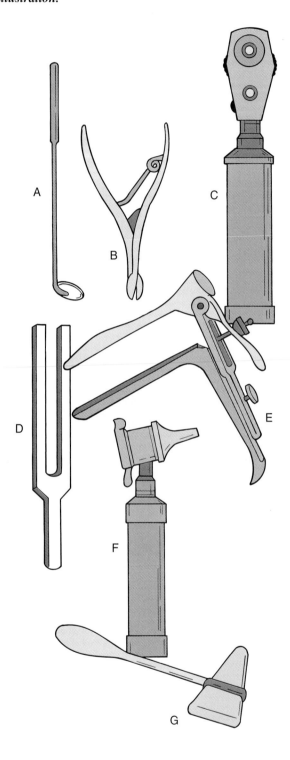

28. Name each of the examination instruments.

    A. _____

    B. _____

    C. _____

    D. _____

    E. _____

    F. _____

    G. _____

29. Which instrument is used to examine the nose?

    _____

30. When the eye is examined, the examiner uses the

    _____.

31. If a person has a sore throat, the examiner will look

    at the throat with the

    _____.

32. The reflexes are examined by using the

    _____.

Answer Questions 33 through 36 using the following illustration.

33. Name each position.

   A. _____

   B. _____

   C. _____

   D. _____

A

34. Which positions may be used when a rectal exami-
    nation is done?

   A. _____

   B. _____

B

35. When the abdomen, chest, and breasts are exam-

    ined, the person is placed in

    _____.

36. The _____ is used

    for a vaginal examination.

C

D

Optional Learning Exercises

37. When you are delegated the job of preparing a person for an exam, why do you need the following information?

    A. What time is the examination?

    _____

    _____

    B. What are two reasons it would be helpful to know which examinations will be done?

    _____

    _____

    C. What equipment will you need if you are assigned to take vital signs?

    _____

    _____

38. You are a female nursing assistant who is assisting a male examiner with an examination of a female resident. The nurse tells you to stay in the examination room during the entire procedure. Why is this important to the examiner and to the woman?

    _____

    _____

Independent Learning Activities

1. You probably have had a physical examination at some time. Perhaps you needed one to be a student in this class. Answer these questions about your experience when you had the physical done to you.
   - Who explained what to expect during the examination? What were you told about any discomfort?
   - What steps were taken to give you privacy? While you changed clothes? During the examination?
   - Who was present during the examination? Were you given a choice of having another person in the room with you and the examiner? How did you feel about having (or not having) another person in the room?
   - How did you know what was being done? How much information were you given about procedures? Positions? Tests?
   - What positions were used during the examination? Which positions shown in this chapter were used? How comfortable did you feel? How did the examiner and assistant help make you more comfortable with the positions?
   - What questions did you have during the examination? Who was able to answer these questions? How well were the questions answered to make you understand what was being done?
   - How comfortable did you feel about the examination? What might have been done to make you more comfortable physically and psychologically?
   - How did this experience help you understand the feelings of persons you may assist during an examination?

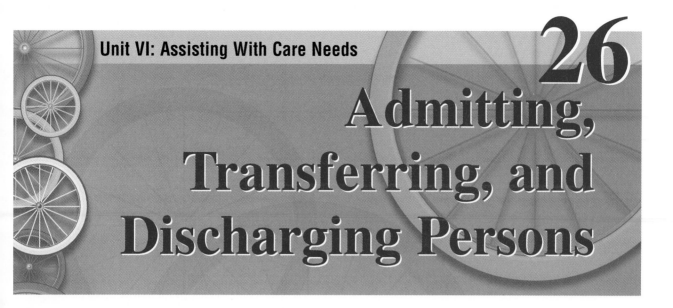

26

Admitting, Transferring, and Discharging Persons

Admission
Discharge
Transfer

Fill in the Blanks: Key Terms

Select your answers from the Key Terms listed above.

1. _____ is

   moving a person from one room or nursing unit to

   another.

2. The official entry of a person into a nursing center is

   _____.

3. _____ occurs with

   the official departure of a person from a nursing

   center or nursing unit.

Circle the BEST Answer

4. Usually, _____ is a happy time.
   A. Admission
   B. Discharge
   C. Transfer
   D. Home care

5. What staff member starts the admissions process?
   A. The physician
   B. The nurse
   C. The admissions coordinator
   D. The activities director

6. When a person with dementia is admitted to a nursing center, the person
   A. Is usually depressed
   B. May have an increase in confusion
   C. May have a decrease in confusion
   D. Usually feels safer in the new setting

7. Persons who are admitted to rehabilitation and sub-acute care units are
   A. Always admitted by the RN
   B. Usually admitted by the nursing assistant
   C. May be admitted by the nursing assistant if the person's condition is stable and the person has no discomfort or distress
   D. Never admitted by the nursing assistant

8. If a person being admitted is arriving by stretcher, you should
   A. Raise the bed to its highest level.
   B. Leave the bed closed.
   C. Raise the head of the bed to Fowler's position.
   D. Lower the bed to its lowest level.

9. During admission, you can help the person feel more comfortable by
   A. Offering the person and the family beverages to drink
   B. Write down names of roommates and other nearby residents
   C. Assist the person with hanging pictures or displaying photos
   D. All of the above

10. When weighing a resident, have the person
    A. Wear socks and shoes and bathrobe.
    B. Remove regular clothes and wear a gown or pajamas.
    C. Wear regular street clothes.
    D. Remove clothing after weighing and then weigh the clothes.

11. A chair scale is used when
    A. A person can transfer from a wheelchair to the chair scale.
    B. A person cannot stand and needs to be lifted into the chair.
    C. A person can stand and walk independently.
    D. A person is in the supine position.

12. When a person cannot stand on the scale to have the height measured,
    A. Ask the person or the family the height of the person.
    B. Have the person sit in a chair and use a tape measure from head to toe to measure the person.
    C. Position the person in supine position and measure with a tape measure.
    D. Estimate the height of the person by observing him or her.

13. When a person is being transferred, who is notified?
    A. Physician
    B. Social worker
    C. Family and business office
    D. Person's roommate

14. When you are transferring a person, you should do all of the following *except*
    A. Identify the person by checking the identification bracelet with the transfer slip.
    B. Explain the reasons for the transfer.
    C. Collect the person's personal belongings and bedside equipment.
    D. Introduce the person to the receiving nurse.

15. If a person wishes to leave the center without the physician's permission, you should
    A. Tell the person that this is not allowed.
    B. Prevent the person from leaving.
    C. Tell the nurse immediately.
    D. Try to convince the person to stay.

16. When you are assisting a person who is being discharged, you should
    A. Check all drawers and closet.
    B. Check off the clothing list.
    C. Help the person dress as needed.
    D. All of the above are true.

Fill in the Blanks

17. OBRA has standards for transfers and discharges. List the ways that these standards affect the person's rights.

    A. Documentation gives reasons for

    _____

    _____

    to protect the person's rights.

    B. The person and family are told of

    _____.

    C. A procedure is followed if the person

    _____.

    D. An _____ often

    works with the person and family to ensure that

    the _____.

18. When you are delegated to assist with admissions, transfers, or discharges, what information should you have from the nurse?

    A. _____

    B. _____

    C. _____

    D. _____

    E. _____

19. When a person is being admitted, what identifying information is obtained?

    A. _____

    B. _____

    C. _____

    D. _____

    E. _____

    F. _____

20. Why is it important to have a person urinate before being weighed?

    _____

    _____

21. What is done to the balance scale before having the person step on?

    A. _____

    B. _____

    C. _____

22. When using a lift scale, the person should be raised

    about _____ off

    the bed.

23. When measuring a person in the supine position, the

    ruler is placed _____

    _____.

24. If you transfer a person to a new unit, you can help

    the person by introducing the person to

    _____.

25. When a person on a rehabilitation or subacute care unit is discharged, what staff members are involved in discharge teaching?

    A. _____

    B. _____

    C. _____

    D. _____

    E. _____

    F. _____

    G. _____

26. When you assist with discharging a person, you should report and record:

    A. _____

    B. _____

    C. _____

    D. _____

    E. _____

27. To help the person and family cope with admission, transfer, and discharge, you should:

    A. Be _____.

    B. Be _____.

    C. Handle _____.

    D. Treat _____.

Nursing Assistant Skills Video Exercise

View the portions of the **Measurements** *video that apply to this chapter and answer these questions.*

28. Before weighing a person, you should empty any

_____

_____.

29. You can provide balance for the person who is

standing on a scale by keeping your

_____

_____.

Optional Learning Exercises

Answer the questions about the following person and situation.

Rosa Romirez, age 65, had a stroke (cerebrovascular accident [CVA]) last week and is being admitted to a rehabilitation unit in the nursing care center in which you work.

30. Because you know Mrs. Romirez is arriving by

wheelchair, you leave the bed

_____

and _____ the level.

31. The nurse instructs you to collect the needed equipment to admit a new person. You collect:

A. _____

B. _____

C. _____

D. _____

E. _____

F. _____

G. _____

32. When Mrs. Romirez arrives with her husband, it may help them feel more comfortable if you offer them _____.

33. You greet Mrs. Romirez by name and ask her if a

certain _____

_____.

34. You orient Mrs. Romirez to the room and equipment and also explain

_____

and the location of

_____.

35. Mrs. Romirez has some weakness on her left side but can safely transfer from the wheelchair to chairs or the bed. The nurse tells you to weigh Mrs. Romirez with the

_____ scale.

When you arrive at work one day, you are told that Mrs. Romirez is being transferred to another unit, and you are asked to assist. Answer these questions about transferring her.

36. When you transport Mrs. Romirez in a wheelchair,

she is covered with a

_____.

37. What items are taken with Mrs. Romirez to the new unit?

_____

_____

38. What information is recorded and reported about the transfer?

   A. _____

   B. _____

   C. _____

   D. _____

   E. _____

   F. _____

Several weeks later, you are sent to the unit in which Mrs. Romirez is living, and find that she is going home. Answer these questions about her discharge.

39. Mrs. Romirez tells you that the therapists visited her home yesterday to ensure that the home setting is

   _____.

   The home was also assessed for

   _____.

40. Good communication skills should be used when assisting with the discharge. When Mrs. Romirez and her family leave, you should

   _____

   _____.

Independent Learning Activities

1. Have a discussion with three or four classmates to share experiences you have had with admissions to care facilities. You may have had personal experience or you may have observed a friend or family member being admitted. If you have not had this experience, perhaps you can relate the feelings you have had when visiting a physician's office. Use these questions during the discussion.
   • Who was the first person you met when you arrived to be admitted? How were you greeted? Did you feel welcome?
   • How did you arrive at your room? Were you escorted or did you have to find your way?
   • How long did you wait in the room before a staff member came to admit you? How did this affect your feelings about the place?
   • How were you addressed? First name? Last name? Did anyone ask you what you preferred?
   • What information were you given to make you feel more comfortable? What printed information was provided?
   • Overall, how did the admission procedure affect your feelings about the facility? Negative? Positive?
   • How will your personal experience and the experiences of others in this group affect your approach to new persons in a care facility?

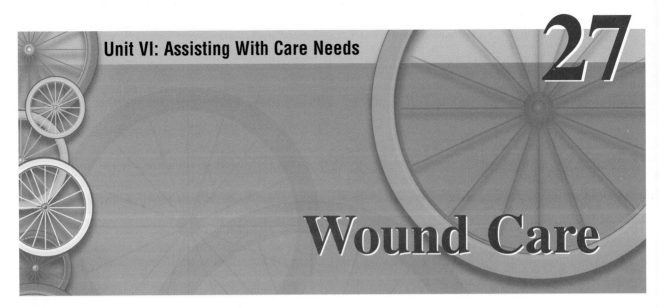

Wound Care

Abrasion	Embolus	Puncture wound
Arterial ulcer	Evisceration	Purulent drainage
Bedsore	Full-thickness wound	Sanguineous drainage
Chronic wound	Gangrene	Serosanguineous drainage
Circulatory ulcer	Incision	Serous drainage
Clean wound	Infected wound	Skin tear
Clean-contaminated wound	Intentional wound	Stasis ulcer
Closed wound	Laceration	Thrombus
Contaminated wound	Open wound	Trauma
Contusion	Partial-thickness wound	Unintentional wound
Decubitus ulcer	Penetrating wound	Vascular ulcer
Dehiscence	Phlebitis	Venous ulcer
Dirty wound	Pressure sore	Wound
Edema	Pressure ulcer	

Fill in the Blanks: Key Terms

Select your answers from the Key Terms listed above.

1. A _____ is a break or rip in the epidermis that separates it from the underlying tissue.

2. An open wound with clean, straight edges, usually produced with a sharp instrument, is an

   _____.

3. _____ is another name for a pressure ulcer, pressure sore, or decubitus ulcer.

4. A wound in which tissues are injured but the skin is not broken is a

   _____.

5. _____ is thick green, yellow, or brown drainage.

6. A wound in which the dermis and epidermis of the skin are broken is called a

   _____.

7. A _____ is a break in the skin or mucous membrane.

8. A wound that is not infected and microbes have not entered the wound is a

   _____.

9. An _____ is a partial-thickness wound caused by the scraping away or rubbing of the skin.

10. Another name for a pressure ulcer, pressure sore, or bedsore is a _____.

11. Thin, watery drainage that is blood-tinged is called

    _____.

12. An _____ is a wound containing large amounts of bacteria and that shows signs of infection; it is also called a dirty wound.

13. A vascular wound or a _____ is an open wound on the lower legs and feet caused by decreased blood flow through arteries and veins.

14. Another name for a blood clot is a

    _____.

15. _____ is an inflammation of a vein.

16. A wound with a high risk of infection is a

    _____.

17. A condition in which there is death of tissue is

    _____.

18. Any injury caused by unrelieved pressure is a

    _____,

    or a decubitus ulcer, bedsore, or pressure sore.

19. A _____ is an open wound with torn tissues and jagged edges.

20. A wound resulting from trauma is an

    _____.

21. An _____ is an open wound on the lower legs and feet caused by decreased blood flow through the arteries.

22. Clear, watery fluid is

    _____.

23. A blood clot that travels through the vascular system until it lodges in a distant vessel is called an

    _____.

24. A _____ is also called a bedsore, decubitus ulcer, or a pressure ulcer.

25. An infected wound is a

    _____.

26. A wound occurring from the surgical entry of the urinary, reproductive, respiratory, or gastrointestinal system is a

    _____.

27. A _____ is a

    wound that does not heal easily.

28. A stasis ulcer is also called a

    _____.

29. An open wound made by a sharp object is a

    _____.

    The entry of the skin and underlying tissues may be

    intentional or unintentional.

30. A wound created for therapy is an

    _____.

31. A _____ is an

    open wound in which the skin and underlying tis-

    sues are pierced.

32. _____ is the

    separation of wound layers.

33. A circulatory ulcer is also called a

    _____.

34. Swelling that is caused by fluid collecting in tissues

    is _____.

35. A _____ occurs

    when the dermis, epidermis, and subcutaneous

    tissue are penetrated. Muscle and bone may be

    involved.

36. An accident or violent act that injures the skin, mu-

    cous membranes, bones, and internal organs is

    called _____.

37. The separation of the wound along with the protru-

    sion of abdominal organs is

    _____.

38. A _____ is an

    open wound on the lower legs and feet caused by

    poor blood return through the veins; it is also called

    a venous ulcer.

39. Bloody drainage is called

    _____.

40. A closed wound caused by a blow to the body is a

    _____.

41. An _____ occurs

    when the skin or mucous membrane is broken.

Circle the BEST Answer

42. The skin
    A. Is the body's first line of defense
    B. Protects the body from microbes
    C. Is easily injured in older and disabled persons
    D. All of the above

43. Mrs. Seymour complains that her elbow hurts from
    pushing herself up in bed. When you inspect her
    elbow, you find some of the skin is rubbed away.
    You would report this wound to the nurse as a
    A. Laceration
    B. Abrasion
    C. Contusion
    D. Incision

44. Mr. Telford catches his arm on a chair. When you
    look at his arm, the tissue is torn with jagged edges.
    You report this injury to the nurse and tell him or
    her that Mr. Telford has a
    A. Puncture wound
    B. Abrasion
    C. Penetrating wound
    D. Laceration

45. Which of the following would *not* place a person at risk for skin tears?
    A. The person is obese.
    B. The person requires complete help in moving.
    C. The person has poor nutrition.
    D. The person has altered mental awareness.

46. Applying lotion will help prevent skin breakdown or skin tears because it may prevent
    A. Loss of fatty layer under the skin
    B. General thinning of the skin
    C. Dryness
    D. Moisture in dark areas of the body

47. A pressure ulcer occurs because
    A. The person is restless and moves around in the bed or chair.
    B. Too much fluid is taken in the diet.
    C. Unrelieved pressure occurs between hard surfaces.
    D. The person is repositioned too frequently.

48. The first sign of a pressure ulcer in an area would be
    A. Pale or reddened skin
    B. Swelling in the area
    C. A break in the skin
    D. Exposed tissue and some drainage from the area

49. Mrs. Greene keeps sliding down in bed. The nurse tells you to raise the head of the bed no more than 30 degrees. This position will help prevent tissue damage caused by
    A. Pressure over hard surfaces
    B. Shearing
    C. Poor body mechanics
    D. Poor fluid balance

50. Pressure ulcers can occur
    A. Over bony areas, such as the hips
    B. Underneath the breasts
    C. Between abdominal folds
    D. All of the above

51. When following a repositioning schedule, the person should be repositioned
    A. According to the schedule in the person's care plan
    B. Every 2 hours
    C. Every 15 minutes
    D. As often as you have time

52. One way to prevent friction in the bed is to
    A. Use soap when cleansing the skin.
    B. Rub or massage reddened areas.
    C. Use pillows and blankets to prevent skin from being in contact with skin.
    D. Use pillows for support.

53. Bed cradles are used to
    A. Position the person in good body alignment.
    B. Keep top linens off the legs and feet.
    C. Keep the heels off the bed.
    D. Distribute body weight evenly.

54. When the person is using an eggcrate-like mattress, it is covered with a special cover and
    A. Only a bottom sheet
    B. A bottom sheet and a waterproof pad
    C. A bottom sheet and a draw sheet
    D. Several layers of waterproof materials, a lift pad, and a bottom sheet

55. Ulcers of the feet and legs are caused by
    A. Poorly fitted shoes
    B. Decreased blood flow through arteries or veins
    C. Increased activity
    D. Increased fluid intake

56. A measure to prevent stasis ulcers involves
    A. Using elastic, or rubber band—type garters, to hold the person's socks in place
    B. Keeping the person's feet flat on the floor while sitting in a chair
    C. Applying elastic stockings or elastic wraps to legs
    D. All of the above

57. All of these measures would be helpful in preventing stasis ulcers *except*
    A. Never rubbing or massaging reddened areas
    B. Repositioning the person at least every 2 hours
    C. Reminding the person to cross the legs when sitting
    D. Making sure the person wears comfortable socks and shoes

58. Elastic stockings
    A. Are removed every 8 hours for 30 minutes
    B. Are applied after the person has been out of bed for 30 minutes or more
    C. Normally cause the person to complain of tingling or numbness in the feet
    D. Are removed only at bedtime or for a bath or shower

59. When applying elastic stockings, all of the following are correct *except*
    A. Position the person in the chair.
    B. Turn the stocking inside out down to the heel.
    C. Grasp the stocking top and slip it over the foot and heel.
    D. Remove twist, creases, or wrinkles.

60. Elastic bandages are
    A. Applied loosely to prevent discomfort
    B. Applied starting at the hip
    C. Used with persons with varicose veins
    D. Used with persons with arterial ulcers

61. When applying elastic bandages, you should
    A. Apply the bandage so that it completely covers the fingers or toes.
    B. Apply the bandage to the smallest part of the wrist, foot, ankle, or knee first.
    C. Secure the bandage at the back of the leg with a safety pin.
    D. Remove the bandage only when it becomes loose or falls off the extremity.

62. When caring for a person who is at risk for arterial ulcers, you should do all of the following *except*
    A. Remind the person to sit with the legs uncrossed.
    B. Assist the person with applying garters to hold up socks or hose.
    C. Make sure the shoes fit well.
    D. Encourage the person to stop smoking.

63. When a person is at risk for arterial ulcers, the nursing assistant should *not*
    A. Apply elastic stockings.
    B. Give any foot care.
    C. Cut the person's toenails.
    D. Use protective devices to keep pressure off heels.

64. During wound healing, what phase is happening when the wound is about 1 year in duration?
    A. Initial phase
    B. Inflammatory phase
    C. Maturation phase
    D. Proliferative phase

65. The nurse tells you to make sure that Mrs. Reynolds supports her abdominal wound when she coughs. The nurse wants this procedure done to protect against
    A. Secondary intention healing
    B. Infection
    C. Scarring
    D. Dehiscence

66. When you are caring for Mrs. Reynolds, you notice thin, watery drainage that is blood-tinged. When you report your observations, you would tell the nurse that the wound has which kind of drainage?
    A. Purulent
    B. Serosanguineous
    C. Serous
    D. Sanguineous

67. Which of these methods used in wound care will prevent microbes from entering a draining wound?
    A. Wet-to-dry dressings
    B. A Hemovac suction device
    C. A Penrose drain
    D. Nonadherent gauze

68. When wet-to-dry dressings are used, they
    A. Are removed when dry
    B. Are kept moist
    C. Allow air to reach the wound but fluids and bacteria cannot
    D. Do not stick to the wound

69. Plastic and paper tape may be used to secure a dressing
    A. Because they allow movement of the body part
    B. When the dressing must be changed frequently
    C. If the person is allergic to adhesive tape
    D. Because they stick well to the skin

70. If you are caring for a person who has Montgomery straps to secure a dressing, you should
    A. Replace the cloth ties when you give care.
    B. Tell the nurse if the adhesive strips are soiled.
    C. Replace the adhesive strips each time you give care.
    D. Retie the cloth ties when you reposition the person.

71. If you are assigned to change a dressing, what information is important to have?
    A. What kind of medication the person receives
    B. The person's diagnosis
    C. When pain medication was given and how long until it takes effect
    D. All of the above

72. You can make the person more comfortable when changing a dressing by doing all of the following *except*
    A. Control your nonverbal communication when looking at the wound.
    B. Avoid body language that indicates the wound is unpleasant.
    C. Encourage the person to look at the wound.
    D. Make sure the person does not see the old dressing when it is removed.

73. When you are assigned to change dressings, you should
    A. Follow Bloodborne Pathogen Standards.
    B. Use sterile technique.
    C. Wear gloves to remove old dressings.
    D. Use one pair of gloves throughout the dressing change.

74. A binder may be used when the person has a dressing to
    A. Prevent infection
    B. Prevent drainage
    C. Reduce or prevent swelling by promoting circulation
    D. Prevent bleeding

75. Which of these measures will *not* be helpful when a person has a wound?
    A. Tell the person that the wound looks fine and he or she should not be upset.
    B. Encourage the person to eat well so that the body can heal better.
    C. Remove any soiled dressings from the room as soon as possible.
    D. Allow pain medications to take effect before giving wound care.

Fill in the Blanks

76. When a wound is created for therapy, it is called an

    _____ wound.

77. A wound caused by a bruise, twist, or sprain is a

    _____ wound.

78. Identify the wounds described here:

    A. Pressure sores and circulatory ulcers are

       _____ wounds

       because they do not heal easily.

    B. When a surgical entry is made into body systems

       that are not sterile and contain normal flora, it

       creates a _____

       wound.

    C. When the dermis and epidermis of the

       skin are broken, it causes a

       _____ wound.

    D. If microbes have not entered a wound, it is a

       _____ wound.

    E. When the wound involves muscle and bone, as

       well as the dermis, epidermis, and subcutaneous

       tissue, it is called a

       _____ wound.

    F. When a wound contains large amounts of bac-

       teria and shows signs of infection, it is a

       _____ or

       _____ wound.

    G. A _____ wound

       has a high risk of infection. These wounds are

       often unintentional or result from breaks in sur-

       gical asepsis.

79. You can cause a skin tear when moving, repositioning, and transferring by holding on to a person's arm or leg _____.

80. List ways to prevent skin tears in the following:

   A. Keep the person hydrated by

   _____

   B. What kind of clothing would be helpful?

   _____

   _____

   C. Nail care of the person

   _____

   _____

   D. Lift and turn the person with a

   _____

   E. Support the arms and legs with

   _____

   F. Pad _____.

   G. Your personal hygiene practices

   _____

   and _____.

81. Friction scrapes the skin, and the scrape is a portal of entry for _____.

82. Name the stage of pressure ulcer described in each of these situations.

   A. The skin is gone, and underlying tissues are exposed.

   _____

   B. The skin is red. The color does not return to normal when the skin is relieved of pressure.

   _____

   C. Muscle and bone are exposed and damaged. Drainage is likely.

   _____

   D. The skin cracks, blisters, or peels.

   _____

83. You can help prevent shearing by raising the head of the bed only

   _____.

84. If a person sitting in a chair is able to move, remind the person to shift position every

   _____

   to decrease pressure on

   _____.

85. Explain how these protective devices help prevent pressure ulcers.

   A. Bed cradle prevents pressure on

   _____.

   B. Elbow protectors prevent

   _____

   between _____.

   C. Heel elevators raise

   _____.

   D. Eggcrate-like mattress distributes

   _____.

E. Special beds allow persons to

_____

on the mattress so the body weight is

_____ .

There is little pressure on

_____ .

86. Walking and exercise are measures to prevent stasis ulcers because they increase

_____ .

87. You are caring for a person with a disease that affects venous circulation. You notice her toenails are long and sharp. You should

_____

_____ .

88. Elastic stockings help prevent the development of thrombi because the elastic

_____

_____ .

89. When you are delegated to apply elastic stockings, what observations should you report and record?

A. _____

B. _____

C. _____

D. _____

E. _____

F. _____

90. When you apply elastic bandages, the fingers or toes are exposed to allow

_____ .

91. After applying elastic bandages, you should check the fingers or toes for

_____ .

You should also ask about

_____ .

If any of these problems occur, you should

_____ .

92. What two diseases are common causes of arterial ulcers?

A. _____

B. _____

93. With primary intention healing, the wound edges are held together with

_____ .

94. Secondary intention healing is used for

_____

wounds. Because healing takes longer, the threat of

_____

is great.

95. A transparent adhesive film dressing allows

_____

to reach the wound.

96. What is the difference between wet-to-dry dressings and wet-to-wet dressings?

_____

_____

97. When taping a dressing in place, the tape should not encircle the entire body part because

_____ .

98. When delegated to apply dressings, list the observations that should be reported and recorded.

A. _____

B. _____

C. _____

D. _____

E. _____

F. _____

G. _____

H. _____

I. _____

Labeling

Answer Questions 99 and 100 using the following illustration.

99. Name this position.

_____

100. Place an "X" on each of the five pressure points. Name the bony point for each one.

A. _____

B. _____

C. _____

D. _____

E. _____

Answer Questions 101 and 102 using the following illustration.

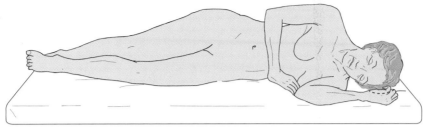

101. Name this position.

_____

102. Place an "X" on each of the seven pressure points. Name the bony point for each one.

A. _____

B. _____

C. _____

D. _____

E. _____

F. _____

G. _____

Answer Questions 103 and 104 using the following illustration.

103. Name this position.

_____

104. Place an "X" on each of the six pressure points. Name the bony point for each one.

A. _____

B. _____

C. _____

D. _____

E. _____

F. _____

Answer Questions 105 and 106 using the following illustration.

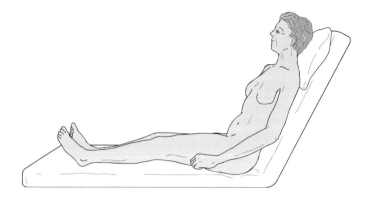

105. Name this position.

_____

106. Place an "X" on each of the three pressure points. Name the bony point for each one.

A. _____

B. _____

C. _____

Answer Questions 107 and 108 using the following illustration.

107. Name this position.

_____

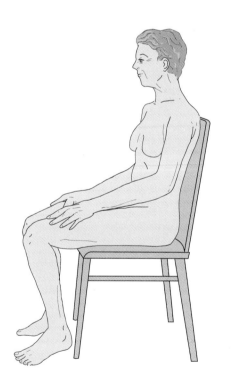

108. Place an "X" on each of the five pressure points.
Name the bony point for each one.

A. _____

B. _____

C. _____

D. _____

E. _____

Crossword

Fill in the crossword puzzle by answering the clues with words from this list.

Adhesive	Bony prominence	Gauze	Infection	Sutures
Anti-embolism	Eggcrate-like	Hemoglobin	Montgomery ties	T-binder
Bed cradle	Footboard	Hemovac	Penrose	Trochanter roll

Note: the words used in this crossword puzzle are found in the chapter but are not in the key terms. Some of the words are defined in other chapters.

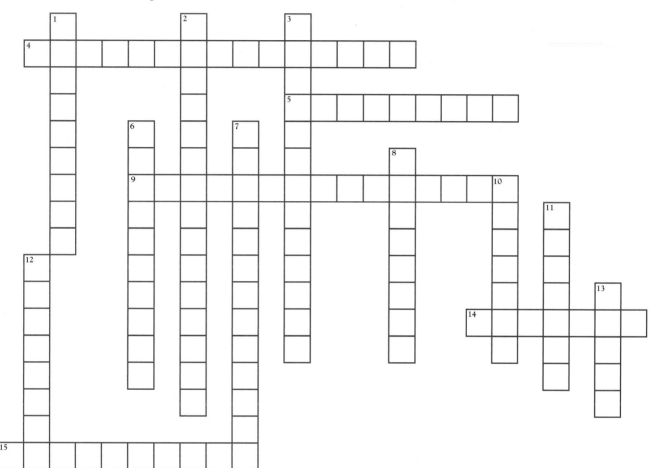

Across

4. Area where the bone sticks out or projects from the flat surface of the body.
5. Disease state resulting from the invasion and growth of microorganisms in the body.
9. Consists of adhesive strips and cloth ties. Designed to hold dressings in place.
14. Closed drainage system that removes drainage from a wound with suction.
15. Metal frame placed on a bed and over the person.

Down

1. Device placed at the foot of the mattress to prevent plantar flexion.
2. Device that prevents the hips and legs from turning outward
3. Stockings that prevent the development of thrombi.
6. Substance in red blood cells that carries oxygen and gives blood its color.
7. Mattress made of foam with peaks in the mattress to distribute the person's weight.
8. Binder that holds dressings in place after rectal or perineal surgeries.
10. Stitches used to close a wound.
11. Rubber tube that drains onto a dressing from a wound.
12. Tape that sticks well to skin but can irritate skin.
13. Type of dressing that absorbs moisture. Comes in rolls, squares, rectangles, and pads.

Nursing Assistant Skills Video Exercise

View the **Preventing and Treating Pressure Ulcers** *video to answer these questions.*

109. What are the basic principles of preventing and treating pressure ulcers?

    A. _____

    B. _____

    C. _____

    D. _____

110. What stage of a pressure ulcer is the most serious?

    _____

    Describe this stage.

    _____

    _____

111. When tissue is squeezed between two hard surfaces,

    oxygen and nutrients cannot get to the tissue, thus

    the tissue _____.

112. Name four pressure sites in obese persons.

    A. _____

    B. _____

    C. _____

    D. _____

113. If the skin is dry, you may apply

    _____,

    but do not _____.

Optional Learning Exercises

You are assigned to care for Mrs. Stevens. She is 87 years of age and has diabetes and high blood pressure. She walks with difficulty and spends most of her day sitting in her chair. She is somewhat overweight and tells you that she had a knee replacement 5 years ago and had phlebitis after surgery. The nurse tells you to watch carefully for signs of circulatory ulcers.

114. What risk factors does Mrs. Stevens have that place her at risk for circulatory ulcers?

    A. _____

    B. _____

    C. _____

    D. _____

    E. _____

    F. _____

    G. _____

115. What signs and symptoms may be present if Mrs. Stevens has stasis ulcers?

    _____

    _____

116. If arterial ulcers develop, they are usually found

    _____

    _____.

Mr. Hawkins, age 74, was in an automobile accident and has a wound on his leg that is large and open. The wound has become infected, and he is being treated with antibiotics. When you are talking with him, Mr. Hawkins tells you that he has smoked for 55 years and has poor circulation in his legs. He lives alone and generally eats take-out foods or eats cereal when he is at home.

117. Why is he receiving antibiotics?

    _____

    _____

118. What side effect of the antibiotics can cause a problem that might interfere with healing?

    _____

    _____

119. What factors would increase Mr. Hawkins' risk for complications?

    A. _____

    B. _____

    C. _____

    D. _____

120. What is missing in Mr. Hawkins' diet that is needed to help in healing the wound?

    _____

You are assisting the nurse with wound care. She is changing dressings for two different persons. Mrs. Henderson has a wound that has a large amount of drainage. Mr. Wendel has a drain in his wound, which is attached to suction.

121. Why does the nurse weigh Mrs. Henderson's new dressings before applying them to the wound and the old dressings when they are removed?

    _____

    _____

122. How does the nurse find out the amount of drainage from Mr. Wendel's wound?

    _____

123. What other ways can be used to measure drainage?

    A. _____

    B. _____

    C. _____

    D. _____

    E. _____

    F. _____

124. When you are changing a nonsterile dressing, why do you need two pairs of gloves?

    _____

    _____

125. When a wound is infected and has poor circulation, the wound may be left open at first and then closed later.

    This type of wound healing is called healing

    through _____.

    This type of healing combines

    _____ and

    _____ intention healing.

Independent Learning Activities

1. Take turns with a classmate and carry out these exercises, which will help you understand how a person who cannot move without help feels when pressure is unrelieved. Note: these exercises work best if the person wears thin clothes so the discomfort is more noticeable.
   - Place a pencil or similar hard object on the seat of a chair and have a classmate sit on the object for 10 minutes. Keep time and remind the person not to move so as to make it more uncomfortable. Remember, persons at risk for pressure ulcers are often unable to change position without assistance.
   - Position a classmate in bed, making sure that the bedclothes are wrinkled to form lumps under bony pressure points. (For example, place a wrinkle under the sacrum in the supine position or under the hip or shoulders in the lateral position.)

2. Answer these questions about the exercises done.
   - How long did it seem when you were waiting for 10 minutes to pass?
   - How many times did you begin to reposition yourself without thinking about it?
   - How did the pressure areas feel when you completed the 10 minutes? What color was the area?
   - How will this exercise affect your care of persons who cannot move?

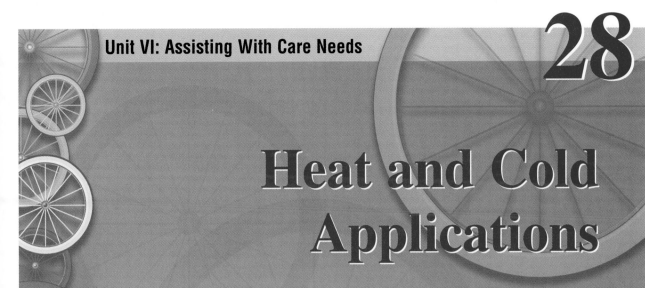

Heat and Cold Applications

28

Compress	Hyperthermia
Constrict	Hypothermia
Dilate	Pack

Fill in the Blanks: Key Terms

Select your answers from the Key Terms listed above.

1. A body temperature that is much higher compared with the person's normal range is

   _____.

2. _____ means

   to narrow.

3. A treatment that involves wrapping a body part with

   a wet or dry application is a

   _____.

4. A _____ is a

   soft pad applied over a body area.

5. _____

   means to expand or open wider.

6. _____ occurs

   when the body temperature is very low.

Circle the BEST Answer

7. Before you apply heat applications, it is important to know if
   A. A nurse is available to answer questions and supervise.
   B. Your state allows you to perform the procedure.
   C. The procedure is in your job description.
   D. All of the above are true.

8. Heat applications can be applied
   A. Only to extremities
   B. To areas with metal implants
   C. To almost any body part
   D. To persons who have difficulty sensing heat or pain

9. When heat is applied to the skin,
   A. Blood vessels in the area dilate.
   B. Tissues have less oxygen.
   C. Blood flow decreases.
   D. Blood vessels constrict.

10. When heat is applied too long, a complication that occurs is
    A. Blood vessels dilate.
    B. Blood flow increases.
    C. Blood vessels constrict.
    D. More nutrients reach the area.

11. Moist heat applications have cooler temperatures than do dry heat applications because
    A. Dry heat penetrates more deeply.
    B. Dry heat cannot cause burns.
    C. Heat penetrates deeper with a moist application.
    D. Moist heat has a slower effect than does dry heat.

12. When heat is applied in an area, which of the following is an expected response?
    A. The skin is red and warm.
    B. The skin is pale, white, or gray.
    C. The person begins to shiver.
    D. The area is excessively red.

13. The care plan states that the resident receives a heat application of 110° F. As a nursing assistant, you know that you should
    A. Measure the temperature carefully before applying to the person.
    B. Not apply an application that is above 106° F.
    C. Ask the person if the application is too warm.
    D. Apply the application and remind the person not to remove the application.

14. Heat and cold applications are applied for no longer than
    A. 1 hour
    B. 30 minutes
    C. 15 to 20 minutes
    D. 4 hours

15. When a hot or cold application is in place, you should check the area
    A. Every 15 to 20 minutes
    B. Every 5 minutes
    C. About every 30 minutes
    D. Once an hour

16. When hot compresses are in place, you may apply an aquathermia pad over the compress
    A. To keep the compress wet
    B. To protect the area from injury
    C. To measure the temperature of the compress
    D. To maintain the correct temperature of the compress

17. A hot soak is applied
    A. By placing the body part into water
    B. By applying a soft pad to a body part
    C. And is covered with plastic wrap
    D. Only until the water temperature cools down

18. When giving a sitz bath,
    A. Pad the part of the tub in contact with the person.
    B. Observe for signs of weakness, faintness, or fatigue.
    C. Prevent the person from chills and burns.
    D. All of the above are true.

19. Hot packs may be heated by all of these methods *except*
    A. Boiling in water for a few minutes
    B. Squeezing, kneading, or striking the pack
    C. Sterilizing in an autoclave
    D. Warming in a microwave oven

20. When you use an aquathermia pad,
    A. The pad temperature will cool down after about 20 to 30 minutes.
    B. The temperature is maintained by the flow of water through the pad.
    C. It is a form of moist heat.
    D. You do not need to check the person as often as you do with other heat applications.

21. When a cold application is applied, the numbing effect helps
    A. Reduce or relieve pain in the part.
    B. Constrict blood vessels.
    C. Decrease blood flow.
    D. Cool the body part.

22. Which of these cold applications is moist?
    A. Ice bag
    B. Ice collar
    C. Ice glove
    D. Cold compress

23. If the cover of a cold application becomes moist, you should
    A. Discard the cold pack and get a new one.
    B. Leave it in place and check the person more often.
    C. Remove the wet covering and apply a dry cover.
    D. Remove it immediately and report this to the nurse.

24. When a person has hyperthermia, ice packs are applied to all of these areas *except*
    A. The abdomen
    B. The head
    C. The underarms
    D. The groin

Fill in the Blanks

25. What are the effects of heat applications?

    A. _____

    B. _____

    C. _____

    D. _____

    E. _____

26. When you are caring for a confused person and heat or cold is applied, how can you know if he or she is in pain?

    _____

27. What are the advantages of dry heat applications?

    A. _____

    B. _____

28. Give an example of a dry heat application.

    _____

29. When the nurse delegates you to prepare a warm soak, what is the temperature range that is correct?

    _____

30. When you are giving a sitz bath, what should you do if the person has a rapid pulse?

    _____

31. When using an aquathermia pad, you should make sure the hoses do not have kinks or air bubbles to allow the water to

    _____.

32. List uses for cold applications.

    A. _____

    B. _____

    C. _____

    D. _____

    E. _____

33. When you prepare an ice bag, collar, or glove, remove the excess air by

    _____.

34. When a cold compress is in place, it usually needs to be changed every 5 minutes because it

    _____.

35. When hyperthermia or hypothermia is present, it is important to check the

    _____ often to

    prevent rapid changes.

Optional Learning Exercises

Situation: Your daughter, Sarah, age 3, falls while out playing and twists her ankle. You take her to the physician, who tells you to apply cold dry applications for the first day. Use the information you learned in this chapter to answer these questions about carrying out this treatment.

36. What is the purpose of the cold application for Sarah's injury?

    _____

    _____

37. What can you use to make a cool dry application to Sarah's ankle?

_____

_____

38. Why do you squeeze the application tightly after filling it with ice?

_____

_____

39. How will you protect Sarah's skin?

_____

What should you do if the covering is wet?

_____

_____

40. How often do you check the application?

_____

41. What signs and symptoms would be important when you check the area?

_____

What should you do if signs and symptoms are present?

_____

42. How long should you leave the application in place?

_____

What happens if you leave the application on too long?

_____

Independent Learning Activities

SITUATION: Mr. Chavez is 45 years of age and has a reddened area on his left calf. The physician has ordered moist warm compresses to the area, and the nurse has delegated this task to you.

1. Role-play this situation with a classmate. One of you should act as Mr. Chavez, and one should act as the nursing assistant. Work together to answer the questions for each role.
   As the nursing assistant:
   • What questions would you ask the nurse before you apply the compresses?
   • What temperature range is used for this compress?
   • How did you check the temperature of the compresses?
   • How did you keep the compress at the correct temperature?
   • How often did you check the compress? What did you observe when you checked the area?
   As Mr. Chavez:
   • How was the treatment explained to you?
   • How were you positioned? How did the nursing assistant check to see if you were comfortable?
   • How did the compress feel? Was the temperature maintained? How?
   • How often was the compress checked?

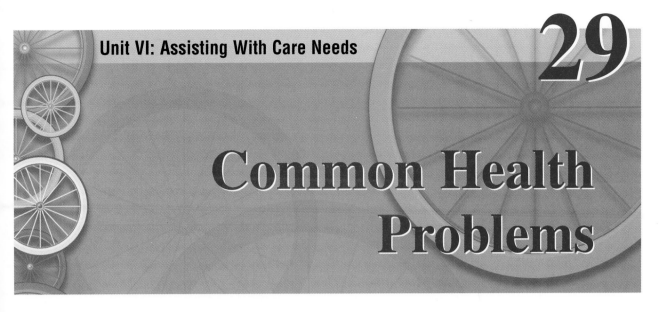

Common Health Problems

29

Amputation	Expressive aphasia	Open fracture
Aphasia	Expressive-receptive aphasia	Paralysis
Arthritis	Fracture	Quadriplegia
Arthroplasty	Gangrene	Receptive aphasia
Benign tumor	Hemiplegia	Simple fracture
Braille	Hyperglycemia	Stomatitis
Cancer	Hypoglycemia	Tinnitus
Closed fracture	Malignant tumor	Tumor
Compound fracture	Metastasis	Vertigo
Dysphagia		

Fill in the Blanks: Key Terms

Select your answers from the Key Terms listed above.

1. Dizziness is also called

   _____.

2. _____ is a

   writing system that uses raised dots. The raised dots

   are arranged for each letter of the alphabet and for

   numbers 0 through 9.

3. Difficulty expressing or sending out thoughts and

   difficulty receiving information is called

   _____.

4. The spread of cancer to other body parts of the body

   is _____.

5. _____

   is ringing in the ears.

6. A new growth of abnormal cells that may be benign

   or malignant is a _____.

7. _____ is a

   condition in which death of tissue occurs.

8. When the bone is broken but the skin is intact, it is called a simple fracture, or a

   _____.

9. _____ is joint inflammation.

10. Low sugar in the blood is

    _____.

11. An inflammation of the mouth is

    _____.

12. A _____ is a tumor that grows slowly and within a local area.

13. When a person has difficulty expressing or sending out thoughts, it is called

    _____.

14. Paralysis of the arms, legs, and trunk is

    _____.

15. An _____ is the surgical replacement of a joint.

16. An open fracture is also called a

    _____.

17. _____ means

    high sugar in the blood.

18. A malignant tumor is

    _____.

19. An _____

    is the removal of all or part of an extremity.

20. A closed fracture is also called a

    _____.

21. _____ means difficulty swallowing.

22. A _____ is a broken bone.

23. A tumor that grows and invades tissues is cancer, or

    a _____.

24. Difficulty receiving information is

    _____.

25. _____

    is paralysis on one side of the body.

26. The inability to speak is

    _____.

27. Paralysis of the legs is

    _____.

28. When a broken bone has come through the skin, it is a compound or _____

    _____.

Circle the BEST Answer

29. Benign tumors
    A. Grow slowly and within a local area
    B. Invade healthy tissue
    C. Spread to other parts of the body
    D. Divide in an orderly and controlled way

30. Risk factors that cause cancer include all of the following *except*
    A. Exposure to sunlight and tanning booth lights
    B. Smoking
    C. A diet high in fresh fruits and vegetables
    D. Close relatives with certain types of cancer

31. If you care for a person who is receiving radiation therapy to treat cancer, you might expect the person to
    A. Have pain related to the therapy
    B. Need extra rest because of fatigue
    C. Be at risk for bleeding and infections
    D. Complain of influenza-like symptoms—chills, fever, muscle aches, for example

32. Chemotherapy involves
    A. X-ray beams aimed at the tumor
    B. Giving drugs that prevent the production of certain hormones
    C. Therapy to help the immune system
    D. Giving drugs that kill cells

33. You are giving care to Mrs. Ferris, a resident who is receiving chemotherapy. She tells you that she is upset because her hair is falling out. You know that
    A. The hair often falls out when a person receives chemotherapy.
    B. This is a result of her illness.
    C. You should report this to the nurse immediately because it means her chemotherapy is not working.
    D. Change the subject to keep Mrs. Ferris from getting upset.

34. When hormone therapy is used to treat cancer, a woman may experience
    A. Loss of sexual desire
    B. Changes in fertility
    C. Weight gain, hot flashes, nausea, and vomiting
    D. All of the above

35. A person with cancer may complain of constipation because of
    A. The side effects of pain relief drugs
    B. Pain
    C. Rest and exercise
    D. Fluids and nutrition

36. When a person who is having treatment for cancer expresses anger, fear, and depression, you can help the most by
    A. Telling the person not to worry or get upset
    B. Giving the person privacy and time alone
    C. Being there when needed and listening to the person
    D. Changing the subject to distract the person

37. Osteoarthritis differs from rheumatoid arthritis because osteoarthritis
    A. Is an inflammatory disease
    B. Occurs with aging
    C. Makes the person not feel well
    D. Occurs on both sides of the body

38. When you are caring for a person with osteoarthritis, which of the following would be most helpful to the person?
    A. Allow the person to stay in bed all day.
    B. Keep the room cool because osteoarthritis improves with cold temperatures.
    C. Give the person time to move slowly when getting up after a period of rest and lack of motion.
    D. Tell the person not to exercise because it will prevent healing.

39. You are caring for a person who has rheumatoid arthritis and the person has a flare-up of the disease. You should do all of the following *except*
    A. Make sure the person exercises more frequently.
    B. Position the person in good body alignment.
    C. Encourage the person to rest more than usual.
    D. Apply splints to support affected joints.

40. Which of the following will help strengthen bones in a person who is at risk for osteoporosis?
    A. Bedrest
    B. Decreased calcium intake
    C. Exercise and activity
    D. Smoking and alcohol

41. Which of the following is *not* a sign or symptom of a fracture?
    A. Full range of motion in the affected limb
    B. Bruising and color change in the skin in the area
    C. Pain and tenderness
    D. Swelling

42. When a person has a newly applied plaster cast, it will dry in
    A. 2 to 4 hours
    B. 3 to 4 days
    C. 24 to 48 hours
    D. 12 to 24 hours

43. You can prevent flat spots on the cast by
    A. Positioning the cast on a hard surface
    B. Supporting the entire cast with pillows
    C. Using your fingertips to lift the cast
    D. Cover the cast with a blanket

44. If a person complains of numbness in a body part that is in a cast, you should
    A. Tell the person to move the limb a little to relieve the numbness.
    B. Reposition the person to help the numbness.
    C. Gently rub the exposed toes or fingers to relieve the numbness.
    D. Report the complaint immediately because it may mean there is pressure on a nerve or reduced blood flow to the body part.

45. If a person is in traction and you are giving care, it would be correct to
    A. Place bottom linens on the bed from the top down.
    B. Remove the weights while you are giving care.
    C. Turn the person from side to side to change the bed and give care.
    D. Assist the person with using the commode chair to avoid walking very far.

46. When caring for a person who has had surgery to repair a hip fracture, the operated leg should be
    A. Abducted at all times
    B. Adducted at all times
    C. Exercised with range-of-motion exercises every 4 hours
    D. Positioned to keep the hip in external rotation

47. If you assist a person with getting up to a chair after hip surgery you should
    A. Place the chair on the affected side.
    B. Have the person stand on the operative side.
    C. Place the person in a low, soft chair.
    D. Remind the person not to cross the legs.

48. If a person complains of pain in the amputated part, you should
    A. Report this immediately to the nurse.
    B. Tell the person that he or she is confused.
    C. Reassure the person that this is a normal reaction.
    D. Tell the person that this feeling will go away shortly.

49. Which of these people are at higher risk for stroke?
    A. A 79-year-old man with hypertension and diabetes
    B. A 50-year-old woman who smokes and is slightly overweight
    C. A 70-year-old African-American man who has high blood pressure and diabetes
    D. A 75-year-old Asian-American man who is inactive, has normal blood pressure, and has diabetes

50. If a person who has had a stroke ignores the weaker side of the body, it is probably because the person has
    A. Lost movement on that side
    B. Lost feeling on that side
    C. A loss of vision on that side
    D. All of the above

51. When a person who has a stroke has urinary incontinence, you can expect that
    A. Bladder training will restore normal function.
    B. The person will always be incontinent.
    C. Bladder training will help the person regain the highest possible level of function.
    D. Bladder training will not help.

52. You are caring for a person who had a stroke. When giving care, the person follows your directions easily but cannot tell you what he wants when he tries to talk. He has
    A. Expressive aphasia
    B. Receptive aphasia
    C. Expressive-receptive aphasia
    D. Depressive aphasia

53. A safety concern for a person with Parkinson's disease would be
    A. Changes in speech
    B. Swallowing and chewing problems
    C. A mask-like expression
    D. Emotional changes

54. A person with relapsing-remitting multiple sclerosis is likely to
    A. Recover quickly from the disease
    B. Have mild symptoms that affect the nervous system
    C. Have a series of attacks that cause more symptoms to occur
    D. Be given medication to cure the disease

55. A person who has a spinal cord injury in the lumbar region will likely have
    A. Quadriplegia
    B. Paraplegia
    C. Hemiplegia
    D. All of the above

56. When you are caring for a person whose speech is impaired, you should
    A. Assume you know what the person said so he or she does not need to repeat a statement.
    B. Avoid asking the person questions.
    C. Tell the person not to talk because it is too difficult to understand the words.
    D. Repeat what the person has said. Ask if your understanding is correct.

57. When caring for hearing aids, you should
    A. Wash them carefully with soap and water.
    B. Soak them in alcohol to remove wax.
    C. Follow the manufacturer's instructions for cleaning.
    D. Wipe them only with cotton or a cleansing tissue.

58. Which of the following would *not* be helpful when communicating with a hearing-impaired person?
    A. Face the person when speaking.
    B. Stand or sit on the side of the better ear.
    C. Speak in a very loud voice.
    D. Write out important names and words.

59. A person with glaucoma is given drugs to
    A. Cure the disease.
    B. Prevent further damage to the optic nerve.
    C. Prevent pain.
    D. Improve the vision.

60. A cataract is treated with
    A. Drugs applied as eye drops
    B. Eyeglasses
    C. Contact lenses
    D. Surgery

61. When you assist a person with caring for an artificial eye, the prostheses is usually cleaned with
    A. Mild soap and warm water
    B. Saline solution
    C. Alcohol
    D. With a cleansing tissue

62. When caring for a blind person, it is important to
    A. Assume the person is totally blind.
    B. Avoid using words that will upset the person, such as "look," "see," or "read."
    C. Identify yourself. Give your name, title, and reason for being there.
    D. Speak loudly so the person can understand you.

63. When assisting a blind person with walking, you should
    A. Offer an arm, and walk slightly ahead of the person.
    B. Take the person by the arm, and guide him or her.
    C. Walk ahead of the person so you can open doors or clear the path.
    D. Walk behind the person with a hand placed on the shoulder to guide him or her.

64. The most common cause of chronic obstructive pulmonary disease (COPD) is
    A. Family history
    B. Infections
    C. Smoking
    D. Exercise

65. When a person has COPD, the body cannot get normal amounts of
    A. Carbon dioxide
    B. Oxygen
    C. Carbon monoxide
    D. Nutrition

66. When a person has pneumonia, fluid intake is increased to
    A. Decrease the amount of bacteria in the lungs.
    B. Dilute medication given to treat the disease.
    C. Thin mucous secretions.
    D. Decrease inflammation of the breathing passages.

67. Breathing is easier for a person with respiratory disorders when the person is positioned in
    A. Semi-Fowler's or Fowler's position
    B. Side-lying position
    C. Supine position
    D. A soft chair

68. When you care for a person with tuberculosis, you should
    A. Wash your hands if you have contact with sputum.
    B. Flush tissues down the toilet.
    C. Remind the person to cover the mouth and nose with tissues when coughing and sneezing.
    D. All of the above are true.

69. Hypertension (high blood pressure) is a condition in which
    A. The systolic pressure is 120 mm Hg or higher and diastolic is 70 mm Hg or higher.
    B. The systolic pressure is 100 mm Hg or higher and diastolic is 60 mm Hg or higher.
    C. The systolic pressure is 140 mm Hg or higher and diastolic is 90 mm Hg or higher.
    D. The systolic pressure is 140 mm Hg or higher and diastolic is 60 mm Hg or higher.

70. A risk factor for hypertension that cannot change is
    A. Stress
    B. Being overweight
    C. Age
    D. Lack of exercise

71. The leading cause of death in the United States is
    A. Coronary artery disease
    B. Hypertension
    C. Cancer
    D. COPD

72. When a person has angina pectoris, the chest pain occurs when
    A. Oxygen does not reach the lungs.
    B. The heart needs more oxygen.
    C. Blood pressure is too high.
    D. The heart muscle dies.

73. If a person has angina pain, it will usually be relieved by
    A. Resting for about 3 to15 minutes
    B. Taking narcotic drugs
    C. Using oxygen therapy
    D. Getting up and walking for exercise

74. If a person takes a nitroglycerin tablet when an angina attack occurs, you should
    A. Give them a large glass of water to swallow the pill.
    B. Take the pills back to the nurse's station.
    C. Make sure the person tells the nurse that a pill was taken.
    D. Encourage the person to walk around.

75. When a myocardial infarction occurs, it means that
    A. A part of the heart muscle dies.
    B. The heart muscle is not receiving enough oxygen.
    C. The pain is relieved by rest.
    D. Blood backs up into the lungs.

76. If a person complains of pain that radiates to the neck, jaw, and teeth, you should get help because the person
    A. Is having an angina attack
    B. Has indigestion
    C. May be having a heart attack
    D. May be having a stroke

77. When heart failure occurs, the person may have
    A. Fluid in the lungs
    B. Swelling in the feet and ankles
    C. Confusion, dizziness, and fainting
    D. All of the above

78. An older person with heart failure is at risk for
    A. Contractures
    B. Skin breakdown
    C. Fractures
    D. Urinary tract infections

79. Women have a higher risk of urinary tract infections because of
    A. Hormone levels in the body
    B. The short female urethra
    C. Bacteria
    D. Prostrate gland secretions

80. If a person has cystitis, you should
    A. Restrict fluid intake.
    B. Assist the person with ambulating frequently.
    C. Keep the person on bedrest.
    D. Encourage the person to drink 2000 ml per day.

81. If you are caring for a person with renal calculi, you will be expected to
    A. Restrict fluids.
    B. Keep the person on bedrest.
    C. Strain all urine.
    D. All of the above are true.

82. When you care for a person with acute renal failure, you will be expected to
    A. Increase fluid intake to 2000 to 3000 cc per day.
    B. Measure and record urine output every hour.
    C. Make sure the person does not drink any fluids.
    D. Measure weight weekly.

83. Chronic renal failure
    A. Occurs suddenly
    B. Generally improves and kidney function returns to normal within 1 year
    C. Occurs when nephrons of the kidney are destroyed over many years
    D. Has very little effect on the person's overall health

84. An obese 50-year-old woman with hypertension is diagnosed with diabetes. She most likely has
    A. Type 1
    B. Type 2
    C. Gestational
    D. None of the above

85. A person with diabetes complains of thirst and frequent urination. You notice that the person has a flushed face and slow, deep, and labored respirations. It is likely that the person has
    A. Hyperglycemia
    B. Hypoglycemia
    C. Diabetic coma
    D. An infection

86. Vomiting can be life threatening when it
    A. Is caused by an infection
    B. Is aspirated and obstructs the airway
    C. Contains undigested food
    D. When it has a bitter taste

87. When hepatitis is contracted by eating or drinking food or water that has been contaminated by feces, it is
    A. Hepatitis A
    B. Hepatitis B
    C. Hepatitis C
    D. Hepatitis D and E

88. A person with hepatitis will need good skin care because
    A. Of muscle aches
    B. The person will have itching and skin rash
    C. Of nausea and vomiting
    D. Of diarrhea or constipation

89. Human immunodeficiency virus (HIV) is *not* spread by
    A. Blood
    B. Semen
    C. Sneezing or coughing
    D. Breast milk

90. To protect yourself from HIV and acquired immunodeficiency syndrome (AIDS), you should
    A. Avoid all body fluids when giving care.
    B. Refuse to care for persons diagnosed with these diseases.
    C. Follow Standard Precautions and the Bloodborne Pathogen Standard when giving care.
    D. Always use sterile technique when giving care.

91. A woman who complains about a frothy, thick, foul-smelling yellow vaginal discharge most likely has
    A. Gonorrhea
    B. Genital warts
    C. Syphilis
    D. Trichomoniasis

Matching

Match the form of COPD with the related symptom.

92. _____ Person develops a barrel chest.

93. _____ Mucus and inflamed breathing passages obstruct airflow.

94. _____ Alveoli become less elastic.

95. _____ Air passages narrow.

96. _____ The first symptom is often a smoker's cough in the morning.

97. _____ Normal oxygen and carbon dioxide exchange cannot occur in affected alveoli.

98. _____ Allergies and emotional stress are common causes.

A. Chronic bronchitis

B. Emphysema

C. Asthma

Match the symptom listed with either hypoglycemia or hyperglycemia.

99. _____ Trembling; shakiness

100. _____ Sweet breath odor

101. _____ Slurred speech

102. _____ Cold, clammy skin

103. _____ Slow, deep, and labored respirations

104. _____ Emotional changes

105. _____ Flushed face

106. _____ Frequent urination

A. Hypoglycemia

B. Hyperglycemia

Match the type of hepatitis with the correct statement.

107. _____ This hepatitis occurs in a person who is infected with Hepatitis B.

108. _____ This hepatitis is caused by poor sanitation, crowded living conditions.

109. _____ This hepatitis is caused by HBV.

110. _____ The person may have the virus but no symptoms.

A. Hepatitis A

B. Hepatitis B

C. Hepatitis C

D. Hepatitis D

Match the sexually transmitted disease (STD) with the correct statement.

111. _____ Surgical removal may be required if ointment is not effective.

112. _____ Sores may have a watery discharge.

113. _____ Vaginal bleeding may occur.

114. _____ Urinary urgency and frequency may occur.

115. _____ The condition is treated with antiviral drugs.

116. _____ The person may not show symptoms.

A. Herpes

B. Genital warts

C. Gonorrhea

D. Chlamydia

Fill in the Blanks

117. Signs and symptoms of cancer include:

A. _____

B. _____

C. _____

D. _____

E. _____

F. _____

G. _____

H. _____

118. When a person has radiation therapy, skin care

measures may be ordered because these side effects

occur:

_____

_____

119. Chemotherapy has the following uses when treating cancer:

A. _____

B. _____

C. _____

120. When a person has cancer, preventing bowel problems is one of the person's needs. Explain why bowel problems occur.

A. Constipation occurs from

_____.

B. Diarrhea occurs from

_____.

121. If you are caring for a person with osteoarthritis, why is exercise important?

    A. _____

    B. _____

    C. _____

122. Rest and joint care are also used to treat osteo-arthritis. Explain how these treatments help.

    A. Regular rest:

    _____.

    B. Cane and walkers:

    _____.

    C. Splints:

    _____.

123. List the risk factors for developing osteoporosis.

    A. _____

    B. _____

    C. _____

    D. _____

    E. _____

    F. _____

    G. _____

124. What diseases increase the risk for stroke?

    A. _____

    B. _____

    C. _____

    D. _____

125. Which risk factors for stroke cannot be controlled?

    A. _____

    B. _____

    C. _____

    D. _____

    E. _____

126. Which risk factors for stroke can be reduced by changes in personal habits?

    A. _____

    B. _____

    C. _____

    D. _____

    E. _____

127. What are the signs and symptoms of Parkinson's disease?

    A. _____

    B. _____

    C. _____

    D. _____

    E. _____

128. Chronic otitis media should be treated to prevent permanent _____.

129. When a person has Meniere's disease, safety is a concern because vertigo can cause

    _____.

130. How do these risk factors increase blood pressure?

    A. Stress: _____

    B. Tobacco: _____

    C. High-salt diet: _____

    D. Excessive alcohol: _____

    E. Lack of exercise: _____

131. List the difference between pain from angina and a myocardial infarction.

    A. _____

    B. _____

132. When left-sided heart failure occurs, blood

    _____.

    What effect does this have on the rest of the body?

    A. Brain: _____

    B. Kidneys: _____

    C. Skin: _____

    D. Blood pressure: _____

133. When right-sided heart failure occurs, the signs and symptoms in the previous question occur. In addition, what happens to these areas?

    Feet and ankles: _____

    Liver: _____

    Abdomen: _____

134. Why are older persons with heart failure at risk for pressure ulcers?

    A. _____

    B. _____

    C. _____

135. What are the risk factors of developing renal calculi?

    A. Age, race, sex: _____

    B. _____

    C. _____

    D. _____

136. A person with renal calculi is encouraged to drink 2000 to 3000 ml of fluid a day to help

    _____.

137. When acute renal failure occurs, two phases occur. Name and explain these phases.

    (1) _____

    (2) _____

    Phase 1: urine output is:

    _____

    Phase 1 lasts:

    _____

    _____

    Phase 2: urine output is:

    _____

    Phase 2 lasts:

    _____

    _____

138. Signs and symptoms of chronic renal failure appear when _____.

139. You may need to assist a person who is in chronic renal failure with nutritional needs. List what is needed in these areas:

    A. Diet: _____

    B. Fluid intake: _____

140. A person with _____ diabetes will be treated with healthy eating, exercise, and sometimes, oral drugs. A person with _____ diabetes will be treated with daily insulin therapy, healthy eating, and exercise.

141. Slow wound healing occurs in diabetes because of this complication:

_____

142. What can you do to make a person more comfortable after the person has vomited?

A. _____

B. _____

C. _____

D. _____

143. How are communicable diseases transmitted from one person to another?

A. _____

B. _____

C. _____

D. _____

E. _____

144. To protect yourself when caring for a person with hepatitis, you should follow _____.

145. AIDS is caused by a _____ that attacks the _____.

146. A threat to the health team when caring for a person with AIDS is from _____.

147. Why are older persons less likely to be tested for HIV and AIDS?

_____

_____

148. STDs are spread by _____.

149. The use of _____ helps prevent the spread of STDs.

Labeling

150. Use the manual alphabet in the textbook to decode the word shown.

_____ _____ _____ _____ _____

151. Use the sign language chart in the textbook to understand what the person is telling you.

_____

_____

Optional Learning Exercises

Mrs. Myers, 62 years of age, is having chemotherapy to treat cancer. She has not been eating well and complains of feeling very tired. When you are assisting her with personal care, you notice a large amount of hair on her pillow. Answer Questions #150 through #152 about Mrs. Myers and her care.

152. Mrs. Myers is probably not eating well because the

chemotherapy_____

the gastrointestinal tract and causes

_____

and _____.

153. She may also have _____,

which is called stomatitis. You can help her relieve

the discomfort and eat better when you provide

good _____.

154. What is causing Mrs. Myers to lose her hair?

_____

What is this condition called?

_____

You are caring for two persons who have arthritis. Read the information about each of them and answer Questions #153 through #155 about these two persons.

Mr. Miller is 78 years of age. He worked in construction for many years during which time he did heavy physical work. He complains about pain in his hips and his right knee. His fingers are deformed by the arthritis and interfere with good range of motion. Ms. Haxton is 40 years of age. She has swelling, warmth, and tenderness in her wrists, several finger joints on both hands, and both knees. She tells you that she has had arthritis for 10 years, and that it "comes and goes." At present, Ms. Haxton is complaining about pain in the affected joints, has a temperature of 100.2° F, and states that she is very tired.

155. Mr. Miller has

_____.

What time of day is he likely to have more joint

stiffness? _____

156. It is cold and raining. Which of these persons is likely to be more affected?

_____

157. Ms. Haxton has

_____.

She is likely to complain of not feeling well because

the arthritis affects

_____,

as well as joints.

You are caring for several persons with diabetes as follows:
  75-year-old African-American man
  45-year-old Caucasian, obese woman
  32-year-old pregnant woman
  60-year-old Hispanic woman with hypertension
  14-year-old girl who has lost 15 pounds
Answer Questions #156 through #160 about these persons.

158. Which of these persons is most likely to have type 2 diabetes?

A. _____

B. _____

C. _____

159. The 32-year-old pregnant woman probably has

_____.

She is at risk for developing

_____

later in life.

160. The 14-year-old girl probably has

_____

161. Which type of diabetes develops rapidly?

_____

162. _____ is treated with

daily insulin therapy. _____

is treated with oral drugs. Both types include healthy

_____ and _____

in treatment.

Independent Learning Activities

1. Many people have had a fracture at some time. If you have had a broken bone, answer these questions about the experience.
   - Did you know the bone was broken right away? Several hours later? Days later? How did you find out?
   - What symptoms did you have? Describe the pain.
   - What treatment was done? A cast? Surgery? Pins, plates, screws, traction?
   - How did the fracture affect your day-to-day life? Work? School? Leisure activities?
   - What changes were needed for you to carry out activities of daily living? How much help did you need from others? How did the need for help make you feel?
   - How was your mobility affected? Walking? Getting out of bed or out of a chair? Driving?
   - What discomfort did you have during the healing process? With the cast or surgical site?
   - What permanent or long-range problems happened? Periodic pain? Limited mobility?

2. If you have never had a fracture, try this experiment to get a small sample of how a fracture may interfere with your life. Make an immobilizer for your leg. Use one of the methods suggested, or devise one of your own.
   - Find four pieces of sturdy cardboard that are long enough to reach from the ankle to mid-thigh. Place them on the front, back, and sides of the leg and secure with elastic bandages or cloth strips. You should not be able to bend your knee.
   - Use several layers of newspaper or magazines and wrap around leg from ankle to knee. Secure with elastic bandages or cloth strips. You should not be able to bend the knee.

3. After the "cast" is in place, leave it on for 1 to 2 hours, and go about your normal routine. Answer these questions about your experience.
   - How much did the "cast" interfere with your routine?
   - How did the cast interfere with your activities of daily living? Driving? Walking? Working?
   - What other problems did you have with the cast?
   - How did you feel when you were in the cast? Awkward? Embarrassed?
   - How do you think this short experience will help you care for someone with a cast?

4. Try these experiments to understand how these diseases affect the body or the person.
   - Osteoporosis: fold a standard 81/2 3 11 piece of paper in half the long way three times. (It will now be about 1 inch by 10 inches.) Now, try to tear it in half along the fold and along the 1-inch edge. What happens? Unfold the paper once (it will be 2 inches by 10 inches), and cut pieces out along all of the edges. This step will make the paper porous, similar to the way in which bone becomes with osteoporosis. Refold the paper to the 1-inch by 10-inch size and try to tear it again. What happens now?
   - Coronary artery disease: use a straw to drink water. Now, put small pieces of a paper towel into the end of the straw and try to drink again. What happens? Add more paper and try to drink again. How does this experiment relate to coronary artery disease?

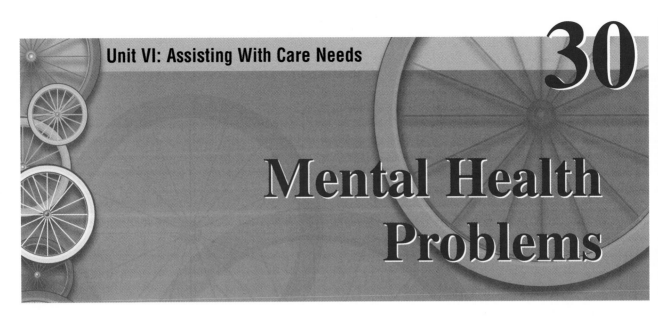

Mental Health Problems

Affect	Hallucination	Phobia
Anxiety	Mental	Psychiatric disorder
Compulsion	Mental disorder	Psychosis
Defense mechanism	Mental health	Schizophrenia
Delusion	Mental illness	Stress
Delusion of grandeur	Obsession	Stressor
Delusion of persecution	Panic	
Emotional illness	Paranoia	

Fill in the Blanks: Key Terms

Select your answers from the Key Terms listed above.

1. When a person has an exaggerated belief about his or her own importance, wealth, power, or talents, it is called _____.

2. Mental illness, emotional disorder, or psychiatric disorder is also a

   _____.

3. A _____ is any factor that causes stress.

4. _____ is feelings and emotions.

5. _____ is relating to the mind; it is something that exists in the mind or is done by the mind.

6. A constant thought or idea is an

   _____.

7. The response or change in the body resulting from any emotional, physical, social, or economic factor is _____.

8. _____ is a
vague, uneasy feeling in response to stress.

9. _____ is
another name for mental illness, mental disorder, or
psychiatric disorder.

10. A _____ is
fear, panic, or dread.

11. A false belief is a _____
_____.

12. _____ is a
disturbance in the ability to cope or adjust to stress;
behavior and functioning are impaired. This condition is also called a mental disorder, emotional illness, or a psychiatric disorder.

13. A serious mental disorder in which the person does
not view or interpret reality correctly is called a
_____.

14. A _____ is
seeing, hearing, or feeling something that is not real.

15. _____ is a
disorder of the mind. The person has false beliefs
and suspicion about a person or situation.

16. The uncontrolled performance of an act is
_____.

17. _____ is
when the person copes with and adjusts to the
stresses of everyday living in ways that are accepted
by society.

18. _____ is
described as a split mind.

19. _____ is
a false belief that one is being mistreated, abused, or
harassed.

20. An intense and sudden feeling of fear, anxiety,
terror, or dread is
_____.

21. _____ is
another name for mental illness, mental disorder, or
emotional disorder.

22. A _____ is an
unconscious reaction that blocks unpleasant or
threatening feelings.

Circle the BEST Answer

23. Which of these statements about anxiety is *not* true?
    A. Anxiety often occurs when needs are not met.
    B. Anxiety is always abnormal.
    C. Increases in pulse, respirations, and blood pres-
       sure may be the result of anxiety.
    D. The anxiety level depends on the stressor.

24. An unhealthy coping mechanism would be
    A. Talking about the problem
    B. Playing music
    C. Smoking
    D. Exercising

25. Panic is
    A. The highest level of anxiety
    B. A disorder that occurs gradually
    C. A psychosis
    D. A condition that continues for many months or years

26. A person in your care tells you that he is the President of the United States. He has a delusion of grandeur, which is a part of
    A. Obsessive-compulsive disorder
    B. Phobias
    C. Bipolar disorders
    D. Schizophrenia

27. A person with bipolar disorder may
    A. Be more depressed than manic
    B. Be more manic than depressed
    C. Alternate between depression and mania
    D. Have any of the above

28. A major risk of depression is that the person
    A. Is very sad
    B. May be a suicide risk
    C. Has depressed body functions
    D. Cannot concentrate

29. A person with an antisocial personality may
    A. Be suspicious and distrust others
    B. Have violent behavior
    C. See, hear, or feel something that is not real
    D. Blame others for actions and behaviors

30. Safety measures are included in the care plan of a person with mental health problems if
    A. Communication is a problem.
    B. The person is anxious.
    C. Suicide is a risk.
    D. The person does not learn from experiences or punishment.

Fill in the Blanks

31. What are causes of mental health disorders?

    A. _____

    B. _____

    C. _____

    D. _____

    E. _____

    F. _____

32. Name the defense mechanism being used in these situations:
    A. A girl fails a test. She blames another girl for not helping her study.

    _____

    B. A man does not like his boss. He buys the boss an expensive Christmas present.

    _____

    C. A girl complains of a stomachache so she will not have to read aloud.

    _____

    D. A child is angry with his teacher. He hits his brother.

    _____

    E. A woman misses work frequently and is often late. She gets a bad evaluation. She says that the boss does not like her.

    _____

33. The following are examples of problems that occur with schizophrenia. Name each one.
    A. A man believes his neighbor is poisoning his water.

    _____

    B. A woman says that voices told her to set fire to her apartment.

    _____

    C. A man believes that he is a physician.

    _____

    D. A woman tells you that she owns three BMW cars and is the president of MacDonald's.

    _____

Optional Learning Exercises

34. Mr. Johnson is very worried about his surgery to-morrow. You notice that he is talking very fast and is sweating. You give him directions to collect a urine specimen. Five minutes later, he turns on his signal light to ask you to repeat the directions. He tells you that he is using the toilet "all the time" because he has diarrhea and frequent urination. The nurse knows that all of these signs and symptoms indicate what?

_____

35. You are assigned to care for Mrs. Grand, a new resident. She is getting ready to go to the dining room. You assist her with getting dressed, and she tells you that she wants to wash her hands before going to the dining room. She goes to the bathroom and washes her hands for several minutes. As she leaves the room, she stops to turn off the light. She then tells you that she must wash her hands again. She repeats washing her hands and turning the lights on and off four or five times. You report this situation to the nurse, who tells you that Mrs. Grand has what?

_____

Independent Learning Activities

1. Try this experiment with a group of classmates. Make up labels with various roles for "staff members" and "mentally ill" persons. A list is provided, but you may add or subtract according to the size of your group. Make sure that the group includes a mixture of people with mental health problems and staff or visitors.

Physician	Recreational therapist	Person with obsessive-compulsive disorder
Nurse	Dietician	Person with schizophrenia with paranoia
Visitor	Person with bipolar disorder	Person with hallucinations
Nursing assistant	Person with delusions of grandeur	Person with anorexia nervosa

2. Attach a label to each person so that he or she cannot read it. (It may be placed on the back or the forehead.) Have everyone move around the group and talk to each other based on how the person thinks he or she should approach the person with a certain "label." Continue the experiment for about 15 minutes, and then use the following questions to guide a group discussion.
   - How did you feel when talking to a person with a mental health disorder?
   - How were the people with a mental health disorder approached? How quickly were the "mentally ill" persons able to sense that this was their label? What cues did they receive from others?
   - How quickly did "staff members" recognize the label they had? What cues did they receive from others?
   - In what ways did the approach of others cause people to respond in a way expected? Did the people with mental health problems show signs of the illness based on the reactions of others?
   - What did the group learn about approaching a person with a mental health problem?

3. Consider the following situation and answer the questions concerning how you would feel about caring for a person with a mental health problem.

   SITUATION: Marion Cross, age 65, is a patient in an acute care hospital with a diagnosis of pneumonia. The nurse tells you that Mrs. Cross has a history of schizophrenia. You are assigned to provide morning care for Mrs. Cross.
   - How would you approach Mrs. Cross when you enter her room? How would your knowledge about her mental health problem affect your initial contact with her?
   - What would you do if Mrs. Cross told you that she sees an elephant in the room? What would you say to her?
   - How would you react if Mrs. Cross told you that she owns Disney World and goes there free anytime she wants? How would you respond?
   - How would you provide good oral hygiene if Mrs. Cross refuses to cooperate because she is sure that the staff is trying to poison her? What might you try that would be helpful?
   - What would you do if Mrs. Cross curls up in a tight ball and refuses to talk or cooperate during morning care? What might you do to maintain her hygiene?
   - How would you feel about caring for a person with abnormal behavior? Why?

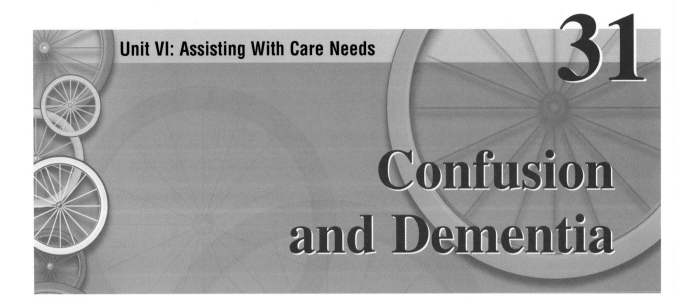

31

Confusion and Dementia

Delirium
Delusion
Dementia

Hallucination
Pseudodementia
Sundowning

Fill in the Blanks: Key Terms

Select your answers from the Key Terms listed above.

1. A false belief is a

   _____.

2. Seeing, hearing, or feeling something that is not real

   is _____.

3. Signs, symptoms, and behavior of Alzheimer's disease (AD) that increase during hours of darkness is

   _____.

4. _____

   is a state of temporary but acute mental confusion .

5. The loss of cognitive function and social function

   caused by changes in the brain is

   _____.

6. _____

   is a false dementia.

Circle the BEST Answer

7. Confusion caused by aging
   A. Occurs suddenly
   B. Is caused by reduced blood flow to the brain
   C. Can be cured
   D. Is usually temporary

8. When a person is confused, it is helpful if you
   A. Repeat the date and time as often as is necessary.
   B. Change the routine each day to stimulate the person.
   C. Keep the drapes pulled during the day.
   D. Give complex answers to questions.

9. Hearing and vision decrease with confusion; therefore you should
   A. Speak in a loud voice.
   B. Write out directions to the person.
   C. Face the person and speak clearly and slowly.
   D. Keep the lighting dim in the room.

10. Dementia can be caused by
    A. Infections
    B. Depression
    C. Trauma and head injury
    D. All of the above

11. Dementia
    A. Is the same as changes in the brain that occur with aging
    B. Causes the person to have difficulty with common tasks
    C. Is always temporary and can be cured
    D. Affects most older people

12. The most common mental health problem for older persons is
    A. AD
    B. Dementia
    C. Depression
    D. Delirium

13. The classic sign of AD is
    A. Forgetting how to use simple, everyday things
    B. Gradual loss of short-term memory
    C. Acute confusion and delirium
    D. Wandering and sundowning

14. In stage 1 of AD, the person may
    A. Walk slowly with a shuffling gait
    B. Be totally incontinent
    C. Blame others for mistakes
    D. Become agitated and may be violent

15. In stage 2 of AD, the person may
    A. Have difficulty performing everyday tasks
    B. Need assistance with activities of daily living
    C. Be disoriented to time and place
    D. Have seizures

16. In stage 3 of AD, the person may
    A. Forget recent events
    B. Lose impulse control and use foul language or have poor table manners
    C. Be less interested in things or be less outgoing
    D. Be disoriented to person, time, and place

17. When a person wanders, the major concern is
    A. The person's comfort
    B. Protecting the person from injury or life-threatening accidents
    C. Inconvenience of the family or facility
    D. Making sure the person gets enough rest and sleep

18. When a person with AD has symptoms of sundowning, it may be the result of
    A. Being tired or hungry
    B. Having poor judgment
    C. Impaired vision or hearing
    D. The person looking for something or someone

19. Too much stimuli from being asked too many questions all at once can overwhelm a person and cause
    A. Delusions
    B. Catastrophic reactions
    C. Hallucinations
    D. Sundowning

20. A caregiver may cause agitation and restlessness by
    A. Calling the person by name
    B. Selecting tasks and activities that are specific to the person's cognitive abilities and interests
    C. Encouraging activity early in the day
    D. Insisting that the person hurry to complete care quickly

21. When you are caring for a person with AD, it is helpful if you
    A. Give the person simple clothing choices, such as choosing between two shirts or blouses.
    B. Play loud familiar television programs during meals and care activities.
    C. Encourage late afternoon or early evening exercise and activity.
    D. Restrain a person who insists on going outside.

22. When a person with AD screams, it may be because the person
    A. Has hearing and vision problems
    B. Is trying to communicate
    C. Has too much stimulation in the environment
    D. All of the above

23. If a person with AD displays sexual behaviors, the nurse may tell you to
    A. Tell the person this behavior is not acceptable.
    B. Make sure the person has good hygiene to prevent itching.
    C. Avoid caring for the person.
    D. Ignore the behavior because the disease causes it.

24. What should you do when a person repeats the same motions or repeats the same words over and over?
    A. Remind the person to stop the repeating.
    B. Report this to the nurse immediately.
    C. Take the person for a walk or distract the person with music or picture books.
    D. Isolate the person in his or her room until the repeating behavior stops.

25. A person with AD is encouraged to take part in therapies and activities that will
    A. Increase the level of confusion.
    B. Help the person feel useful, worthwhile, and active.
    C. Prevent aggressive behaviors.
    D. Improve physical problems such as incontinence and contractures.

26. How do AD special care units differ from other areas of a care facility?
    A. Complete care is provided.
    B. Entrances and exits may be locked.
    C. Meals are served in the person's room.
    D. No activities are provided.

27. A person with AD no longer stays in a secured unit when
    A. The condition improves.
    B. The family requests a move to another unit.
    C. The person cannot sit or walk and is in bed.
    D. Aggressive behaviors disrupt the unit.

28. A family who cares for a person with dementia at home
    A. May feel anger and resentment towards the person
    B. May feel guilty
    C. Needs assistance from others to cope with the person
    D. All of the above

Fill in the Blanks

29. Cognitive function relates to:

    A. _____

    B. _____

    C. _____

    D. _____

    E. _____

    F. _____

30. What senses decrease with changes in the nervous system from aging?

    _____

    _____

31. Give examples of how these areas are affected early in the onset of dementia.

    A. Memory: _____

    B. Doing tasks: _____

    C. Language: _____

    D. Judgment: _____

32. What substances can cause dementia?

    _____

    _____

33. Pseudodementia can occur with

    _____

    and _____.

34. When a person has signs and symptoms that include sadness, inactivity, difficulty thinking, changes in appetite, fatigue, agitation, and withdrawal, it is important to get a correct diagnosis. Why?

    _____

    _____

    These symptoms can be caused by

    _____,

    _____,

    and _____.

35. AD damages brain cells that control these functions:

    A. _____

    B. _____

    C. _____

    D. _____

    E. _____

    F. _____

    G. _____

    H. _____

Optional Learning Exercises

You are caring for Mr. Harris, age 78, who is confused. You know that there are ways to help a person be more oriented. Answer Questions #36 through #38 about ways to help a confused person.

36. How can you help orient Mr. Harris toward who he is every time you are in contact with him?

   _____

   _____

37. What are two ways you can help orient Mr. Harris toward time?

   A. _____

   B. _____

38. What are ways you can maintain the day-night cycle?

   _____

   _____

You are caring for Mrs. Matthews, an 82-year-old resident. The nurse tells you that Mrs. Matthews lived with her daughter for the last 2 years, but the family is now concerned for her safety. She left the house when the temperature was 35° and was found 2 miles away, wearing a light sweater. On another occasion, she turned on the gas stove and was unable to remember how to turn it off. Sometimes, she did not recognize her daughter and resisted getting a bath or changing clothes. Since admission to the care facility, she tells everyone that she must leave to go to her birthday party. She brushes her arms and legs and tells you that "bugs" are crawling on her. Answer Questions 39 through 43 about Mrs. Matthews and her care.

39. Why would Mrs. Matthews most likely be in a special care unit in the nursing facility?

   _____

   _____

40. It is likely that Mrs. Matthews has what disease?

   _____

41. Mrs. Matthews is probably in stage _____ of the disease. What activities would indicate that she is in this stage?

   A. _____

   B. _____

   C. _____

   D. _____

   E. _____

42. How often will the health team review Mrs. Matthew's need to stay on this unit?

   _____

   Why is this review done?

   _____

   _____

43. The nurse may encourage Mrs. Matthew's daughter to join a _____

   group. How can this group be helpful to the daughter?

   _____

   _____

Independent Learning Activities

1. Consider the following situation and answer the questions about how you would feel.

   SITUATION: Imagine that you are in a strange country in which people talk to you, but you do not understand what they are saying. They use strange tools to eat, and you cannot figure out how to use them. They try to feed you food that you do not recognize. Sometimes, these people seem friendly and caring; but at other times, they become angry because you are not doing what they ask you to do. You become frightened when they try to remove your clothes and take you in a room to shower you. You become frightened and upset because you do not know what will happen next. At times, other strangers come to your room and bring gifts. They talk kindly to you, but you do not know them. They seem upset when you do not respond to their gifts and gestures. The doors and windows in this country are all locked and you cannot find a way out so that you can go home.
   - How does this situation relate to the information in this chapter?
   - How would you react if you were the person in this situation? Why?
   - What methods might you use to communicate with the person in this situation?
   - Why would the person want to go home? What does "home" mean to him or her?
   - How will this exercise help you when you care for a person who is confused?

2. Consider the following situation and answer the questions about how you would care for a person who has dementia.

   SITUATION: You are assigned to care for Ronald Myers, age 85, who has AD. He often wanders from room to room and tries to open the outside doors. He frequently becomes agitated and restless, especially in the evening. Most of the time, Mr. Myers is unable to feed himself and is often incontinent. He keeps repeating, "Help me, help me" all day.
   - How do you feel about caring for a person such as this? Frightened? Angry? Impatient? How do you deal with your feelings so that you can give care to the person?
   - At what stage of AD is Mr. Myers? What signs and symptoms support your answer?
   - Why would it be ineffective to remind Mr. Myers of the date and time during your shift? Why is this technique effective with some confused persons and not with others?
   - Why does Mr. Myers become more agitated toward the evening? What is this increased agitation called?
   - What methods might you use to make sure Mr. Myers receives the care needed to maintain good personal hygiene? How might you get him to cooperate or participate in his care?
   - What parts of Mr. Myers behavior would be most difficult for you to tolerate? What would you do if you found yourself becoming irritated and angry with Mr. Myers?
   - What information in this chapter has helped you understand persons such as Mr. Myers better? How will this information help you give better care to these persons and maintain their quality of life?

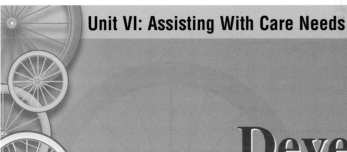

Unit VI: Assisting With Care Needs

Developmental Disabilities

32

Cerebral palsy	Epilepsy
Convulsion	Seizure
Developmental disability	Spastic
Diplegia	

Fill in the Blanks: Key Terms

Select your answers from the Key Terms listed above.

1. When similar body parts are affected on both sides of the body, it is called

   _____.

2. The uncontrolled contraction of skeletal muscles is

   _____.

3. Another name for a seizure is a

   _____.

4. _____

   is a chronic condition produced by temporary

   changes in the brain's electrical function.

5. _____

   is a term applied to a group of disorders involving

   muscle weakness or poor muscle control; the defect

   is in the motor region of the brain.

6. A disability that occurs before 22 years of age is

   _____.

7. A _____

   or a convulsion is the violent and sudden contrac-

   tions or tremors of muscle groups.

Circle the BEST Answer

8. A developmental disability
   A. Always occurs at birth
   B. Is usually temporary
   C. Limits function in three or more life skills
   D. Is present before the age of 12

9. Developmentally disabled adults
   A. Need lifelong assistance, support, and special services
   B. Can usually live independently after they become adults
   C. Always need to be in long-term care in special centers
   D. Generally outgrow the problems as they mature

10. A person is considered to have mental retardation if
   A. The intelligence quotient (IQ) score is below 70 to 75.
   B. The person has difficulty understanding the behavior of others.
   C. The person is limited in the skills needed to live, work, and play.
   D. All of the above are true.

11. The Arc of the United States is a national organization
   A. Related to Alzheimer's disease
   B. Dealing with mental retardation
   C. That provides care for people with physical disability
   D. For persons with cerebral palsy

12. Down syndrome (DS) is caused by
   A. An extra 21st chromosome
   B. Head injury during birth
   C. Diseases of the mother during pregnancy
   D. Lack of oxygen to the brain

13. A person with Down syndrome is at risk for
   A. Cerebral palsy
   B. Diplegia
   C. Alzheimer's disease after age 35
   D. Poor nutrition

14. Cerebral palsy is a group of disorders involving
   A. Mental retardation
   B. Muscle weakness or poor muscle control
   C. Abnormal genes from one or both parents
   D. An increased risk of developing leukemia

15. When a person has spastic cerebral palsy, the symptoms include
   A. Constant, slow weaving or writhing motions
   B. Uncontrolled contractions of skeletal muscles
   C. Using little or no eye contact
   D. A strong attachment to a single item, idea, activity, or person

16. A person with autism may have
   A. Frequent tantrums for no apparent reason
   B. Bladder and bowel control problems
   C. Generalized seizures
   D. Hemiplegia

17. An adult with autism may
   A. Need help with developing social and work skills
   B. Work and live independently
   C. Live in group homes or residential care centers
   D. All of the above

18. Seizures are caused by
   A. Diplegia
   B. Bursts of electrical energy in the brain
   C. Mental illness
   D. Spinal abnormalities

19. When epilepsy can be controlled, it usually
   A. Does not affect learning and activities of daily living
   B. Is easily controlled with drugs
   C. Can be cured with medications
   D. Requires the person to have assistance with developing social and work skills

20. Spina bifida occurs
   A. At birth as a result of injury during delivery
   B. Because of traumatic injury in childhood
   C. During the first month of pregnancy
   D. As a result of child abuse

21. Which of these types of spina bifida causes the person to have leg paralysis and lack of bowel and bladder control?
   A. Spina bifida cystica
   B. Myelomeningocele
   C. Spina bifida occulta
   D. Meningocele

22. A shunt placed in the brain of a child with hydrocephalus will
   A. Relieve pressure on the brain.
   B. Drain fluid from the brain to the abdomen.
   C. Reduce the mental retardation or neurological damage that may occur with hydrocephalus.
   D. All of the above are true.

23. Which of these statements about persons with a developmental disability is *not* true?
    A. All persons with a disability will always need to live with family or in a nursing care center.
    B. The Americans with Disabilities Act of 1990 protects the rights of persons with developmental disabilities.
    C. When a person with a developmental disability needs care in a nursing center, OBRA protects his or her rights.
    D. The developmental disability will affect the person and the family throughout life.

Fill in the Blanks

24. A developmental disability is present when function is limited in three or more of these life skills:

    A. _____

    B. _____

    C. _____

    D. _____

    E. _____

    F. _____

    G. _____

25. What genetic conditions can cause mental retardation?

    A. _____

    B. _____

    C. _____

    D. _____

26. Mental retardation may be caused after birth by:

    A. _____

    B. _____

    C. _____

    D. _____

    E. _____

    F. _____

    G. _____

27. According to the Arc of the United States, mental retardation involves the condition being present before _____.

28. The Arc of the United States believes the following about persons with mental retardation:

    A. _____

    B. _____

    C. _____

    D. _____

29. If a child has Down syndrome, how are these areas affected?

    A. Head: _____

    B. Eyes: _____

    C. Tongue: _____

    D. Nose: _____

    E. Hands and fingers: _____

30. Persons with Down syndrome need therapy in these areas:

    A. _____

    B. _____

    C. _____

    D. _____

31. The usual cause of cerebral palsy is a lack of

    _____

    _____.

32. The goal for a person with cerebral palsy is to be

    _____

    _____.

33. What skills are impaired with autism?

    A. _____

    B. _____

    C. _____

    D. _____

    E. _____

34. A partial seizure occurs in

    _____.

    A generalized seizure involves the

    _____.

35. Spina bifida is a defect of the

    _____.

36. Children with spina bifida may have learning problems with the following:

    A. _____

    B. _____

    C. _____

    D. _____

37. Spina bifida may place the person at risk for these other problems:

    A. _____

    B. _____

    C. _____

    D. _____

    E. _____

    F. _____

    G. _____

38. When a person has hydrocephalus, it can lead to these problems:

    A. _____

    B. _____

    C. _____

Optional Learning Exercises

Mr. Murphy is one of the residents in your care. He has Down syndrome. Answer Questions #39 through #41 that relate to this person.

39. Mr. Murphy is 40 years of age. What disease is a risk for persons with Down syndrome past the age of 35?

    _____

40. Mr. Murphy is encouraged to eat a well-balanced diet and to attend regular exercise classes. Why are these activities important for a person with Down syndrome?

    _____

    _____

41. What types of therapies may help Mr. Murphy communicate more clearly?

    A. _____

    B. _____

You care for Mary Reynolds who has cerebral palsy. Answer Questions #42 and #43 about Ms. Reynolds.

42. It is difficult to feed Ms. Reynolds because she

    drools, grimaces, and moves her head constantly.

    You know that she displays these signs because she

    has a type of cerebral palsy called

    _____.

43. Because Ms. Reynolds remains in bed or a special

    chair all the time, she is at special risk for

    _____

    because of immobility. She needs to be repositioned

    at least every

    _____ .

Mr. Calhoun was in an automobile accident and now has epilepsy. Answer Questions #44 through #46 about his care.

44. Mr. Calhoun has frequent seizures. He asks you how long he will continue to have these. You report this question to the nurse, who tells Mr. Calhoun that, at this time, seizures cannot be

    _____ .

    What may be done to control his seizures?

    _____

45. What limits can be placed on a person who has seizures at any time?

    A. _____

    B. _____

46. Safety measures are needed for the:

    A. _____

    B. _____

    C. _____

    D. _____

Independent Learning Activities

1. Many communities have services available to families with children and adults who are developmentally disabled. Some communities have sheltered workshops, day-care centers, sheltered living centers, or physical and occupational therapy programs available. If your community has these services, ask permission to visit them and observe the persons being served there. Answer these questions when you observe the agency.
   - What age groups are served in this program?
   - What activities are available to the group?
   - What training is required for the people who work there?
   - How do the persons in the program act? Happy? Bored? Withdrawn? Other reactions?
   - What other services are available to these individuals in the agency? In the community?
   - Where do the persons in this program live? With family? Group homes? Other?

2. Do you know a family who has a developmentally disabled family member? Ask the family if they will answer these questions about living with this person.
   - How old is the developmentally disabled person? Where does the person live?
   - What abilities does the person have? What disabilities interfere with the activities of daily living for the person?
   - What therapies are being done to help the person reach his or her highest level of function?
   - What community programs have been helpful for the person?
   - How does this person's disability affect the family? Physical? Emotional? Financial? Day-to-day activities?

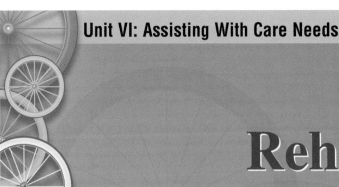

Rehabilitation and Restorative Care

Activities of daily living (ADL)	Prosthesis	Restorative aide
Disability	Rehabilitation	Restorative nursing care

Fill in the Blanks: Key Terms

Select your answers from the Key Terms listed above.

1. A nursing assistant with special training in restorative nursing and rehabilitation skills is a

   _____.

2. _____

   are specific self-care activities done daily to remain

   independent and to function in society.

3. An artificial replacement for a missing body part is a

   _____.

4. Care that helps persons regain their health, strength,

   and independence is

   _____.

5. A _____

   is any lost, absent, or impaired physical or mental

   function.

6. The process of restoring the disabled person to the

   highest possible level of physical, psychological,

   social, and economic functioning is

   _____.

Circle the BEST Answer

7. The focus of rehabilitation is to
   A. Improve the person's abilities.
   B. Restore function to normal.
   C. Help the person regain health and strength.
   D. Prevent injury.

8. Restorative nursing promotes
   A. Self-care, elimination, and positioning
   B. Mobility, communication, and cognitive function
   C. Helping regain health, strength, and independence
   D. All of the above

9. If you are a restorative aide, it means that you have
   A. Special training in restorative nursing and rehabilitation skills
   B. Taken the required training for restorative aides
   C. Passed a special test to show that you can perform these duties
   D. The most seniority at the facility

10. When assisting with rehabilitation and restorative care, it is important to
    A. Give complete care to prevent exertion by the person.
    B. Make sure you do everything for the person.
    C. Encourage the person to perform ADL to the greatest extent possible.
    D. Complete care quickly.

11. Which of the following would be most helpful for a person who is receiving rehabilitative care?
    A. Give the person pity or sympathy when tasks are difficult.
    B. Remind the person not to try new skills or those that are difficult.
    C. Give praise when even a little progress is made.
    D. Encourage the person to perform ADL quickly.

12. Complications can be prevented by
    A. Prolonged bedrest
    B. Incontinence
    C. Good alignment, turning and repositioning, and range-of-motion exercises
    D. Prolonged illnesses

13. Self-help devices help meet the goal of
    A. Recovery of all normal abilities
    B. Self-care
    C. Living alone
    D. Dependence on others

14. When dysphagia occurs after a stroke, a person may need
    A. Exercises to improve swallowing
    B. A gastrostomy tube
    C. Assistance in feeding
    D. All of the above

15. The care plan for a person in rehabilitation gives information to meet
    A. Only physical care needs
    B. Only ambulation needs
    C. All needs, including psychological and social needs
    D. Only psychological and social needs

16. The rehabilitation team meets to evaluate the person's progress
    A. Every 90 days
    B. As often as is necessary to change the plan when needed
    C. Every week
    D. Only when requested by the family or person

17. When do rehabilitation services begin?
    A. When the person first needs health care
    B. After discharge from the hospital
    C. Only when ordered by the physician
    D. When the person returns home

18. OBRA requires that nursing centers
    A. Have a full-time physical therapist.
    B. Provide rehabilitation services.
    C. Provide physical care only.
    D. Employ full-time occupational and speech therapists.

Fill in the Blanks

19. Rehabilitation and restorative nursing programs do the following:

    A. _____

    B. _____

20. A person with a disability needs to adjust in these areas:

    A. _____

    B. _____

    C. _____

    D. _____

21. Rehabilitation takes longer in which age-group?

_____

What are reasons for this increase?

A. _____

B. _____

C. _____

22. What are some self-help devices that will assist in self-feeding?

A. _____

B. _____

C. _____

23. The goal for a prosthesis is to

_____

_____

_____

24. When you are assisting with rehabilitation and restorative care, why should you practice the task that the person must perform?

_____

_____

_____

25. When assisting with rehabilitation and restorative care, what complications can be prevented if you report early signs and symptoms?

_____

_____

26. What measures can you take to promote the person's quality of life?

A. _____

B. _____

C. _____

D. _____

E. _____

F. _____

G. _____

H. _____

I. _____

Optional Learning Exercises

Mrs. Mercer is 82 years of age. She is a resident in a rehabilitation unit because she had a stroke that has caused weakness on her left side. Although she is right-handed, she needs to learn to use several self-help devices as she relearns ways to carry out ADL. She often becomes angry or depressed. Answer Questions #27 through #32 about Mrs. Mercer and her care.

27. Mrs. Mercer is having difficulty with controlling urinary and bowel elimination. What would be the goal of her care for these problems?

_____

Her plan of care would include programs for

_____.

28. What should you do to prepare Mrs. Mercer's food at mealtime so she can feed herself?

_____

_____

_____

29. Mrs. Mercer can brush her teeth but needs help getting prepared. What should you do to get her ready to brush her teeth?

_____

_____

_____

30. Why does Mrs. Mercer need help at mealtime and to brush her teeth?

_____

_____

_____

31. Mrs. Mercer needs help to get in and out of bed.

When helping her transfer, you remember to

position the chair on her

_____ side.

32. When Mrs. Mercer becomes discouraged because

progress is slow, how can you help her? You can

stress _____

and focus on _____.

Independent Learning Activities

1. Role-play the following situation with a classmate. Answer the questions about how you felt when you played Mrs. Leeds to understand how a person with a disability feels. Use your nondominant hand to attempt the activities she must do.

   SITUATION: Mary Leeds, age 62, had a stroke last month. She has weakness on her dominant side and has been admitted to a rehabilitation unit to relearn ADL. She is practicing eating by using a spoon to place fluids and food in her mouth. She is also learning to button clothing. How well might you hold the spoon with your non-dominant hand?
   * What problems did you have controlling the spoon?
   * How rapidly were you able to eat? What type of food was easier to eat?
   * How well were you able to button your clothing? What techniques did you find that increased your success?
   * How did this experience make you feel? How will it affect the way you interact with persons who have similar disabilities?

2. With your instructor's permission, borrow a wheelchair from your school to use for 1 to 2 hours. While you are in the chair, have a classmate push you around a grocery store, shopping mall, or in your school. You must stay in the chair for the entire time to experience the feelings of a person who must use a wheelchair. Use a handicap-equipped bathroom during this experience.
   * How comfortable was the wheelchair? Did you use any special padding or cushion in the seat?
   * What difficulties were encountered moving about? Doorways? Steps? Aisles? Crowds? How did you deal with any difficulties?
   * How accessible was the handicap-equipped bathroom? How much room was available for you to transfer from the wheelchair to the toilet?
   * How did other people treat you? How many spoke to you? How many talked to your classmate and avoided you?
   * How did this experience make you feel? How will it affect the way you interact with a person in a wheelchair?

34

Basic Emergency Care

Cardiac arrest	First aid	Seizure
Convulsion	Hemorrhage	Shock
Fainting	Respiratory arrest	

Fill in the Blanks: Key Terms

Select your answers from the Key Terms listed above.

1. In _____,
   breathing stops, but the heart action continues for
   several minutes.

2. The sudden loss of consciousness from an inade-
   quate blood supply to the brain is
   _____.

3. When the heart and breathing stops suddenly and
   without warning, it is
   _____.

4. _____ results
   when organs and tissues do not get enough blood.

5. Emergency care given to an ill or injured person before medical help arrives is
   _____.

6. A convulsion may also be called a
   _____.

7. _____
   is the excessive loss of blood in a short period.

8. Violent and sudden contractions or tremors of muscles comprise a seizure, or a
   _____.

Circle the BEST Answer

9. When an emergency occurs, the nurse will
   A. Call the physician for orders.
   B. Activate the emergency medical service (EMS) system.
   C. Call the supervisor.
   D. Assist the person to bed.

10. If you find a person lying on the floor, you should
   A. Keep the person lying down.
   B. Help the person back to bed.
   C. Elevate the head.
   D. Help the person to a chair.

11. If the nurse instructs you to activate the EMS system, you should do all of the following *except*
   A. Tell the operator your location.
   B. Explain to the operator what has happened.
   C. Describe aid that is being given.
   D. Hang up as soon as you have finished giving the information.

12. It is important to restore breathing and circulation quickly because
   A. The lungs will be damaged.
   B. The person will lose consciousness.
   C. Permanent brain damage occurs.
   D. Hemorrhage will occur.

13. Which of the following is *not* a major sign of cardiac arrest?
   A. Complaints of chest pain
   B. No pulse
   C. No breathing
   D. Unconsciousness

14. The purpose of the head-tilt/chin-lift maneuver is to
   A. Make the person more comfortable.
   B. Open the airway.
   C. Practice Standard Precautions.
   D. Stimulate the heart to beat.

15. To determine breathlessness, you
   A. Ask the person if he or she can take a deep breath.
   B. Pinch the person's nostrils shut with your thumb and index finger.
   C. Look to see if the person's chest rises and falls.
   D. Remove the dentures.

16. When you use mouth-to-mouth breathing, you should
   A. Allow the person's chin to relax against the neck.
   B. Place your mouth loosely over the person's mouth.
   C. Blow into the person's mouth slowly. You should see the chest rise.
   D. Apply pressure on the chin to close the mouth.

17. Mouth-to-nose breathing is used when
   A. You cannot ventilate through the person's mouth.
   B. You want to avoid contact with body fluids.
   C. Giving rescue breaths to a child.
   D. Chest compressions are not needed.

18. When cardiopulmonary resuscitation (CPR) is started, you first give
   A. Five chest compressions
   B. Two breaths
   C. Five breaths
   D. Fifteen chest compressions

19. The purpose of chest compressions is to
   A. Deflate the lungs.
   B. Increase oxygen in the blood.
   C. Force blood through the circulatory system.
   D. Help the heart work more effectively.

20. For chest compressions to be effective, the person must be
   A. In a prone position
   B. On a soft surface
   C. Supine on a hard, flat surface
   D. In a semi-Fowler's position

21. When preparing to give chest compressions, locate the hands
   A. Midway on the sternum
   B. On the lower one-half of the sternum
   C. Side by side over the sternum
   D. Slightly below the end of the sternum

22. When giving chest compressions to an adult, depress the sternum
   A. About 1 to $1^{1}/2$ inches
   B. About $^{1}/2$ to 1 inch
   C. About $1^{1}/2$ to 2 inches
   D. About 2 to $2^{1}/2$ inches

23. CPR is done when the person
   A. Does not respond when you shout, "Are you OK?"
   B. Is not breathing
   C. Is unconscious
   D. Does not respond, is not breathing, and has no pulse

24. If the person is not breathing or not breathing adequately, give two breaths that
    A. Last about 2 seconds each
    B. Last about 5 seconds each
    C. Last 5 to 10 seconds each
    D. Last 15 seconds each

25. When performing one-rescuer CPR, chest compressions are at a rate of
    A. 15 compressions per minute
    B. 100 compressions per minute
    C. 60 compressions per minute
    D. 12 compressions per minute

26. When performing one-rescuer CPR, check for a carotid pulse, breathing, coughing, and moving after
    A. 5 minutes
    B. 100 compressions
    C. One cycle of 15 compressions and two breaths
    D. Four cycles of 15 compressions and two breaths

27. A person with a foreign-body obstructed airway (FBOA)
    A. Can move some air in and out of the lungs
    B. Can remove the object with forceful coughing
    C. Cannot breathe, speak, or cough
    D. Does not lose consciousness

28. The Heimlich maneuver is used when
    A. The person is standing, sitting, or lying.
    B. The person is conscious.
    C. The person is unconscious.
    D. All of the above are true.

29. If a person is very obese or pregnant, an FBOA is relieved with
    A. The Heimlich maneuver
    B. Chest thrusts
    C. CPR
    D. A finger sweep

30. When performing the Heimlich maneuver, a fist is placed
    A. In the middle of the abdomen above the navel and below the end of the sternum
    B. On the lower part of the sternum
    C. In the middle of the sternum
    D. On the lower part of the abdomen below the navel

31. If a person with an FBOA is unresponsive, activate the EMS system, and then
    A. Perform the Heimlich maneuver.
    B. Do the finger sweep maneuver to check for a foreign object.
    C. Give two slow rescue breaths.
    D. Open the airway using the head-tilt/chin-lift method.

32. If you find an unconscious adult, you should
    A. Assume that the person is choking and perform the Heimlich maneuver.
    B. Begin CPR immediately.
    C. Open the airway and check for breathing.
    D. Do the finger sweep maneuver to check for foreign objects.

33. The side-lying position is the recovery position that is used when the person is breathing and has a pulse but is not responding because
    A. The position helps keep the airway open.
    B. It allows fluids to drain from the mouth.
    C. It prevents the tongue from falling toward the back of the throat.
    D. All of the above are true.

34. When an automated external defibrillator (AED) is used, it
    A. Stops the heart
    B. Slows the heart rate
    C. Stops ventricular fibrillation and restores a regular heartbeat
    D. Starts the heart beating

35. Which of the following is a sign of internal hemorrhage?
    A. Steady flow of blood from a wound
    B. Pain, shock, vomiting blood, or coughing up blood
    C. Bleeding that occurs in spurts
    D. Dried blood at the site of an injury

36. To control external bleeding, you should do all of the following *except*
    A. Remove any objects that have pierced or stabbed the person.
    B. Place a sterile dressing directly over the wound.
    C. Apply pressure with your hand directly over the bleeding site.
    D. Bind the wound when bleeding stops.

37. If a person is in shock, it is helpful if you
    A. Have the person sit in a chair.
    B. Keep the person cool by removing some of the clothing.
    C. Stay calm, which helps the person feel more secure.
    D. Give the person something to drink or eat.

38. If a person has a seizure, you should
    A. Place an object between the teeth.
    B. Distract the person so as to stop the seizure.
    C. Position the person in bed.
    D. Move furniture, equipment, and sharp objects away from the person.

39. If you are assisting a person with burns, it is correct to
    A. Remove burnt clothing.
    B. Cover the burn wounds with a clean, cool, moist covering.
    C. Give the person plenty of fluids.
    D. Apply oils or ointments to the burns.

40. If a person tells you that he or she feels faint, it is best if you
    A. Have the person lie down in a supine position.
    B. Let the person walk around to increase circulation.
    C. Have the person sit or lie down before fainting occurs.
    D. Raise the head with pillows if the person is lying down.

41. When a stroke occurs, position the person in the recovery position
    A. On the affected side
    B. On the unaffected side
    C. In the supine position
    D. In a semi-Fowler's position

Fill in the Blanks

42. If you activate the EMS system, what information should you give to the operator?

    A. _____

    B. _____

    C. _____

    D. _____

    E. _____

    F. _____

43. Chain-of-Survival actions are as follows:

    A. _____

    B. _____

    C. _____

    D. _____

44. CPR means _____.

45. CPR has three basic parts:

    A. _____

    B. _____

    C. _____

46. When performing the head-tilt/chin-lift maneuver, explain how you tilt the head and lift the chin.

    A. Tilt _____.

    B. Place _____.

    C. Lift _____.

47. When you are trying to determine breathlessness, explain what you do when you:

    A. Look: _____

    B. Listen: _____

    C. Feel: _____

48. When you perform mouth-to-mouth breathing, it is likely that you will have contact with

    _____.

49. If a person has a mouth that is severely injured and you need to perform rescue breathing, you will use

    _____.

50. To find the carotid pulse, place

    _____.

    Slide your fingers down

    _____.

51. Common causes of choking that place older persons at risk are:

    A. _____

    B. _____

    C. _____

    D. _____

52. If you choke, you can perform the Heimlich maneuver on yourself by:

    A. _____

    B. _____

    C. _____

    D. _____

    E. _____

    F. _____

53. If the choking person is obese or pregnant, your fist

    is placed on the _____

    _____ .

54. List the signs and symptoms of shock.

    A. _____

    B. _____

    C. _____

    D. _____

    E. _____

    F. _____

    G. _____

55. Describe the two phases of a generalized tonic-clonic seizure.

    A. Tonic phase: _____

    B. Clonic phase: _____

56. Partial-thickness burns involve the

    _____ .

    Full-thickness burns involve

    _____ .

57. A _____

    burn is very painful because

    _____ .

58. Common causes of fainting are:

    A. _____

    B. _____

    C. _____

    D. _____

59. When a person has a stroke, the affected side is

    _____

    _____ .

Optional Learning Exercises

You are eating in a fast-food restaurant when a man at the next table begins choking and gasping for air. Answer Questions #60 through #65 about this situation.

60. What should you do first?

    _____

    _____

61. You determine the man is not able to breathe in air. What would you do?

    _____

    _____

62. You are unsuccessful in dislodging the food and the man becomes unresponsive. After you lower the man to the floor, you should first

    _____

    _____ .

63. Before beginning rescue breathing, you need to

    _____

    _____ .

64. Open the airway with the

    _____ .

65. Give _____ rescue breaths and _____ abdominal thrusts.

You are visiting a neighbor and she is washing dishes. As she washes a glass, it shatters and she sustains a deep cut on her wrist. Answer Questions #66 through #71 about how you would respond.

66. How would you determine whether the bleeding was from an artery or vein?

    _____

    _____

67. Your neighbor is crying and walking around the room. What is the best thing you can do to help her?

    _____

    _____

68. Clean rubber gloves are lying on the counter. How can they be useful to you?

    _____

    _____

69. What materials in the home can be used to place over the wound?

    _____

    _____

70. Your neighbor is restless and has a rapid and weak pulse. You notice that her skin is cold, moist, and pale. These signs indicate that she may be in

    _____ .

71. Her wound is still bleeding, and she loses consciousness. What should you do before you continue to give first aid?

    _____

    _____

Independent Learning Activities

1. You have learned some basic emergency care in this chapter. Find out where a more advanced first aid course is available in your community. Answer these questions about the course.
   - What agency or agencies offer a course in first aid?
   - How long does the course last? How much does it cost?
   - Who may take the course? The public? Medical personnel? Others, such as police, firefighters, and so forth?
   - What subjects are covered in the course?
   - Would taking this course help you on your job? In your family? In your community?

2. Most health care facilities require employees to take a course in basic CPR. You may be required to take CPR as part of this course. Answer these questions about CPR training in your community.
   - What agency or agencies offer CPR courses?
   - How long does the course take? How much does it cost?
   - Who can take the courses? The public? Medical personnel? Are different classes offered to the medical personnel? If so, what is the difference?
   - How often does the person need to be re-certified? How does the re-certification course differ from the beginning class?

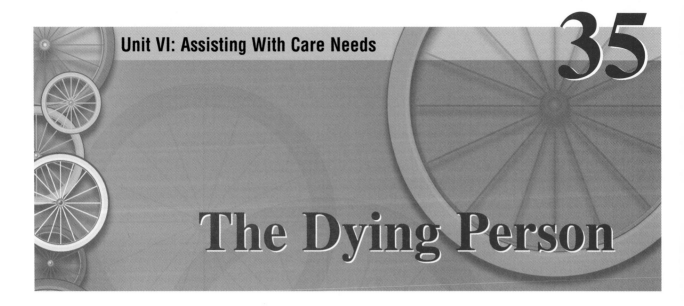

The Dying Person

Advance directive

Postmortem

Reincarnation

Rigor mortis

Terminal illness

Fill in the Blanks: Key Terms

Select your answers from the Key Terms listed above.

1. The stiffness or rigidity of skeletal muscles that

    occurs after death is _____.

2. An _____

    is a document stating a person's wishes about health

    care when that person cannot make his or her own

    decisions.

3. After death is _____.

4. An illness or injury for which there is no reasonable

    expectation of recovery is a

    _____.

5. _____

    is the belief that the spirit or soul is reborn in an-

    other human body or in another form of life.

Circle the BEST Answer

6. When a person has a terminal illness,
    A. The physician is able to accurately predict when
       the person will die.
    B. Modern medicine can cure the disease.
    C. He or she often lives longer than expected be-
       cause of a strong will to live.
    D. He or she will die when expected.

7. Practices and attitudes among people from India
    include
    A. Placing small pillows under the person's neck,
       feet, and wrists
    B. White clothing that is worn for mourning
    C. A time and place for prayer that are essential for
       the family and the person
    D. Having an aversion to death

8. A group that believes in reincarnation would be
   A. Hindus
   B. Chinese
   C. Christians
   D. Jewish people

9. Children between ages 3 and 5 years see death as
   A. Final
   B. Punishment for being bad
   C. Suffering and pain
   D. A reunion with those who have died

10. Older persons see death as
    A. A temporary state
    B. Freedom from pain, suffering, and disability
    C. Something that happens to other people
    D. Something that affects plans, hopes, dreams, and ambitions

11. In which stage of dying does the person make promises and make "just one more" request?
    A. Acceptance
    B. Anger
    C. Depression
    D. Bargaining

12. If a dying person begins to talk about worries and concerns, you should
    A. Call a spiritual leader.
    B. Tell the nurse.
    C. Be there and listen quietly.
    D. Change the subject to more pleasant topics.

13. When a person is dying, care should be given
    A. Only if the person requests it
    B. To meet basic needs
    C. Often so as to keep the person active
    D. Only while the person is conscious

14. Because vision fails as death approaches, you should
    A. Explain what you are doing to the person when you are in the room.
    B. Have the room very brightly lit.
    C. Turn out all the lights.
    D. Keep the eyes covered at all times.

15. Hearing is one of the last functions lost; therefore it is important to
    A. Speak in a normal voice.
    B. Offer words of comfort.
    C. Provide reassurance and explanations about care.
    D. All of the above are true.

16. As death nears, oral hygiene is
    A. Given routinely
    B. Given more frequently when taking oral fluids is difficult
    C. Given very infrequently to avoid disturbing the person
    D. Never given because the person cannot swallow

17. Which of the following does *not* occur as death nears?
    A. Body temperature rises.
    B. The skin is cool, pale, and mottled.
    C. Perspiration decreases.
    D. Circulation fails.

18. Because of breathing difficulties, the dying person is generally more comfortable in
    A. A supine position
    B. A side-lying position
    C. A prone position
    D. A semi-Fowler's position

19. When a person is dying, you can help the family by
    A. Allowing the family to stay as long as they wish
    B. Staying away from the room and delay giving care
    C. Telling the family that they need to leave so you can give care
    D. Telling the family that the person who is dying is not in pain

20. The goal of hospice is to
    A. Cure the person.
    B. Improve the dying person's quality of life.
    C. Provide life-saving measures.
    D. Help the family seek hospitals or clinics that specialize in the disease of the dying person.

21. If a person has a living will, it instructs physicians
    A. Not to start measures that will save the person's life
    B. To start CPR whenever necessary
    C. Not to start measures that prolong dying
    D. Never to activate the EMS system for a person

22. If the physician writes a "do not resuscitate" (DNR) order, it means that
    A. The person will not be resuscitated.
    B. The person will be resuscitated if it is an emergency.
    C. The physician will decide whether to resuscitate.
    D. The RN may decide that, in a particular situation, resuscitation is needed.

23. A sign that death is near would be
    A. Deep, rapid respirations
    B. Blood pressure beginning to fall
    C. Muscles that tense and contract in spasms
    D. Peristalsis that increases

24. When the family wishes to see the body after death, it should be
    A. Positioned in normal alignment
    B. Positioned to appear comfortable and natural
    C. Bathed and cleaned
    D. All of the above

25. When you are assisting with postmortem care, you should do all of these *except*
    A. Place the body in good alignment in a supine position without pillows.
    B. Tape wedding ring in place.
    C. Gently pull eyelids over the eyes.
    D. Dress the person in his or her regular clothing.

26. An identification tag is attached to the big toe or the
    A. Wrist
    B. Ankle
    C. Upper arm
    D. Upper leg

27. The Dying Person's Bill of Rights includes all of the following *except*
    A. Freedom from restraint
    B. The right to visit with others in private
    C. The right to participate in resident and family groups
    D. The right to personal choice

Fill in the Blanks

28. It is important to examine your own feelings about

    death because they will affect

    _____.

29. When you understand the dying process, you can

    approach the dying person with

    _____.

30. Religious beliefs strengthen when dying, and they

    often provide _____.

31. Adults fear death because they fear:

    A. _____

    B. _____

    C. _____

    D. _____

    E. _____

    F. _____

32. Name the five stages of dying.

    A. _____

    B. _____

    C. _____

    D. _____

    E. _____

33. When caring for a dying person, do not ask questions that need long answers because

    _____

    _____.

34. Because crusting and irritation of the nostrils can

    occur, you should _____

    _____.

35. What kinds of elimination problems are common in the dying person?

    _____

    _____

36. You can promote comfort by providing:

    A. _____

    B. _____

    C. _____

    D. _____

    E. _____

37. List the service that a hospice provides to these persons or groups:

    A. Dying person: _____

    B. Survivors: _____

    C. Health team: _____

38. The Patient Self-Determination Act and OBRA give two rights that affect the rights of a dying person:

    A. _____

    B. _____

39. A living will instructs physicians:

    A. _____

    B. _____

40. When a person cannot make health care decisions, the authority to do so is given to the person with

    _____.

41. What are the signs that death is near?

    A. _____

    _____

    B. _____

    _____

    C. _____

    _____

    D. _____

    _____

    E. _____

    _____

    F. _____

    _____

42. The signs of death include no

    _____.

    The pupils are _____

    and _____.

43. When assisting with postmortem care, what information do you need from the nurse?

    A. _____

    B. _____

    C. _____

    D. _____

44. The right to confidentiality before and after death

    provides that _____

    _____

    _____.

Optional Learning Exercises

You are assigned to care for Mrs. Adams, who is dying. Answer Questions #45 through #52 regarding this situation.

45. You find Mrs. Adams crying in her room. When you ask her what is wrong, she tells you that no one gave her fresh water this morning and that she has not had her bath yet. She tells you to just go away. What stage of dying is she displaying?

    _____

46. Later in the day, Mrs. Adams tells you that she cannot wait until she is better to go home and plant her garden. She states that she knows the tests done last week were wrong and she will recover quickly from her illness. What stage is she now displaying?

_____

Why is she displaying two different stages so rapidly?

_____

_____

47. A minister comes to visit Mrs. Adams while you are giving care. What should you do?

_____

48. You are working one night and find Mrs. Adams awake during the night. She asks you to sit with her. She begins to talk about her fears, worries, and anxieties. What are two things you can do to convey caring to her?

_____

_____

49. As Mrs. Adams becomes weaker, a family member is always at her bedside. When they ask to assist with her care, you know that this is acceptable.

Why?

_____

_____

50. Mrs. Adams has very irregular breathing that becomes deeper and then stops for a period.

This pattern of breathing is called

_____,

and occurs because the

_____

fails as death nears.

51. Mrs. Adams dies while you are working, and the nurse asks you to assist with postmortem care. As you clean soiled areas, you assist the nurse with turning the body, and air is expelled.

Why did this event occur?

_____

_____

52. You wear gloves during postmortem care because

they will _____

_____.

Independent Learning Activities

1. It is important to explore your own beliefs about death and dying before you care for persons who are dying. Answer these questions to understand your own feelings.
    • Have you attended a funeral or visited a funeral home? How did you feel?
    • Has anyone close to you died? How did you assist with any of the funeral arrangements? What kinds of preparation did the family do?
    • What cultural or religious practices in your family affect death and funeral arrangements? How do you think these practices will affect you when you care for persons who are dying?
    • Have you ever been present when someone died? In your personal life? As a student? At your job? How did you react? What were you asked to do in this situation?
    • What is your personal belief about a living will? How will you respond if a person or family refuses a feeding tube or a ventilator? How will you respond if they ask to have these measures discontinued and the person dies?
    • What is your personal belief about a DNR order? How would you feel if a person in your care has this order? How will you respond when the person dies and no effort is made to help the person?

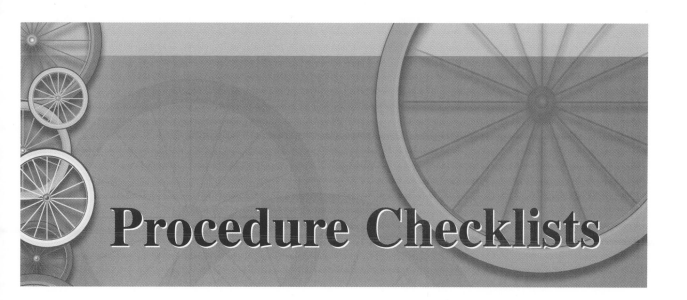

Procedure Checklists

Using a Fire Extinguisher

QUALITY OF LIFE

Remember to:
- Knock before entering the person's room
- Address the person by name
- Introduce yourself by name and title

Name: _____

Date: _____

Pre-Procedure

	S	U	Comments
1. Pulled the fire alarm.	____	____	_____
2. Got the nearest fire extinguisher.	____	____	_____
3. Carried the extinguisher upright.	____	____	_____
4. Took the extinguisher to the fire.	____	____	_____

Procedure

5. Removed the safety pin.	____	____	_____
6. Pushed the handle down.	____	____	_____
7. Directed the hose at the base of the fire.	____	____	_____

Post-Procedure

8. Followed agency policy for used extinguisher.	____	____	_____

Applying Restraints

QUALITY OF LIFE

Name: _____

Date: _____

Remember to:
- Knock before entering the person's room
- Address the person by name
- Introduce yourself by name and title

Pre-Procedure

	S	U	Comments

1. Obtained the correct restraint.
2. Decontaminated hands.
3. Identified the person.
4. Explained the procedure to the person.
5. Provided for privacy.

Procedure

6. Made sure the person was comfortable and in good body alignment.
7. Applied bed rail pads or gap protectors, if needed.
8. Padded bony areas as directed by nurse.
9. Read the manufacturer's instructions.
10. *For wrist restraints:*
    a. Applied the restraint correctly.
    b. Secured the restraint so that it was snug but not tight. Made sure two fingers could be slid under restraint.
    c. Tied the ends to the movable part of the bed or bedspring. Used an agency-approved knot. Left 1 to 2 inches of slack in straps.
    d. Repeated steps 10 a, b, and c for other wrist.
11. *For mitt restraints:*
    a. Used hand rolls, if needed.
    b. Decontaminated person's hands.
    c. Placed hand roll, if not using padded mitts.
    d. Applied the mitt. Followed manufacturer's instructions.
    e. Tied the ends to the movable part of the bed or bedspring. Used an agency-approved knot. Left 1 to 2 inches of slack in straps.
    f. Secured the restraint so that it was snug but not tight. Made sure two fingers could be slid between the restraint and wrist.
    g. Repeated steps 11 a, b, c, d, e, and f for the other hand.

Procedure—cont'd	**S**	**U**	**Comments**

12. *For a vest restraint:*
   a. Assisted the person to a sitting position.
   b. Applied the restraint correctly. Followed the manufacturer's instructions.
   c. Made sure the vest was free of wrinkles.
   d. Helped the person to lie down in bed.
   e. Brought the straps through the slots.
   f. Made sure the person was comfortable and in good body alignment.
   g. Tied the straps to the movable part of the bed or bedspring. Used an agency-approved knot. Left 1 to 2 inches of slack in straps. Or secured the straps to a chair that is out of person's reach.
   h. Made sure vest was snug. Slid an open hand between the restraint and the person.

13. *For jacket restraint:*
   a. Assisted the person into a sitting position.
   b. Applied the restraint. Followed the manufacturer's instructions.
   c. Closed the back of the jacket.
   d. Made sure side seams were under the arms, and made sure jacket was free of wrinkles.
   e. Helped the person lie down, if in bed, or sit back, if in chair.
   f. Made sure the person was comfortable and in good body alignment.
   g. Tied the straps to the movable part of the bed frame or chair. Used an agency-approved knot. Left 1 to 2 inches of slack in straps.
   h. Made sure jacket was snug. Slid an open hand between the restraint and the person.

14. *For belt restraint:*
   a. Assisted the person to a sitting position.
   b. Applied the restraint. followed manufacturer's instructions.
   c. Removed wrinkles from restraint.
   d. Brought the ties through the slots in the belt.
   e. Helped the person lie down or sit.
   f. Made sure person was comfortable and in good body alignment.
   g. Secured the straps to the movable part of the bed frame or to a chair that is out of the person's reach. Used an center-approved knot.

Post-Procedure   S   U   Comments

15. Placed the signal light within the person's reach.   _____ _____ _____

16. Unscreened the person.   _____ _____ _____

17. Used bed rails as indicated in person's plan of care.   _____ _____ _____

18. Decontaminated hands.   _____ _____ _____

19. Checked the person and the restraint at least every 15 minutes.   _____ _____ _____
    Reported observations to the nurse.

    a. For wrist and mitt restraints: checked the pulse, color, and   _____ _____ _____
        temperature of the extremity.

    b. For vest, jacket, and belt restraints: checked person's   _____ _____ _____
        breathing and position of restraint.

20. Did the following at least every 2 hours:

    • Removed the restraint.   _____ _____ _____

    • Repositioned the person.   _____ _____ _____

    • Met the person's needs for food, fluids, hygiene, and   _____ _____ _____
      elimination.

    • Gave skin care.   _____ _____ _____

    • Performed range-of-motion exercises or ambulated the   _____ _____ _____
      person. Followed the care plan.

    • Reapplied the restraints.   _____ _____ _____

21. Reported and recorded observations and the care given.   _____ _____ _____

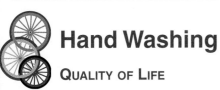

Hand Washing

QUALITY OF LIFE

Name: _____

Date: _____

Remember to:
- Knock before entering the person's room
- Address the person by name
- Introduce yourself by name and title

Pre-Procedure	S	U	Comments
1. Made sure to have soap, paper towels, orange stick or nail file, and wastebasket.	___	___	_____
2. Pushed watch up 4 to 5 inches. Also, pushed up uniform sleeves.	___	___	_____
3. Stood away from the sink so that clothes did not touch the sink. Stood so that the soap and faucet were easy to reach.	___	___	_____
4. Turned on the faucet. Adjusted the water temperature.	___	___	_____
5. Wet wrists and hands. Kept hands lower than elbows.	___	___	_____
6. Applied about 1 teaspoon of soap to hands.	___	___	_____
7. Worked up lather, taking at least 10 seconds.	___	___	_____
8. Washed each hand and wrist thoroughly. Cleaned under fingernails.	___	___	_____
9. Used a nail file or orange stick to clean under fingernails.	___	___	_____
10. Rinsed wrists and hands well. Water flowed from arms to hands.	___	___	_____
11. Repeated following steps if needed:			
• Applied about 1 teaspoon of soap to hands.	___	___	_____
• Worked up lather, taking at least 10 seconds.	___	___	_____
• Washed each hand and wrist thoroughly.	___	___	_____
• Cleaned under fingernails.	___	___	_____
• Used a nail file or orange stick to clean under fingernails.	___	___	_____
12. Rinsed wrists and hands well. Water flowed from arms to hands.	___	___	_____
13. Dried wrists and hands with paper towels. Patted dry. Started at fingertips.	___	___	_____
14. Discarded paper towels.	___	___	_____
15. Turned off faucets with clean paper towels. Used a clean paper towel for each faucet.	___	___	_____
16. Discarded paper towels.	___	___	_____

Removing Gloves

QUALITY OF LIFE

Name: _____

Date: _____

Remember to:
- Knock before entering the person's room
- Address the person by name
- Introduce yourself by name and title

Procedure

	S	U	Comments
1. Made sure that glove touched only glove.	_____	_____	_____
2. Grasped a glove just below the cuff.	_____	_____	_____
3. Pulled the glove down over hand so that it was inside out.	_____	_____	_____
4. Held the removed glove with other gloved hand.	_____	_____	_____
5. Reached inside the other glove with the first two fingers of un-gloved hand.	_____	_____	_____
6. Pulled the glove down over hand and the other glove.	_____	_____	_____
7. Discarded the gloves.	_____	_____	_____
8. Decontaminated hands.	_____	_____	_____

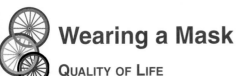

Wearing a Mask

QUALITY OF LIFE

Remember to:
- Knock before entering the person's room
- Address the person by name
- Introduce yourself by name and title

Name: _____

Date: _____

Procedure

	S	U	Comments
1. Decontaminated hands.	____	____	_____
2. Picked up the mask by its upper ties. Did not touch part that covers face.	____	____	_____
3. Placed the mask over nose and mouth.	____	____	_____
4. Placed the upper strings over ears. Tied the strings.	____	____	_____
5. Tied the lower strings at the back of the neck. Lower part of the mask was under chin.	____	____	_____
6. Pinched the metal band around nose so that it was snug and under the glasses.	____	____	_____
7. Decontaminated hands.	____	____	_____
8. Provided necessary care. Avoided coughing, sneezing, and unnecessary talking.	____	____	_____
9. Changed the mask if it became moist or contaminated.	____	____	_____
10. Removed the mask as follows:			
a. Removed the gloves.	____	____	_____
b. Untied the lower strings.	____	____	_____
c. Untied the top strings.	____	____	_____
d. Held the top strings and removed the mask.	____	____	_____
e. Brought the strings together. The inside of the mask folded together.	____	____	_____
11. Discarded the mask. Followed center policy.	____	____	_____
12. Decontaminated hands.	____	____	_____

Donning and Removing a Gown

QUALITY OF LIFE

Name: _____

Remember to:
- Knock before entering the person's room
- Address the person by name
- Introduce yourself by name and title

Date: _____

Procedure	S	U	Comments
1. Removed watch and all jewelry.	____	____	_____
2. Rolled up uniform sleeves.	____	____	_____
3. Decontaminated hands.	____	____	_____
4. Put on a facemask if required.	____	____	_____
5. Picked up a clean gown. Held it out and allowed it to unfold; did not shake the gown.	____	____	_____
6. Put hands and arms through the sleeves.	____	____	_____
7. Made sure the gown covered the front of uniform. Made sure it was snug at neck.	____	____	_____
8. Tied the strings at the back of the neck.	____	____	_____
9. Overlapped the back of the gown. Made sure the gown covered uniform snugly.	____	____	_____
10. Tied the waist strings at the back.	____	____	_____
11. Put on the gloves.	____	____	_____
12. Provided necessary person care.	____	____	_____
13. Removed and discarded the gloves.	____	____	_____
14. Removed the gown as follows:			
a. Untied the waist strings.	____	____	_____
b. Decontaminated hands.	____	____	_____
c. Untied the neck strings. Did not touch the outside of the gown.	____	____	_____
d. Pulled the gown down from the shoulder.	____	____	_____
e. Turned the gown inside out as it was removed.	____	____	_____
15. Rolled up the gown away from self. Kept it inside out.	____	____	_____
16. Discarded the gown.	____	____	_____
17. Decontaminated hands.	____	____	_____
18. Removed the facemask. Discarded it following center policy.	____	____	_____
19. Decontaminated hands.	____	____	_____
20. Opened the door using a paper towel. Discarded the paper towel when leaving.	____	____	_____

Donning and Removing Sterile Gloves

QUALITY OF LIFE

Name: _____

Date: _____

Remember to:
- Knock before entering the person's room
- Address the person by name
- Introduce yourself by name and title

Procedure	**S**	**U**	**Comments**
1. Inspected the package for sterility:			
a. Checked the expiration date.	_____	_____	_____
b. Made sure the package was dry.	_____	_____	_____
c. Checked for tears, holes, punctures, and watermarks.	_____	_____	_____
2. Arranged a work surface:			
a. Made sure enough room was available.	_____	_____	_____
b. Arranged the work surface at waist level and within vision.	_____	_____	_____
c. Made sure the work surface was clean and dry.	_____	_____	_____
d. Did not reach over or turned your back on the work surface.	_____	_____	_____
3. Opened the package by grasping the flaps and peeling the flaps back.	_____	_____	_____
4. Removed the inner package. Placed it on a clean work surface.	_____	_____	_____
5. Read the manufacturer's instructions.	_____	_____	_____
6. Arranged the inner package for left, right, up, and down. Had the cuffs near self with the fingers pointing away.	_____	_____	_____
7. Used the thumb and index finger of each hand to grasp the folded edges of the inner packaging.	_____	_____	_____
8. Folded back the inner packaging to expose the gloves. Did not contaminate the inside of the package or the gloves.	_____	_____	_____
9. Noted that the cuffs and insides of the gloves are not sterile.	_____	_____	_____
10. Put on the right glove if right-handed or the left glove if left-handed:			
a. Picked up the glove with other hand. Used thumb and index and middle fingers.	_____	_____	_____
b. Touched only the cuff and the inside of the glove.	_____	_____	_____
c. Turned the hand to be gloved palm side up.	_____	_____	_____
d. Lifted the cuff up. Slid fingers and hand into the glove.	_____	_____	_____
e. Pulled the glove up over hand. If some fingers got stuck, left them that way until the other glove was on. Did not let the outside of the glove touch any nonsterile surface.	_____	_____	_____
f. Left the cuff turned down.	_____	_____	_____
11. Put on the other glove with gloved hand:			
a. Reached under the cuff of the second glove with the four fingers of gloved hand.	_____	_____	_____
b. Kept gloved thumb close to gloved palm.	_____	_____	_____
c. Pulled on the second glove. Gloved hand did not touch the cuff or any other surface.	_____	_____	_____
d. Held the thumb of first gloved hand away from the gloved palm.	_____	_____	_____

Procedure—cont'd	S	U	Comments
12. Adjusted each glove with the other hand. Gloves were smooth and comfortable.	_____	_____	_____
13. Slid fingers under the cuffs to pull them up.	_____	_____	_____
14. Touched only sterile items.	_____	_____	_____
15. Removed the gloves properly.	_____	_____	_____

Raising the Person's Head and Shoulders

QUALITY OF LIFE

Remember to:
- Knock before entering the person's room
- Address the person by name
- Introduce yourself by name and title

Name: _____

Date: _____

Pre-Procedure

	S	U	Comments
1. Asked a co-worker for help if needed.	_____	_____	_____
2. Decontaminated hands.	_____	_____	_____
3. Identified the person.	_____	_____	_____
4. Explained what would be done.	_____	_____	_____
5. Provided for privacy.	_____	_____	_____
6. Locked the bed wheels.	_____	_____	_____
7. Raised the bed to the best level for good body mechanics. Made sure the bed rails were up.	_____	_____	_____

Procedure

	S	U	Comments
8. Asked helper to stand on the other side of the bed. Lowered the bed rails.	_____	_____	_____
9. Asked the person to put his or her near arm under worker's arm and behind shoulder. Person's hand rested on top of worker's shoulder. Asked person to do the same with helper.	_____	_____	_____
10. Put arm nearest to the person under his or her arm.Put hand on the person's shoulder. Had helper do the same.	_____	_____	_____
11. Put free arm under the person's neck and shoulders. Asked helper to do the same.	_____	_____	_____
12. Helped the person pull up to a sitting or semi-sitting position on the count of "3."	_____	_____	_____
13. Used the arm and hand that supported the person's neck and shoulders to straighten or support the person.	_____	_____	_____
14. Helped the person lie down. Provided support with locked arms. Supported his or her neck and shoulders with other arms.	_____	_____	_____

Post-Procedure

	S	U	Comments
15. Provided for comfort. Positioned the person in good body alignment.	_____	_____	_____
16. Placed the signal light within reach.	_____	_____	_____
17. Raised or lowered bed rails. Followed the care plan.	_____	_____	_____
18. Lowered the bed to lowest position.	_____	_____	_____
19. Unscreened the person.	_____	_____	_____
20. Decontaminated hands.	_____	_____	_____

Moving the Person Up in Bed

QUALITY OF LIFE

Name: _____

Date: _____

Remember to:
- Knock before entering the person's room
- Address the person by name
- Introduce yourself by name and title

Pre-Procedure

	S	U	Comments
1. Decontaminated hands.	___	___	_____
2. Identified the person.	___	___	_____
3. Explained what would be done.	___	___	_____
4. Provided for privacy.	___	___	_____
5. Locked the bed wheels.	___	___	_____
6. Raised the bed to the best level for good body mechanics. Made sure the bed rails were up.	___	___	_____

Procedure

	S	U	Comments
7. Lowered the head of the bed to a level appropriate for the person. Kept the bed as flat as possible.	___	___	_____
8. Lowered the nearest bed rail.	___	___	_____
9. Placed the pillow against the headboard if person could be without it.	___	___	_____
10. Stood with feet about 12 inches apart. Pointed the foot nearest the head of the bed toward the head of the bed. Faced the head of the bed.	___	___	_____
11. Bent hips and knees. Kept back straight.	___	___	_____
12. Placed one arm under the person's shoulders and the other under his or her thighs.	___	___	_____
13. Asked the person to grasp the trapeze bar and to flex both knees.	___	___	_____
14. Explained that both of you moved on the count of "3."	___	___	_____
15 Moved the person to the head of the bed on the count of "3." Shifted weight from rear leg to front leg.	___	___	_____
16. Place the pillow under the person's head and shoulders.	___	___	_____

Post-Procedure

	S	U	Comments
17. Straightened linens.	___	___	_____
18. Provided for comfort. Positioned the person in good body alignment.	___	___	_____
19. Placed the signal light within reach.	___	___	_____
20. Raised or lowered the bed rails. Followed the care plan.	___	___	_____
21. Raised the head of the bed to a level appropriate for the person.	___	___	_____
22. Lowered the bed to its lowest position.	___	___	_____
23. Unscreened the person.	___	___	_____
24. Decontaminated hands.	___	___	_____

Moving the Person Up in Bed With a Lift Sheet

QUALITY OF LIFE

Name: _____

Date: _____

Remember to:
● Knock before entering the person's room
● Address the person by name
● Introduce yourself by name and title

Pre-Procedure

	S	U	Comments
1. Asked a co-worker to help.	___	___	_____
2. Decontaminated hands.	___	___	_____
3. Identified the person.	___	___	_____
4. Explained the procedure to the person.	___	___	_____
5. Provided for privacy.	___	___	_____
6. Locked the bed wheels.	___	___	_____
7. Raised the bed to the best level for good body mechanics. Made sure the bed rails were up.	___	___	_____

Procedure

8. Lowered the head of the bed to a level appropriate for the person. It was as flat as possible.	___	___	_____
9. Stood on one side of the bed with helper on the other side.	___	___	_____
10. Lowered the bed rails.	___	___	_____
11. Placed the pillow against the headboard if the person could be without it.	___	___	_____
12. Stood with a broad base of support. Pointed the foot nearest the head of the bed toward the head of the bed. Faced that direction.	___	___	_____
13. Rolled the sides of the lift sheet up close to the person.	___	___	_____
14. Grasped the rolled-up lift sheet firmly near the person's shoulders and buttocks. Made sure you supported the head.	___	___	_____
15. Bent hips and knees.	___	___	_____
16. Slid the person up in bed on the count of "3." Shifted weight from rear leg to front leg.	___	___	_____
17. Unrolled the lift sheet.	___	___	_____

Post-Procedure

18. Put the pillow under the person's head and shoulders. Straightened linens.	___	___	_____
19. Provided for comfort. Positioned the person in good body alignment.	___	___	_____
20. Placed the signal light within reach.	___	___	_____
21. Raised or lowered bed rails. Followed the care plan.	___	___	_____
22. Raised the head of the bed to a level appropriate for the person.	___	___	_____
23. Lowered the bed to its lowest position.	___	___	_____
24. Unscreened the person.	___	___	_____
25. Decontaminated hands.	___	___	_____

Moving the Person to the Side of the Bed

QUALITY OF LIFE

Remember to:
- Knock before entering the person's room
- Address the person by name
- Introduce yourself by name and title

Name: _____

Date: _____

Pre-Procedure	S	U	Comments

1. Asked a co-worker to help if using a lift sheet.   ____ ____ _____
2. Decontaminated hands.   ____ ____ _____
3. Identified the person.   ____ ____ _____
4. Explained the procedure to the person.   ____ ____ _____
5. Provided for privacy.   ____ ____ _____
6. Locked the bed wheels.   ____ ____ _____
7. Raised the bed to the best level for good body mechanics. Made sure the bed rails were up.   ____ ____ _____

Procedure

8. Lowered the head of the bed to a level appropriate for the person. It was as flat as possible.   ____ ____ _____
9. Stood on the side of the bed to which the person would be moved.   ____ ____ _____
10. Lowered the near bed rail.   ____ ____ _____
11. Stood with feet about 12 inches apart and with one foot in front of the other. Flexed knees.   ____ ____ _____
12. Crossed the person's arms over the person's chest.   ____ ____ _____
13. Method 1: Moving the person in segments:
    a. Placed arm under the person's neck and shoulders. Grasped the far shoulder.   ____ ____ _____
    b. Placed other arm under the mid-back.   ____ ____ _____
    c. Moved the upper part of the person's body toward self. Rocked backward, and shifted your weight to your rear leg.   ____ ____ _____
    d. Placed one arm under the person's waist and one under the thighs.   ____ ____ _____
    e. Rocked backward to move the lower part of the person toward you.   ____ ____ _____
    f. Repeated the procedure for the legs and feet. Arms were under the person's thighs and calves.   ____ ____ _____
14. Method 2: Moving the person with a lift sheet:
    a. Rolled up the lift sheet close to the person.   ____ ____ _____
    b. Grasped the rolled-up lift sheet near the person's shoulders and buttocks. Made sure to support the head.   ____ ____ _____
    c. Rocked backward. On the count of "3," moved the person toward you. Co-worker rocked backward slightly and then forward toward you while keeping the arms straight.   ____ ____ _____
    d. Unrolled the lift sheet.   ____ ____ _____

Post-Procedure

	S	U	Comments
15. Provided for comfort.	_____	_____	_____
16. Positioned the person in good body alignment. Followed the nurse's directions and the care plan. Repositioned the pillow under the person's head and shoulders.	_____	_____	_____
17. Placed the signal light within the person's reach.	_____	_____	_____
18. Raised or lowered bed rails. Followed the care plan.	_____	_____	_____
19. Lowered the bed to its lowest position.	_____	_____	_____
20. Unscreened the person.	_____	_____	_____
21. Decontaminated hands.	_____	_____	_____

Turning and Positioning the Person

QUALITY OF LIFE

Remember to:
- Knock before entering the person's room
- Address the person by name
- Introduce yourself by name and title

Name: _____

Date: _____

Pre-Procedure

	S	U	Comments

1. Decontaminated hands.   _____ _____ _____
2. Identified the person.   _____ _____ _____
3. Explained the procedure to the person.   _____ _____ _____
4. Provided for privacy.   _____ _____ _____
5. Locked the bed wheels.   _____ _____ _____
6. Raised the bed to the best level for good body mechanics. Made   _____ _____ _____
   sure the bed rails were up.

Procedure

7. Lowered the head of the bed to a level appropriate for the   _____ _____ _____
   person. The bed was as flat as possible.
8. Stood on the side of the bed opposite to where you would turn   _____ _____ _____
   the person. The far bed rail was up.
9. Lowered the bed rail near you.   _____ _____ _____
10. Moved the person to the side near you.   _____ _____ _____
11. Crossed the person's arms over his or her chest. Crossed the leg   _____ _____ _____
    near you over the far leg.
12. Method 1: Moving the person away from you:
    a. Stood with a wide base of support. Flexed knees.   _____ _____ _____
    b. Placed one hand on the person's shoulder and the other on   _____ _____ _____
       the buttock near you.
    c. Pushed the person gently toward the other side of the bed.   _____ _____ _____
       Shifted weight from rear leg to front leg.
13. Method 2: Moving the person toward you:
    a. Raised the bed rail.   _____ _____ _____
    b. Went to the other side. Lowered the bed rail.   _____ _____ _____
    c. Stood with a wide base of support. Flexed knees.   _____ _____ _____
    d. Placed one hand on the person's far shoulder and the other   _____ _____ _____
       on the far hip.
    e. Rolled the person gently toward you.   _____ _____ _____

Post-Procedure

14. Provided for comfort. Positioned the person in good body   _____ _____ _____
    alignment.
15. Placed the signal light within reach.   _____ _____ _____
16. Raised or lowered bed rails. Followed the care plan.   _____ _____ _____
17. Lowered the bed to its lowest position.   _____ _____ _____
18. Unscreened the person.   _____ _____ _____
19. Decontaminated hands.   _____ _____ _____

Logrolling the Person

QUALITY OF LIFE

Name: _____

Date: _____

Remember to:
- Knock before entering the person's room
- Address the person by name
- Introduce yourself by name and title

Pre-Procedure

	S	U	Comments
1. Asked a co-worker to help.	___	___	_____
2. Decontaminated hands.	___	___	_____
3. Identified the person.	___	___	_____
4. Explained the procedure to the person.	___	___	_____
5. Provided for privacy.	___	___	_____
6. Locked the bed wheels.	___	___	_____
7. Raised the bed to the best level for good body mechanics. Made sure the bed rails were up.	___	___	_____

Procedure

	S	U	Comments
8. Made sure the bed was flat.	___	___	_____
9. Stood on the opposite side to which the person would be turned.	___	___	_____
10. Lowered the bed rail.	___	___	_____
11. Moved the person as a unit to the side of the bed near you. Used the lift sheet.	___	___	_____
12. Placed the person's arms across the chest. Placed a pillow between the knees.	___	___	_____
13. Raised the bed rail. Went to the other side and lowered the bed rail.	___	___	_____
14. Positioned yourself near the shoulders and chest. Co-worker stood near the buttocks and thighs.	___	___	_____
15. Stood with a broad base of support. One foot was in front of the other.	___	___	_____
16. Asked the person to hold his or her body rigid.	___	___	_____
17. Rolled the person toward self or used a turn sheet. Turned the person as a unit.	___	___	_____

Post-Procedure

	S	U	Comments
18. Provided for comfort. Positioned the person in good alignment. Used pillows as directed by the nurse and the care plan. Used:	___	___	_____
a. One pillow against the back for support.	___	___	_____
b. One pillow under the head and neck if allowed.	___	___	_____
c. One pillow or folded bath blanket between the legs.	___	___	_____
d. A small pillow under the arm and hand.	___	___	_____
19. Placed the signal light within reach.	___	___	_____
20. Raised or lowered bed rails. Followed the care plan.	___	___	_____
21. Lowered the bed to its lowest position.	___	___	_____
22. Unscreened the person.	___	___	_____
23. Decontaminated hands.	___	___	_____

Helping the Person Sit on the Side of the Bed (Dangle)

QUALITY OF LIFE

Name: _____

Date: _____

Remember to:
- Knock before entering the person's room
- Address the person by name
- Introduce yourself by name and title

Pre-Procedure

	S	U	Comments
1. Explained the procedure to the person.	_____	_____	_____
2. Decontaminated hands.	_____	_____	_____
3. Identified the person.	_____	_____	_____
4. Decided which side of the bed to use.	_____	_____	_____
5. Moved furniture to provide moving space.	_____	_____	_____
6. Provided for privacy.	_____	_____	_____
7. Positioned the person in a sidelying position facing you.	_____	_____	_____
8. Locked the bed wheels.	_____	_____	_____
9. Raised the bed to the best level for body mechanics. Made sure the bed rails were up.	_____	_____	_____

Procedure

	S	U	Comments
10. Raised the head of the bed so that the person was in a sitting position.	_____	_____	_____
11. Stood near the person's waist.	_____	_____	_____
12. Lowered the bed rail.	_____	_____	_____
13. Stood by the person's hips. Turned so that you faced the far corner of the foot of the bed.	_____	_____	_____
14. Stood with feet apart. The foot closest to the head of the bed was in front of the other foot.	_____	_____	_____
15. Placed one arm under the person's shoulders. Placed the other arm over the person's thighs.	_____	_____	_____
16. Pivoted toward the foot of the bed while moving the person's lower legs and feet over the side of the bed.	_____	_____	_____
17. Let the person's upper legs swing downward. Kept the trunk upright.	_____	_____	_____
18. Asked the person to hold onto the edge of the mattress.	_____	_____	_____
19. Did not leave the person alone. Provided support, if necessary.	_____	_____	_____
20. Asked how the person felt. Checked pulse and respirations. Helped the person lie down, if necessary.	_____	_____	_____
21. Reversed the procedure to return the person to bed.	_____	_____	_____
22. Lowered the head of the bed after the person returned to bed. Helped him or her move to the center of the bed.	_____	_____	_____

Post-Procedure

	S	U	Comments
23. Provided for comfort. Positioned the person in good body alignment.	___	___	_____
24. Placed the signal light within reach.	___	___	_____
25. Lowered the bed to its lowest position.	___	___	_____
26. Raised or lowered bed rails. Followed the care plan.	___	___	_____
27. Returned furniture to its proper place.	___	___	_____
28. Unscreened the person.	___	___	_____
29. Decontaminated hands.	___	___	_____
30. Reported the following to the nurse:			
• How well the activity was tolerated	___	___	_____
• The length of time the person dangled	___	___	_____
• Pulse and respiratory rates	___	___	_____
• The amount of assistance needed	___	___	_____
• Other observations or person's complaints	___	___	_____

Applying a Transfer Belt

Name: _____

Date: _____

Remember to:
- Knock before entering the person's room
- Address the person by name
- Introduce yourself by name and title

Procedure	S	U	Comments
1. Decontaminated hands.	____	____	_____
2. Identified the person.	____	____	_____
3. Explained the procedure to the person.	____	____	_____
4. Provided for privacy.	____	____	_____
5. Assisted the person to a sitting position.	____	____	_____
6. Applied the belt around the person's waist over clothing. Did not apply it over bare skin.	____	____	_____
7. Tightened the belt so that it was snug. It did not cause discomfort or impair breathing.	____	____	_____
8. Made sure that a woman's breasts were not caught under the belt.	____	____	_____
9. Placed the buckle off center in the front or in the back.	____	____	_____

Transferring the Person to a Chair or Wheelchair

QUALITY OF LIFE

Name: _____

Date: _____

Remember to:
- ● Knock before entering the person's room
- ● Address the person by name
- ● Introduce yourself by name and title

	S	U	Comments

Pre-Procedure

1. Explained the procedure to the person.   _____ _____ _____
2. Collected:
   - Wheelchair or armchair   _____ _____ _____
   - One or two bath blankets   _____ _____ _____
   - Robe and nonskid shoes   _____ _____ _____
   - Paper or sheet   _____ _____ _____
   - Transfer belt, if needed   _____ _____ _____
3. Decontaminated hands.   _____ _____ _____
4. Identified the person.   _____ _____ _____
5. Provided for privacy.   _____ _____ _____
6. Decided which side of the bed to use. Moved furniture to provide moving space.   _____ _____ _____

Procedure

7. Placed the chair at the head of the bed. The chair back was even with the headboard.   _____ _____ _____
8. Placed a cushion on the seat. Locked the wheelchair wheels and raised the footrests.   _____ _____ _____
9. Lowered the bed to its lowest position. Locked the bed wheels.   _____ _____ _____
10. Fanfolded top linens to the foot of the bed.   _____ _____ _____
11. Placed the paper or sheet under the person's feet. Put shoes on the person.   _____ _____ _____
12. Helped the person dangle. Made sure his or her feet touched the floor.   _____ _____ _____
13. Helped the person put on a robe.   _____ _____ _____
14. Applied the transfer belt, if needed.   _____ _____ _____
15. Helped the person stand. Used this method, if using a transfer belt:
    a. Stood in front of the person.   _____ _____ _____
    b. Had the person hold onto the mattress, or asked the person to place his or her fists on the bed by the thighs.   _____ _____ _____
    c. Made sure the person's feet were flat on the floor.   _____ _____ _____
    d. Had the person lean forward.   _____ _____ _____
    e. Grasped the transfer belt at each side.   _____ _____ _____

Procedure—cont'd   S   U   Comments

   f. Braced one knee against the person's knee. Blocked his or her foot with foot. ___ ___ _____

   g. Asked the person to push down on the mattress and to stand on the count of "3." Pulled the person into a standing position as you straightened your knees. ___ ___ _____

16. Used this method if a transfer belt was not used:

   a. Stood in front of the person. ___ ___ _____

   b. Had the person hold onto the mattress, or asked the person to place his or her fists on the bed by the thighs. ___ ___ _____

   c. Made sure the person's feet were flat on the floor. ___ ___ _____

   d. Placed hands under the person's arms. Hands were around the person's shoulder blades. ___ ___ _____

   e. Had the person lean forward. ___ ___ _____

   f. Braced one knee against the person's knee. Blocked his or her foot with your foot. Placed your other foot slightly behind you for balance. ___ ___ _____

   g. Asked the person to push down on the mattress and to stand on the count of "3." Pulled the person up into a standing position as you straightened your knees. ___ ___ _____

17. Supported the person in the standing position. Held the transfer belt or kept hands around the person's shoulder blades. Continued to block the person's feet and knees with your feet and knees. ___ ___ _____

18. Turned the person so that he or she could grasp the far arm of the chair. The person's legs touched the edge of the chair. ___ ___ _____

19. Continued to turn the person until the other armrest was grasped. ___ ___ _____

20. Lowered him or her into the chair as you bent your hips and knees. ___ ___ _____

21. Made sure the buttocks were to the back of the seat. ___ ___ _____

22. Positioned the person in good body alignment. ___ ___ _____

23. Positioned the person's feet on the wheelchair footrests. ___ ___ _____

24. Covered the person's lap and legs with a bath blanket. Kept the blanket off the floor and the wheels. ___ ___ _____

25. Removed the transfer belt, if used. ___ ___ _____

26. Positioned the chair as the person preferred. ___ ___ _____

Post-Procedure

27. Made sure the signal light and other necessary items were within reach. ___ ___ _____

28. Unscreened the person. ___ ___ _____

29. Decontaminated hands. ___ ___ _____

30. Reported the following to the nurse:

   • The pulse rate, if taken ___ ___ _____

   • How well the activity was tolerated ___ ___ _____

   • Complaints of lightheadedness, pain, discomfort, difficulty breathing, weakness, or fatigue ___ ___ _____

Transferring the Person From the Chair or Wheelchair to Bed

QUALITY OF LIFE

Remember to:
- Knock before entering the person's room
- Address the person by name
- Introduce yourself by name and title

Name: _____

Date: _____

Pre-Procedure

	S	U	Comments
1. Followed Delegation Guidelines.	___	___	_____
2. Explained the procedure to the person.	___	___	_____
3. Collected:			
• Paper or sheet	___	___	_____
• Transfer belt, if needed	___	___	_____
4. Decontaminated hands.	___	___	_____
5. Identified the person, checked the identification bracelet against the assignment sheet. Called the person by name.	___	___	_____
6. Provided for privacy.	___	___	_____

Procedure

	S	U	Comments
7. Moved furniture for moving space.	___	___	_____
8. Raised the head of the bed to a sitting position, making sure bed was in lowest position.	___	___	_____
9. Moved the signal light to the strong side when the person was in bed.	___	___	_____
10. Positioned chair or wheelchair so person's strong side was next to bed.	___	___	_____
11. Locked wheelchair wheels and made sure bed wheels were locked.	___	___	_____
12. Removed and folded lap blanket.	___	___	_____
13. Removed person's feet from footrests, raised footrests, and removed or swung footrests out of way.	___	___	_____
14. Applied transfer belt, if needed.	___	___	_____
15. Made sure person's feet were flat on floor.	___	___	_____
16. Stood in front of the person.	___	___	_____
17. Asked the person to hold armrests, or placed your arms under person's arms. Placed arms around shoulder blades.	___	___	_____
18. Had person lean forward.	___	___	_____
19. Grasped transfer belt on each side, if used.	___	___	_____
20. Braced your knees against person's knees, blocked his or her feet with your feet, or used your knee and foot of one leg to block person's weak foot. Placed your other foot slightly behind you for balance.	___	___	_____
21. Asked person to push down on armrests on count of "3," pulled person into standing position as you straighten your knees.	___	___	_____

Procedure—cont'd

	S	U	Comments

22. Supported person in standing position, held transfer belt or kept hands around person's shoulder blades. Continued to block person's feet and knees with your feet and knees.

23. Turned person so he or she can reach edge of mattress, with person's legs touching the mattress.

24. Continued to turn person until he or she could reach mattress with both hands.

25. Lowered person onto the bed while bending your hips and knees and person leaning forward bending elbows and knees.

26. Removed transfer belt.

27. Removed robe and shoes.

28. Helped person lie down.

Post-Procedure

29. Provided comfort. Covered the person as needed.

30. Placed signal light and other necessary items within reach.

31. Arranged room furniture to meet the person's needs.

32. Unscreened the person.

33. Decontaminated your hands.

34. Reported and recording your observations.

Transferring the Person to a Wheelchair With Assistance

QUALITY OF LIFE

Remember to:
- Knock before entering the person's room
- Address the person by name
- Introduce yourself by name and title

Name: _____

Date: _____

Pre-Procedure

	S	U	Comments

1. Asked a co-worker to help.
2. Explained the procedure to the person.
3. Collected:
   - Wheelchair with removable armrests
   - Bath blankets
   - Shoes
   - Cushion, if used
4. Decontaminated hands.
5. Identified the person.
6. Provided for privacy.
7. Decided which side of the bed to use. Moved furniture to provide moving space.

Procedure

8. Fanfolded top linens to the foot of the bed.
9. Assisted the person to the near side of the bed. Helped him or her to a sitting position by raising the head of the bed.
10. Placed the wheelchair at the side of the bed, even with the person's hips.
11. Removed the armrest near the bed. Places the cushion or a folded bath blanket on the seat.
12. Locked wheelchair and bed wheels.
13. Stood behind the wheelchair. Put arms under the person's arms and grasped the person's forearms.
14. Had co-worker grasp the person's thighs and calves.
15. Brought the person toward the chair on the count of "3." Lowered him or her into the chair.
16. Made sure the person's buttocks were to the back of the seat. Positioned the person in good alignment.
17. Replaced the armrest back on the wheelchair.
18. Put the shoes on the person. Positioned the person's feet on the footrests.
19. Covered the person's lap and legs with a blanket. Kept the blanket off the floor and wheels.
20. Positioned the chair as the person preferred.

Post-Procedure

	S	U	Comments

21. Made sure the signal light and other necessary items were within reach.

22. Unscreened the person.

23. Decontaminated hands.

24. Reported the following to the nurse:

   • Pulse rate, if taken

   • Complaints of lightheadedness, pain, discomfort, difficulty breathing, weakness, or fatigue

   • How well the activity was tolerated

25. Reversed the procedure to return the person to bed.

Transferring the Person Using a Mechanical Lift

QUALITY OF LIFE

Remember to:
- Knock before entering the person's room
- Address the person by name
- Introduce yourself by name and title

Name: _____

Date: _____

Pre-Procedure

	S	U	Comments
1. Asked a co-worker to help.	___	___	_____
2. Explained the procedure to the person.	___	___	_____
3. Collected:			
• Mechanical lift	___	___	_____
• Armchair or wheelchair	___	___	_____
• Slippers	___	___	_____
• Bath blanket or cushion	___	___	_____
4. Decontaminated hands.	___	___	_____
5. Identified the person.	___	___	_____
6. Provided for privacy.	___	___	_____

Procedure

	S	U	Comments
7. Centered the sling under the person. Turned person from side to side to position the sling.	___	___	_____
8. Placed the chair at the head of the bed, even with the headboard and about 1 foot away from the bed. Placed a folded bath blanket or cushion in the chair.	___	___	_____
9. Locked the bed wheels and lowered the bed to its lowest position.	___	___	_____
10. Raised the lift so that it could be positioned over the person.	___	___	_____
11. Positioned the lift over the person.	___	___	_____
12. Locked the lift wheels in position.	___	___	_____
13. Attached the sling to the swivel bar.	___	___	_____
14. Raised the head of the bed to a sitting position.	___	___	_____
15. Crossed the person's arms over the chest. Let him or her hold onto the straps or chains, but not the swivel bar.	___	___	_____
16. Pumped the lift high enough until the person and sling were free of the bed.	___	___	_____
17. Asked co-worker to support the person's legs as you moved the lift and person away from the bed.	___	___	_____
18. Positioned the lift so that the person's back was toward the chair.	___	___	_____
19. Lowered the person into the chair.	___	___	_____
20. Lowered the swivel bar to unhook the sling. Left the sling under the person, unless otherwise indicated.	___	___	_____
21. Put footwear on the person. Positioned the person's feet on wheelchair footrests.	___	___	_____
22. Covered the person's lap and legs with a blanket. Kept the blanket off the floor and wheels.	___	___	_____

Procedure—cont'd   S   U   Comments

23. Positioned the chair as the person prefers.   _____ _____ _____

24. Placed the signal light and other necessary items within reach.   _____ _____ _____

25. Decontaminated hands.   _____ _____ _____

26. Reported the following to the nurse:

    • The pulse rate, if taken   _____ _____ _____

    • Complaints of lightheadedness, pain, discomfort, difficulty   _____ _____ _____
      breathing, weakness, or fatigue

    • How well the activity was tolerated   _____ _____ _____

27. Reversed the procedure to return the person to bed.   _____ _____ _____

Transferring a Person to and From the Toilet

QUALITY OF LIFE

Name: _____

Date: _____

Remember to:
- Knock before entering the person's room
- Address the person by name
- Introduce yourself by name and title

Pre-Procedure

	S	U	Comments
1. Made sure the person had an elevated toilet seat.	____	____	_____
2. Checked grab bars by toilet. If loose, did not transfer person and told nurse.	____	____	_____

Procedure

	S	U	Comments
3. Had person wear nonskid footwear.	____	____	_____
4. Positioned wheelchair next to toilet. If not enough room, positioned wheelchair at a right angle to the toilet with person's strong side near the toilet.	____	____	_____
5. Locked wheelchair brakes.	____	____	_____
6. Raised foot rests, removing or swinging them out of the way.	____	____	_____
7. Applied transfer belt.	____	____	_____
8. Helped person unfasten clothing.	____	____	_____
9. Used transfer belt to help person stand and turn to toilet.	____	____	_____
10. Supported person with transfer belt while person lowered clothing. Or had person hold grab bars for support. Lowered person's pants and undergarment.	____	____	_____
11. Used transfer belt to lower person onto toilet seat.	____	____	_____
12. Removed transfer belt.	____	____	_____
13. Told person you would be near by. Reminded person to use signal light or call for help.	____	____	_____
14. Closed bathroom door.	____	____	_____
15. Stayed near bathroom, completing other tasks in person's room.	____	____	_____
16. Knocked on bathroom door after person called.	____	____	_____
17. Helped with wiping, perineal care, flushing, and hand hygiene as needed.	____	____	_____
18. Applied transfer belt.	____	____	_____
19. Used transfer belt to help person stand.	____	____	_____
20. Helped person raise and secure clothing.	____	____	_____
21. Used transfer belt to transfer person to the wheelchair.	____	____	_____
22. Made sure person's buttocks were to back of seat. Positioned person in good alignment.	____	____	_____
23. Positioned person's feet on footrests.	____	____	_____
24. Covered person's lap and legs with blanket. Kept blanket off floor and wheels.	____	____	_____
25. Positioned chair. Locked wheelchair wheels.	____	____	_____

Post-Procedure

	S	U	Comments
26. Placed signal light and necessary items within reach.	_____	_____	_____
27. Unscreened person.	_____	_____	_____
28. Decontaminated hands.	_____	_____	_____
29. Reported and recorded observations.	_____	_____	_____

Transferring the Person to a Stretcher

QUALITY OF LIFE

Remember to:
- Knock before entering the person's room
- Address the person by name
- Introduce yourself by name and title

Name: _____

Date: _____

Pre-Procedure

	S	U	Comments
1. Asked two co-workers to help.	___	___	_____
2. Explained the procedure to the person.	___	___	_____
3. Collected:			
• Stretcher covered with a sheet or bath blanket	___	___	_____
• Bath blanket	___	___	_____
• Pillows, if needed	___	___	_____
4. Decontaminated hands.	___	___	_____
5. Identified the person.	___	___	_____
6. Provided for privacy.	___	___	_____
7. Raised the bed to its highest level.	___	___	_____

Procedure

	S	U	Comments
8. Covered the person with a bath blanket. Fanfolded top linens to the foot of the bed.	___	___	_____
9. Loosened the cotton drawsheet on each side.	___	___	_____
10. Lowered the head of the bed so it was as flat as possible.	___	___	_____
11. Lowered the bed rail on the side to which the person would be moved.	___	___	_____
12. Asked co-workers to help move the person to the side of the bed. Used the drawsheet.	___	___	_____
13. Went to the other side of the bed. Lowered the bed rail. Protected the person from falling by holding the far arm and leg.	___	___	_____
14. Had co-workers position the stretcher next to the bed and stood behind the stretcher.	___	___	_____
15. Locked bed and stretcher wheels.	___	___	_____
16. Rolled up and grasped the drawsheet at the hip and mid-chest levels.	___	___	_____
17. Asked co-workers to roll up and grasp the drawsheet.	___	___	_____
18. Transferred the person to the stretcher on the count of "3" by lifting and pulling him or her. Made sure the person was centered on the stretcher.	___	___	_____
19. Placed a pillow or pillows under the person's head and shoulders, if allowed.	___	___	_____
20. Covered the person. Provided for comfort.	___	___	_____
21. Fastened safety straps. Raised the rails.	___	___	_____
22. Unlocked the stretcher's wheels. Transported the person.	___	___	_____

Post-Procedure

	S	U	Comments
23. Decontaminated hands.	_____	_____	_____
24. Reported the following to the nurse:			
• The time of the transport	_____	_____	_____
• Where the person was transported	_____	_____	_____
• Who went with him or her	_____	_____	_____
• How the transfer was tolerated	_____	_____	_____
25. Reversed the procedure to return the person to bed.	_____	_____	_____

Making a Closed Bed

QUALITY OF LIFE

Remember to:
- Knock before entering the person's room
- Address the person by name
- Introduce yourself by name and title

Name: _____

Date: _____

Pre-Procedure

	S	U	Comments
1. Decontaminated hands.	___	___	_____
2. Collected clean linen:			
• Mattress pad	___	___	_____
• Bottom sheet	___	___	_____
• Plastic drawsheet (optional)	___	___	_____
• Cotton drawsheet	___	___	_____
• Top sheet	___	___	_____
• Blanket	___	___	_____
• Bedspread	___	___	_____
• Two pillowcases	___	___	_____
• Bath towel(s)	___	___	_____
• Hand towel	___	___	_____
• Washcloth	___	___	_____
• Hospital gown	___	___	_____
• Bath blanket	___	___	_____
3. Placed linen on a clean surface.	___	___	_____
4. Raised the bed for good body mechanics.	___	___	_____
5. Made sure the bed and bed frame were cleaned if the person was discharged. Rolled linen away from you so that the surface touched by the person was inside the roll. Wore gloves if linens were soiled. Removed and discarded gloves after removing soiled linen. Decontaminated hands.	___	___	_____

Procedure

	S	U	Comments
6. Moved the mattress to the head of the bed.	___	___	_____
7. Put the mattress pad on the mattress. It was even with the top of the mattress.	___	___	_____
8. Placed the bottom sheet on the mattress pad:			
a. Unfolded it lengthwise.	___	___	_____
b. Placed the center crease in the middle of the bed.	___	___	_____
c. Positioned the lower edge even with the bottom of the mattress.	___	___	_____
d. Placed the large hem at the top and the small hem at the bottom.	___	___	_____
e. Faced hemstitching downward.	___	___	_____
9. Picked the sheet up from the side to open it. Fanfolded it toward the other side of the bed.	___	___	_____

Procedure—cont'd   S   U   Comments

10. Went to the head of the bed. Tucked the top of the sheet under the mattress. Made sure the sheet was tight and smooth. _____ _____ _____

11. Made a mitered corner. _____ _____ _____

12. Placed the plastic drawsheet on the bed about 14 inches from the top of the mattress. _____ _____ _____

13. Opened the plastic drawsheet and fanfolded it toward the other side of the bed. _____ _____ _____

14. Placed a cotton drawsheet over the plastic drawsheet. It covered the entire plastic drawsheet. _____ _____ _____

15. Opened the cotton drawsheet and fanfolded it toward the other side of the bed. _____ _____ _____

16. Tucked both drawsheets under the mattress, or tucked each in separately. _____ _____ _____

17. Went to the other side of the bed. _____ _____ _____

18. Mitered the top corner of the bottom sheet. _____ _____ _____

19. Pulled the bottom sheet tight so that there were no wrinkles. Tucked in the sheet. _____ _____ _____

20. Pulled the drawsheets tight so that there were no wrinkles. Tucked both in together or pulled each tight and tucked them in separately. _____ _____ _____

21. Went to the other side of the bed. _____ _____ _____

22. Put the top sheet on the bed:
    a. Unfolded it lengthwise. _____ _____ _____
    b. Placed the center crease in the middle. _____ _____ _____
    c. Placed the large hem at the top, even with the top of the mattress. _____ _____ _____
    d. Opened the sheet and fanfolded the extra part toward the other side. _____ _____ _____
    e. Faced hem with stitching outward. _____ _____ _____

23. Placed the blanket on the bed:
    a. Unfolded it so that the center crease was in the middle. _____ _____ _____
    b. Put the upper hem about 6 to 8 inches from the top of the mattress. _____ _____ _____
    c. Opened the blanket and fanfolded the extra part toward the other side. _____ _____ _____
    d. If steps 28 and 29 would not be done, turned the top sheet down over the blanket. Hemstitching was down. _____ _____ _____

24. Placed the bedspread on the bed:
    a. Unfolded it so that the center crease was in the middle. _____ _____ _____
    b. Placed the upper hem even with the top of the mattress. _____ _____ _____
    c. Opened the bedspread and fanfolded the extra part toward the other side. _____ _____ _____
    d. Made sure the bedspread facing the door was even and covered all the top linens. _____ _____ _____

25. Tucked in top linens together at the foot of the bed so that they were smooth and tight. Made a mitered corner. _____ _____ _____

Procedure—cont'd	S	U	Comments

26. Went to the other side of the bed. ____ ____ _____

27. Straightened all top linens, working from the head of the bed to the foot. ____ ____ _____

28. Tucked in the top linens together. Made a mitered corner. ____ ____ _____

29. Turned the top hem of the bedspread under the blanket to make a cuff. ____ ____ _____

30. Turned the top sheet down over the spread. Hemstitching was down. ____ ____ _____

31. Placed the pillow on the bed. ____ ____ _____

32. Opened the pillowcase so that it was flat on the bed. ____ ____ _____

33. Put the pillowcase on. Folded extra pillowcase material under the pillow at the seam end of the pillowcase. ____ ____ _____

34. Placed the pillow on the bed so that the open end was away from the door. The seam of the pillowcase was toward the head of the bed. ____ ____ _____

Post-Procedure

35. Attached the signal light to the bed. ____ ____ _____

36. Lowered the bed to its lowest position. ____ ____ _____

37. Put towels, washcloth, gown, and bath blanket in the bedside stand. ____ ____ _____

38. Decontaminated hands. ____ ____ _____

Making an Open Bed

QUALITY OF LIFE

Name: _____

Date: _____

Remember to:
- ● Knock before entering the person's room
- ● Address the person by name
- ● Introduce yourself by name and title

Procedure	**S**	**U**	**Comments**
1. Decontaminated hands.	_____	_____	_____
2. Collected linen for a closed bed.	_____	_____	_____
3. Made a closed bed.	_____	_____	_____
4. Fanfolded top linens to the foot of the bed.	_____	_____	_____
5. Attached the signal light to the bed.	_____	_____	_____
6. Lowered the bed to its lowest position.	_____	_____	_____
7. Put towels, washcloth, gown, and bath blanket in the bedside stand.	_____	_____	_____
8. Disposed of dirty linen properly.	_____	_____	_____
9. Decontaminated hands.	_____	_____	_____

Making an Occupied Bed

QUALITY OF LIFE

Remember to: ● Knock before entering the person's room
               ● Address the person by name
               ● Introduce yourself by name and title

Name: _____

Date: _____

Pre-Procedure	S	U	Comments

1. Explained the procedure to the person.   ___ ___ _____
2. Decontaminated hands.   ___ ___ _____
3. Collected the following:
   • Gloves   ___ ___ _____
   • Linen bag   ___ ___ _____
   • Clean linen   ___ ___ _____
4. Placed linen on a clean surface.   ___ ___ _____
5. Provided for privacy.   ___ ___ _____
6. Removed the signal light.   ___ ___ _____
7. Raised the bed for good body mechanics. Made sure the bed rails were up.   ___ ___ _____
8. Lowered the head of the bed to an appropriate working level. It was as flat as possible.   ___ ___ _____
9. Lowered the bed rail near you.   ___ ___ _____
10. Put on gloves.   ___ ___ _____
11. Loosened top linens at the foot of the bed.   ___ ___ _____
12. Removed the bedspread and blanket separately. Folded them as if they would be reused.   ___ ___ _____
13. Covered the person with a bath blanket:
    a. Unfolded a bath blanket over the top sheet.   ___ ___ _____
    b. Asked the person to hold onto the bath blanket. If he or she could not, tucked the top part under the person's shoulders.   ___ ___ _____
    c. Grasped the top sheet under the bath blanket at the shoulders. Brought the sheet down to the foot of the bed. Removed the sheet from under the blanket.   ___ ___ _____

Procedure

14. Moved the mattress to the head of the bed.   ___ ___ _____
15. Positioned the person on the side of the bed away from you. Moved the pillow to the far side of the bed. Adjusted the pillow for the person's comfort.   ___ ___ _____
16. Loosened bottom linens from the head to the foot of the bed.   ___ ___ _____
17. Fanfolded bottom linens one at a time toward the person: cotton drawsheet, plastic drawsheet, bottom sheet, and mattress pad. Did not fanfold the mattress pad if it was to be reused.   ___ ___ _____
18. Placed a clean mattress pad on the bed. Unfolded it lengthwise so that the center crease was in the middle. Fanfolded the top part toward the person. If reusing mattress pad, straightened and smoothed any wrinkles.   ___ ___ _____

Procedure—cont'd

	S	U	Comments

19. Placed the bottom sheet on the mattress pad so that hemstitching was away from the person. Unfolded the sheet so that the crease was in the middle. The small hem was even with the bottom of the mattress. Fanfolded the top part toward the person.

20. Made a mitered corner at the head of the bed. Tucked the sheet under the mattress from the head to the foot.

21. Pulled the fanfolded plastic drawsheet back toward self over the bottom sheet. Tucked excess material under the mattress. Did the following if using a clean plastic drawsheet:

   a. Placed the plastic drawsheet on the bed about 14 inches from the mattress top.

   b. Fanfolded the top part toward the person.

   c. Tucked in the excess material.

22. Placed the cotton drawsheet over the plastic drawsheet. It covered the entire plastic drawsheet. Fanfolded the top part toward the person. Tucked in excess material.

23. Raised the bed rail. Went to the other side and lowered the bed rail.

24. Positioned the person on the side of the bed away from you. Explained that he or she would roll over a bump. As you rolled the person, you assured the person that he or she would not fall. Adjusted the pillow for the person's comfort.

25. Loosened bottom linens. Removed soiled linen one piece at a time. Removed and discarded the gloves.

26. Straightened and smoothed the mattress pad.

27. Pulled the clean bottom sheet toward self. Made a mitered corner at the top. Tucked the sheet under the mattress from the head to the foot of the bed.

28. Pulled the drawsheets tightly toward self. Tucked both under together or tucked each in separately.

29. Positioned the person supine in the center of the bed. Adjusted the pillow for comfort.

30. Put the top sheet on the bed. Unfolded it lengthwise. Made sure the crease was in the middle, the large hem was even with the top of the mattress, and hemstitching was on the outside.

31. Asked the person to hold onto the top sheet while removing the bath blanket. If the person could not do so, tucked the top sheet under the person's shoulders.

32. Placed the blanket on the bed. Unfolded it so that the crease was in the middle. Unfolded the blanket so that it covered the person. The upper hem was 6 to 8 inches from the top of the mattress.

33. Placed the bedspread on the bed. Unfolded it so that the center crease was in the middle and it covered the person. The top hem was even with the mattress top.

Procedure—cont'd

	S	U	Comments
34. Turned the top hem of the bedspread under the blanket to make a cuff.			
35. Brought the top sheet down over the bedspread to form a cuff.			
36. Went to the foot of the bed.			
37. Lifted the mattress corner with one arm. Tucked all top linens under the mattress together. Made sure linens were loose enough to allow for movement of the person's feet. Made a mitered corner.			
38. Raised the bed rail. Went to the other side and lowered the bed rail.			
39. Straightened and smoothed top linens.			
40. Tucked the top linens under the mattress as in step 37. Made a mitered corner.			
41. Changed the pillowcase(s).			
42. Placed the signal light within reach.			
43. Raised or lowered bed rails. Followed the care plan.			

Post-Procedure

	S	U	Comments
44. Raised the head of the bed to a level appropriate for the person. Made sure the person was comfortable.			
45. Lowered the bed to its lowest position.			
46. Placed towels, washcloth, gown, and bath blanket in the bedside stand.			
47. Unscreened the person. Thanked him or her for cooperating.			
48. Followed center policy for dirty linen.			
49. Decontaminated hands.			

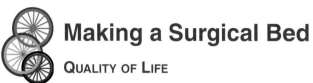

Making a Surgical Bed

QUALITY OF LIFE

Remember to:
- Knock before entering the person's room
- Address the person by name
- Introduce yourself by name and title

Name: _____

Date: _____

Pre-Procedure	S	U	Comments
1. Decontaminated hands.	___	___	_____
2. Collected the following:			
• Clean linen	___	___	_____
• IV pole	___	___	_____
• Tissues	___	___	_____
• Kidney basin	___	___	_____
• Gloves	___	___	_____
• Laundry bag	___	___	_____
• Other equipment as requested by the nurse	___	___	_____
3. Placed linen on a clean surface.	___	___	_____
4. Removed the signal light.	___	___	_____
5. Raised the bed for good body mechanics.	___	___	_____

Procedure

	S	U	Comments
6. Removed all linen from the bed. Wore gloves as needed.	___	___	_____
7. Made a closed bed. Did not tuck the top linens under the mattress.	___	___	_____
8. Folded all top linens at the foot of the bed back onto the bed. The fold was even with the edge of the mattress.	___	___	_____
9. Fanfolded linen lengthwise to the side of the bed farthest from the door.	___	___	_____
10. Put the pillowcase(s) on the pillow(s).	___	___	_____
11. Placed the pillow(s) on a clean surface.	___	___	_____
12. Left the bed in its highest position.	___	___	_____
13. Made sure both bed rails were down.	___	___	_____

Post-Procedure

	S	U	Comments
14. Put the towels, washcloth, gown, and bath blanket in the bedside stand.	___	___	_____
15. Placed the tissues and the kidney basin on the bedside stand. Placed the IV pole near the head of the bed.	___	___	_____
16. Moved all furniture away from the bed. Allowed enough room for the stretcher and staff.	___	___	_____
17. Did not attach the signal light to the bed.	___	___	_____
18. Followed center policy for soiled linen.	___	___	_____
19. Decontaminated hands.	___	___	_____

Assisting the Person to Brush the Teeth

QUALITY OF LIFE

Remember to:
- Knock before entering the person's room
- Address the person by name
- Introduce yourself by name and title

Name: _____

Date: _____

	S	U	Comments

Pre-Procedure

1. Explained the procedure to the person.   ___ ___ _____
2. Decontaminated hands.   ___ ___ _____
3. Collected the following:
   - Toothbrush   ___ ___ _____
   - Toothpaste or dentifrice   ___ ___ _____
   - Mouthwash   ___ ___ _____
   - Water glass with cool water   ___ ___ _____
   - Straw   ___ ___ _____
   - Kidney basin   ___ ___ _____
   - Face towel   ___ ___ _____
   - Paper towels   ___ ___ _____
4. Placed the paper towels on the overbed table. Arranged items on top of them.   ___ ___ _____
5. Identified the person.   ___ ___ _____
6. Provided for privacy.   ___ ___ _____
7. Raised the person's head.   ___ ___ _____

Procedure

8. Lowered the bed rail, if used.   ___ ___ _____
9. Placed the towel over the person's chest.   ___ ___ _____
10. Placed the overbed table in front of the person. Adjusted table height for the person.   ___ ___ _____
11. Allowed the person to perform oral hygiene.   ___ ___ _____
12. Removed the towel when the person was done.   ___ ___ _____
13. Moved the overbed table next to the bed. Lowered it to a level appropriate for the person.   ___ ___ _____

Post-Procedure

14. Provided for comfort.   ___ ___ _____
15. Placed the signal light within reach.   ___ ___ _____
16. Raised or lowered the bed rails. Followed the care plan.   ___ ___ _____
17. Cleaned and returned items to their proper place. Wore gloves for this step   ___ ___ _____
18. Wiped off overbed table with paper towels and discarded them.   ___ ___ _____
19. Unscreened the person.   ___ ___ _____
20. Followed center policy for dirty linen.   ___ ___ _____
21. Decontaminated hands.   ___ ___ _____
22. Reported observations to the nurse.   ___ ___ _____

Brushing the Person's Teeth

QUALITY OF LIFE

Remember to:
- Knock before entering the person's room
- Address the person by name
- Introduce yourself by name and title

Name: _____

Date: _____

Pre-Procedure

	S	U	Comments

1. Explained the procedure to the person.
2. Decontaminated hands.
3. Collected the following:
   - Toothbrush
   - Toothpaste or dentifrice
   - Mouthwash
   - Floss
   - Water glass with cool water
   - Straw
   - Kidney basin
   - Face towel
   - Paper towels
4. Placed the paper towels on the overbed table. Arranged items on top of them.
5. Identified the person.
6. Provided for privacy.
7. Raised the bed to the best level for good body mechanics.

Procedure

8. Lowered the bed rail near you.
9. Raised the head of the bed. If the person could not sit up, positioned in a sidelying position on the side near you.
10. Placed the towel over the person's chest.
11. Positioned the overbed table within easy reach. Adjusted the height as needed.
12. Put on the gloves.
13. Applied toothpaste to the toothbrush.
14. Held the toothbrush over the kidney basin. Poured some water over the brush.
15. Brushed the person's teeth gently.
16. Brushed the person's tongue gently, if needed.
17. Let the person rinse the mouth with water. Held the kidney basin under the person's chin.
18. Flossed the person's teeth.
19. Let the person use mouthwash or other specified solution. Held the kidney basin under the person's chin.
20. Removed the towel when done.
21. Removed and discarded the gloves.

Post-Procedure   S   U   **Comments**

22. Provided for comfort.

23. Placed the signal light within reach.

24. Lowered the bed to its lowest position.

25. Raised or lowered bed rails. Followed the care plan.

26. Cleaned and returned equipment to its proper place. Wore gloves for this step.

27. Wiped off the overbed table with the paper towels and discarded them.

28. Lowered the overbed table to a level appropriate for the person.

29. Unscreened the person.

30. Followed center policy for dirty linen.

31. Decontaminated hands.

32. Reported observations to the nurse.

Flossing the Person's Teeth

QUALITY OF LIFE

Remember to: ● Knock before entering the person's room
               ● Address the person by name
               ● Introduce yourself by name and title

Name: _____

Date: _____

Pre-Procedure

	S	U	Comments
1. Explained the procedure to the person.	___	___	_____
2. Decontaminated hands.	___	___	_____
3. Collected the following:			
• Kidney basin	___	___	_____
• Water glass with cool water	___	___	_____
• Dental floss	___	___	_____
• Face towel	___	___	_____
• Paper towels	___	___	_____
• Gloves	___	___	_____
4. Placed the paper towels on the overbed table. Arranged items on top of them.	___	___	_____
5. Identified the person.	___	___	_____
6. Provided for privacy.	___	___	_____
7. Raised the bed to the best level for good body mechanics. Made sure bed rails were up.	___	___	_____

Procedure

	S	U	Comments
8. Lowered the bed rail near you.			
9. Raised the head of the bed so that the person could sit comfortably. If the person could not sit up, positioned him or her in a sidelying position near you.	___	___	_____
10. Placed the towel over the person's chest.	___	___	_____
11. Positioned the overbed table within easy reach. Adjusted the height as needed.	___	___	_____
12. Put on the gloves.	___	___	_____
13. Broke off an 18-inch piece of floss from the dispenser.	___	___	_____
14. Held the floss between the middle fingers of each hand.	___	___	_____
15. Stretched the floss with thumbs.	___	___	_____
16. Started at the upper back tooth on the right side and worked around to the left side.	___	___	_____
17. Moved the floss gently up and down between the teeth. Moved floss up and down from the top of the crown to the gum line.	___	___	_____
18. Moved to a new section of floss after every second tooth.	___	___	_____
19. Flossed the lower teeth. Held the floss with index fingers. Used up and down motions and went under the gums as for the upper teeth. Started on the right side and worked around to the left side.	___	___	_____

Procedure—cont'd   S   U   **Comments**

20. Let the person rinse his or her mouth. Held the kidney basin _____ _____ _____
    under the chin. Repeated rinsing as necessary.

21. Removed the towel when done.   _____ _____ _____

22. Removed and discarded the gloves.   _____ _____ _____

Post-Procedure

23. Provided for comfort.   _____ _____ _____

24. Placed the signal light within reach.   _____ _____ _____

25. Lowered the bed to its lowest position.   _____ _____ _____

26. Raised or lowered bed rails. Followed the care plan. _____ _____ _____

27. Cleaned and returned equipment to its proper place. Wore _____ _____ _____
    gloves for this step.

28. Wiped off the overbed table with the paper towels and discarded _____ _____ _____
    them.

29. Lowered the overbed table to a level appropriate for the person. _____ _____ _____

30. Unscreened the person.   _____ _____ _____

31. Followed center policy for dirty linen.   _____ _____ _____

32. Decontaminated hands.   _____ _____ _____

33. Reported observations to the nurse.   _____ _____ _____

Providing Mouth Care for an Unconscious Person

QUALITY OF LIFE

Remember to: ● Knock before entering the person's room
              ● Address the person by name
              ● Introduce yourself by name and title

Name: _____

Date: _____

Pre-Procedure	S	U	Comments
1. Decontaminated hands.	_____	_____	_____
2. Collected the following:			
• Cleaning agent (checked the care plan)	_____	_____	_____
• Sponge swabs	_____	_____	_____
• Padded tongue blade	_____	_____	_____
• Water glass with cool water	_____	_____	_____
• Face towel	_____	_____	_____
• Kidney basin	_____	_____	_____
• Lubricant for lips	_____	_____	_____
• Paper towels	_____	_____	_____
• Gloves	_____	_____	_____
3. Placed the paper towels on the overbed table. Arranged items on top of them.	_____	_____	_____
4. Identified the person.	_____	_____	_____
5. Explained the procedure to the person.	_____	_____	_____
6. Provided for privacy.	_____	_____	_____
7. Raised the bed to the best level for good body mechanics. Made sure bed rails were up.	_____	_____	_____

Procedure

	S	U	Comments
8. Lowered the bed rail near you.	_____	_____	_____
9. Put on the gloves.	_____	_____	_____
10. Positioned the person in a sidelying position on the side toward you. Turned his or her head well to the side.	_____	_____	_____
11. Placed the towel under the person's face.	_____	_____	_____
12. Placed the kidney basin under the chin.	_____	_____	_____
13. Positioned the overbed table within easy reach. Adjusted the height as needed.	_____	_____	_____
14. Separated the upper and lower teeth with the padded tongue blade. Did not use force. Asked the nurse for assistance if you had problems.	_____	_____	_____
15. Cleansed the mouth. Used the sponge swabs moistened with the cleaning agent.	_____	_____	_____
a. Cleaned the chewing and inner surfaces of the teeth.	_____	_____	_____
b. Cleaned the outer surfaces of the teeth.	_____	_____	_____
c. Swabbed the roof of the mouth, inside of the cheeks, and the lips.	_____	_____	_____
d. Swabbed the tongue.	_____	_____	_____

Procedure—cont'd	S	U	Comments
e. Moistened a clean swab with water and swabbed the mouth to rinse.	_____	_____	_____
f. Placed used swabs in the kidney basin.	_____	_____	_____
16. Applied lubricant to the lips.	_____	_____	_____
17. Removed the towel.	_____	_____	_____
18. Removed and discarded the gloves.	_____	_____	_____
19. Explained that the procedure was done and that the person would be repositioned.	_____	_____	_____
20. Repositioned the person.	_____	_____	_____
21. Raised the bed rail. Made sure both bed rails were up.	_____	_____	_____

Post-Procedure

	S	U	Comments
22. Placed the signal light within reach.	_____	_____	_____
23. Lowered the bed to its lowest position.	_____	_____	_____
24. Cleaned and returned equipment to its proper place. Discarded disposable items.	_____	_____	_____
25. Unscreened the person.	_____	_____	_____
26. Told the person that you were leaving the room.	_____	_____	_____
27. Followed center policy for dirty linen.	_____	_____	_____
28. Decontaminated hands.	_____	_____	_____
29. Reported observations to the nurse.	_____	_____	_____

Providing Denture Care

QUALITY OF LIFE

Remember to:
- Knock before entering the person's room
- Address the person by name
- Introduce yourself by name and title

Name: _____

Date: _____

	S	U	Comments

Pre-Procedure

1. Explained the procedure to the person.
2. Decontaminated hands.
3. Collected the following:
   - Denture brush or toothbrush
   - Denture cup labeled with the person's name and room number
   - Denture cleaner or toothpaste
   - Water glass with cool water
   - Straw
   - Mouthwash (or other specified solution)
   - Kidney basin
   - Two face towels
   - Gauze squares
   - Gloves
4. Identified the person.
5. Provided for privacy.

Procedure

6. Lowered the bed rail (if used).
7. Placed a towel over the person's chest.
8. Put on the gloves.
9. Asked the person to remove the dentures. Carefully placed them in the kidney basin.
10. Removed the dentures using gauze if person could not do so.
    a. Grasped the upper denture with thumb and index finger. Moved the denture up and down slightly to break the seal. Gently removed the denture once the seal was broken. Placed it in the kidney basin.
    b. Removed the lower denture by grasping it with thumb and forefinger. Turned it slightly and lifted it out of the person's mouth. Placed it in the kidney basin.
11. Followed the care plan for raising bed rails.
12. Took the kidney basin, denture cup, brush, and denture cleaner or toothpaste to the sink.
13. Lined the sink with a towel and filled it with water.
14. Rinsed each denture under warm running water. Returned them to the denture cup.
15. Applied denture cleaner or toothpaste to the brush.
16. Brushed the dentures.

Procedure—cont'd | S | U | Comments

17. Rinsed dentures under cool running water. Handled them carefully.

18. Placed them in the denture cup. Filled it with cool water until the dentures were covered.

19. Cleaned the kidney basin.

20. Brought the denture cup and kidney basin to the bedside table.

21. Lowered the bed rail if up.

22. Positioned the person for oral hygiene.

23. Assisted the person to rinse his or her mouth with mouthwash (or specified solution). Held the kidney basin under the chin.

24. Asked the person to insert the dentures. Inserted them if the person could not.

    a. Grasped the upper denture firmly with thumb and index finger. Raised the upper lip with the other hand and inserted the denture. Used index fingers to gently press on the denture to make sure it was securely in place.

    b. Grasped the lower denture securely with thumb and index finger. Pulled down slightly on the lower lip and inserted the denture. Gently pressed down on it to make sure it was in place.

25. Put the denture cup in the top drawer of the bedside stand if the dentures were not reinserted.

26. Removed the towel.

27. Removed the gloves.

Post-Procedure

28. Provided for comfort.

29. Placed the signal light within reach.

30. Raised or lowered bed rails. Followed the care plan.

31. Unscreened the person.

32. Cleaned and returned equipment to its proper place. Discarded disposable items. Wore gloves for this step.

33. Disposed of dirty linens.

34. Decontaminated hands.

35. Reported observations to the nurse.

Giving a Complete Bed Bath

QUALITY OF LIFE

Remember to: ● Knock before entering the person's room
               ● Address the person by name
               ● Introduce yourself by name and title

Name: _____

Date: _____

Pre-Procedure

	S	U	Comments
1. Identified the person.	___	___	_____
2. Explained the procedure to the person.	___	___	_____
3. Offered the bedpan or urinal. Provided for privacy.	___	___	_____
4. Decontaminated hands.	___	___	_____
5. Collected clean linen for a closed bed. Placed linen on a clean surface.	___	___	_____
6. Collected the following:			
• Washbasin	___	___	_____
• Soap dish with bar or liquid soap	___	___	_____
• Bath thermometer	___	___	_____
• Orange stick or nail file	___	___	_____
• Washcloth	___	___	_____
• Two bath towels and two face towels	___	___	_____
• Bath blanket	___	___	_____
• Gown or pajamas	___	___	_____
• Items for oral hygiene	___	___	_____
• Body lotion	___	___	_____
• Talcum powder	___	___	_____
• Deodorant or antiperspirant	___	___	_____
• Brush and comb	___	___	_____
• Other toilet articles if requested	___	___	_____
• Paper towels	___	___	_____
• Gloves	___	___	_____
7. Arranged items on the overbed table. Adjusted the height as needed. Used the bedside stand if necessary.	___	___	_____
8. Closed doors and windows to prevent drafts.	___	___	_____
9. Provided for privacy.	___	___	_____
10. Raised the bed to the best level for good body mechanics. Made sure bed rails were up.	___	___	_____
11. Removed the signal light and lowered the nearest bed rail.	___	___	_____
12. Provided oral hygiene.	___	___	_____

Procedure

	S	U	Comments
13. Removed top linens and covered the person with a bath blanket.	___	___	_____
14. Lowered the head of the bed to a level appropriate for the person. Kept it as flat as possible. Let the person have at least one pillow.	___	___	_____
15. Placed paper towels on the overbed table.	___	___	_____

Procedure—cont'd   S   U   Comments

16. Raised the nearest bed rail.   ____ ____ _____

17. Filled the washbasin two thirds full with water. Water temperature was between 110° to 115° Fahrenheit (43° to 46° Celsius) for adults. Measured the water temperature with a bath thermometer.   ____ ____ _____

18. Placed the basin on the overbed table on top of the paper towels.   ____ ____ _____

19. Lowered the bed rail.   ____ ____ _____

20. Placed a face towel over the person's chest.   ____ ____ _____

21. Made a mitt with the washcloth. Used a mitt throughout the procedure.   ____ ____ _____

22. Washed the person's eyes with water. Did not use soap. Gently wiped from the inner aspect with a corner of the mitt. Cleansed the far eye first. Repeated this step for the near eye.   ____ ____ _____

23. Asked the person whether you should use soap to wash the face.   ____ ____ _____

24. Washed the face, ears, and neck. Rinsed and dried the skin well using the towel on the chest.   ____ ____ _____

25. Helped the person move to the side of the bed near you.   ____ ____ _____

26. Removed the gown. Did not expose the person.   ____ ____ _____

27. Placed a bath towel lengthwise under the far arm.   ____ ____ _____

28. Supported the arm with the palm under the person's elbow. His or her arm rested on your forearm.   ____ ____ _____

29. Washed the arm, shoulder, and underarm (axilla) with long, firm strokes. Rinsed and patted dry.   ____ ____ _____

30. Placed the basin on the towel. Placed the person's hand into the water. Washed it well. Cleansed under fingernails with an orange stick or nail file.   ____ ____ _____

31. Encouraged the person to exercise the hand and fingers.   ____ ____ _____

32. Removed the basin and dried the hand well. Covered the arm with the bath blanket.   ____ ____ _____

33. Repeated steps 27 to 32 for the near arm.   ____ ____ _____

34. Placed a bath towel over the chest crosswise. Held the towel in place and pulled the bath blanket from under the towel to the waist.   ____ ____ _____

35. Lifted the towel slightly and washed the chest. Did not expose the person. Rinsed and patted dry, especially under the breasts.   ____ ____ _____

36. Moved the towel lengthwise over the chest and abdomen. Did not expose the person. Pulled the bath blanket down to the pubic area.   ____ ____ _____

37. Lifted the towel slightly and washed the abdomen. Rinsed and patted dry.   ____ ____ _____

38. Pulled the bath blanket up to the shoulders, covering both arms. Removed the towel.   ____ ____ _____

39. Changed the water if it was soapy or cool. Raised the bed rail before leaving the bedside. Lowered it on returning.   ____ ____ _____

40. Uncovered the far leg. Did not expose the genital area. Placed a towel lengthwise under the foot and leg.   ____ ____ _____

41. Bent the knee and supported the leg with your arm. Washed it with long, firm strokes. Rinsed and patted dry.   ____ ____ _____

Procedure—cont'd   S   U   **Comments**

42. Placed the basin on the towel near the foot.   ____ ____ _____

43. Lifted the leg slightly. Slid the basin under the foot.   ____ ____ _____

44. Placed the foot in the basin. Used an orange stick or nail file to clean under toenails, if necessary. Did the following if the person could not bend knees: ____ ____ _____

    • Placed a bath towel under the leg and foot.   ____ ____ _____

    • Washed the leg with long, firm strokes. Rinsed and patted dry.   ____ ____ _____

    • Washed the foot. Carefully separated the toes. Rinsed and patted dry.   ____ ____ _____

    • Cleansed under toenails with an orange stick or nail file, if necessary.   ____ ____ _____

45. Removed the basin and dried the leg. Covered the foot with the bath blanket. Removed the towel.   ____ ____ _____

46. Repeated steps 40 to 45 for the near leg.   ____ ____ _____

47. Changed the water. Raised the bed rail before leaving the bedside. Lowered it after returning.   ____ ____ _____

48. Turned the person onto side facing away. Kept him or her covered with the bath blanket.   ____ ____ _____

49. Uncovered the back and buttocks. Did not expose the person. Placed a towel lengthwise on the bed along the back.   ____ ____ _____

50. Washed the back, working from the back of the neck to the lower end of the buttocks. Used long, firm, continuous strokes. Rinsed and dried well.   ____ ____ _____

51. Gave a back massage.   ____ ____ _____

52. Turned the person onto his or her back.   ____ ____ _____

53. Changed the water for perineal care. Raised the bed rail before leaving. Lowered it when you returned.   ____ ____ _____

54. Let the person wash the genital area. Adjusted the overbed table for easy reach. Placed the signal light within reach. Asked the person to signal when finished.   ____ ____ _____

    Made sure the person understood what to do. Answered the signal light promptly. Provided perineal care if the person could not do so.   ____ ____ _____

55. Gave a back massage, if not already done.   ____ ____ _____

56. Applied deodorant or antiperspirant.   ____ ____ _____

57. Put a clean gown or pajamas on the person.   ____ ____ _____

58. Combed and brushed the hair.   ____ ____ _____

59. Made the bed. Attached the signal light.   ____ ____ _____

Post-Procedure

60. Provided for comfort.   ____ ____ _____

61. Lowered the bed to its lowest position.   ____ ____ _____

62. Raised or lowered bed rails. Followed the care plan.   ____ ____ _____

63. Emptied and cleaned the washbasin. Returned it and other supplies to their proper place.   ____ ____ _____

64. Wiped off the overbed table with the paper towels and discarded them.   ____ ____ _____

Post-Procedure—cont'd   S   U   Comments

65. Unscreened the person.

66. Followed center policy for dirty linen.

67. Decontaminated hands.

68. Reported observations to the nurse.

Giving a Partial Bath

QUALITY OF LIFE

Remember to:
- Knock before entering the person's room
- Address the person by name
- Introduce yourself by name and title

Name: _____

Date: _____

Pre-Procedure	S	U	Comments

1. Identified the person.

2. Explained the procedure to the person.

3. Offered the bedpan or urinal. Provided for privacy.

4. Decontaminated hands.

5. Collected clean linen for a closed bed. Placed linen on a clean surface.

6. Collected the following:
   - Washbasin
   - Soap dish with bar or liquid soap
   - Bath thermometer
   - Orange stick or nail file
   - Washcloth
   - Two bath towels and two face towels
   - Bath blanket
   - Gown or pajamas
   - Items for oral hygiene
   - Body lotion
   - Talcum powder
   - Deodorant or antiperspirant
   - Brush and comb
   - Other toilet articles if requested
   - Paper towels
   - Disposable gloves

7. Arranged items on the overbed table. Adjusted height as needed. Used the bedside stand, if necessary.

8. Closed doors and windows to prevent drafts.

9. Provided for privacy.

Procedure

10. Made sure the bed was in the lowest position.

11. Assisted with oral hygiene. Adjusted the height of the overbed table to an appropriate level.

12. Removed top linen. Covered the person with a bath blanket.

13. Placed the paper towels on the overbed table.

14. Filled the washbasin with water. Water temperature was between 110° and 115° Fahrenheit (43° to 46° Celsius).

15. Placed the basin on the overbed table on top of the paper towels.

Procedure—cont'd	S	U	Comments

16. Raised the head of the bed so that the person could bathe comfortably. Assisted the person to sit at the bedside if allowed in that position.

17. Positioned the overbed table so that the person could easily reach the basin and supplies.

18. Helped the person remove the gown or pajamas.

19. Asked the person to wash easy-to-reach body parts. Explained that you would wash the back and those areas that could not be reached.

20. Placed the signal light within reach. Asked the person to signal if help was needed or when bathing was completed.

21. Left the room after decontaminating hands.

22. Returned when the signal light was on. Knocked before entering.

23. Changed the bath water.

24. Asked what was washed. Washed areas that the person could not reach.

25. Gave a back massage.

26. Applied deodorant or antiperspirant.

27. Helped the person put on clean clothes, gown, or pajamas.

28. Assisted with hair care.

29. Assisted the person to a chair. Otherwise, turned person onto the opposite side.

30. Made the bed.

31. Lowered the bed to its lowest position.

32. Assisted the person to return to bed.

Post-Procedure

33. Provided for comfort.

34. Placed the signal light within reach.

35. Raised or lowered bed rails. Followed the care plan.

36. Emptied and cleansed the basin. Returned the basin and supplies to their proper place.

37. Wiped off the overbed table with the paper towels and discarded them.

38. Unscreened the person.

39. Followed the center policy for dirty linen.

40. Decontaminated hands.

41. Reported observations to the nurse.

Assisting With a Tub Bath or Shower

QUALITY OF LIFE

Remember to:
- Knock before entering the person's room
- Address the person by name
- Introduce yourself by name and title

Name: _____

Date: _____

Pre-Procedure

	S	U	Comments

1. Reserved the bathtub or shower, if necessary.
2. Identified the person.
3. Explained the procedure to the person.
4. Decontaminated hands.
5. Collected the following:
   - Washcloth and two bath towels
   - Bar or liquid soap
   - Bath thermometer (for a tub bath)
   - Clean gown or pajamas
   - Deodorant and other toilet articles as requested
   - Robe and nonskid slippers or shoes
   - Rubber bath mat if needed
   - Disposable bath mat

Procedure

6. Placed items in the bathroom or shower room.
7. Cleaned the tub or shower, if needed.
8. Placed a rubber bath mat in the tub or on the shower floor. Did not block the drain.
9. Placed a disposable bath mat on the floor in front of the tub or shower.
10. Put the "occupied" sign on the door.
11. Returned to the person's room. Provided for privacy.
12. Helped the person sit on the side of the bed.
13. Helped the person put on a robe and slippers.
14. Assisted the person to the bathroom or shower room.
15. *For a tub bath:*
    a. Had the person sit on the chair by the tub.
    b. Filled the tub halfway with warm water (105° Fahrenheit, or 41° Celsius).

    For a shower:
    a. Turned on the shower.
    b. Adjusted water temperature and pressure.
16. Helped the person remove slippers, robe, and gown.
17. Assisted the person into the tub or shower. If using a shower chair, placed it in position and locked the wheels.
18. Assisted with washing if necessary. Remembered that the bath should not last longer than 20 minutes.

Procedure—cont'd   **S**   **U**   **Comments**

19. Did not leave the person unattended in the tub or shower room.

20. Placed a towel across the chair.

21. Turned off the shower.

22. Helped the person out of the tub or shower and onto the chair.

23. Helped the person dry off. Patted gently.

24. Assisted with lotion, deodorant, or antiperspirant as needed.

25. Helped the person to dress.

26. Helped the person return to the room. Assisted the person into bed, if indicated.

27. Provided a back massage if the person returned to bed.

28. Assisted with hair care and other grooming.

Post-Procedure

29. Provided for comfort.

30. Raised or lowered bed rails. Followed the care plan.

31. Placed the signal light within reach.

32. Cleaned the tub or shower. Removed soiled linen and discarded disposable items. Wore gloves for this step. Put the "unoccupied" sign on the door. Returned supplies to their proper place.

33. Followed center policy for dirty linen.

34. Decontaminated hands.

35. Reported observations to the nurse.

Giving a Back Massage

QUALITY OF LIFE

Remember to: ● Knock before entering the person's room
                ● Address the person by name
                ● Introduce yourself by name and title

Name: _____

Date: _____

Pre-Procedure

	S	U	Comments

1. Identified the person.
2. Explained the procedure to the person.
3. Decontaminated hands.
4. Collected the following:
   • Bath blanket
   • Bath towel
   • Lotion
5. Provided for privacy.
6. Raised the bed to the best level for good body mechanics. Made sure side rails were up.

Procedure

7. Lowered the bed rail near you.
8. Positioned the person in the prone or sidelying position with the back toward you.
9. Exposed the back, shoulders, upper arms, and buttocks. Covered the rest of the body with the bath blanket.
10. Laid the towel on the bed along the back.
11. Warmed some lotion in hands.
12. Explained that the lotion might feel cool and wet.
13. Applied lotion to the lower back area.
14. Stroked up from the buttocks to the shoulders, then down over the upper arms. Stroked up the upper arms, across the shoulders, and down the back to the buttocks. Used firm strokes. Kept hands in contact with person's skin.
15. Repeated step 14 for at least 3 minutes.
16. Kneaded one half of the back, starting at the buttocks and moving up to the shoulder, then kneaded down from the shoulder to the buttocks. Repeated on the other half of the back.
17. Applied lotion to bony areas. Used circular motion with the tips of index and middle fingers.
18. Used fast movements to stimulate and slow movements to relax.
19. Stroked with long, firm movements to end the massage. Told the person you were finished.
20. Covered the person. Removed the towel and bath blanket.

Post-Procedure	S	U	Comments
21. Provided for comfort.	_____	_____	_____
22. Lowered the bed to its lowest position.	_____	_____	_____
23. Raised or lowered bed rails. Followed the care plan.	_____	_____	_____
24. Placed the signal light within reach.	_____	_____	_____
25. Returned lotion to its proper place.	_____	_____	_____
26. Unscreened the person.	_____	_____	_____
27. Followed center policy for dirty linen.	_____	_____	_____
28. Decontaminated hands.	_____	_____	_____
29. Reported observations to the nurse.	_____	_____	_____

Giving Female Perineal Care

QUALITY OF LIFE

Name: _____

Date: _____

Remember to:
- Knock before entering the person's room
- Address the person by name
- Introduce yourself by name and title

Pre-Procedure

	S	U	Comments
1. Explained the procedure to the person.	___	___	_____
2. Decontaminated hands.	___	___	_____
3. Collected the following:			
• Soap dish with bar or liquid soap	___	___	_____
• At least four washcloths	___	___	_____
• Bath towel	___	___	_____
• Bath blanket	___	___	_____
• Waterproof pad	___	___	_____
• Disposable gloves	___	___	_____
• Paper towels	___	___	_____
4. Arranged items on the overbed table.	___	___	_____
5. Identified the person.	___	___	_____
6. Provided for privacy.	___	___	_____
7. Raised the bed to the best level for good body mechanics. Made sure bed rails were up.	___	___	_____

Procedure

	S	U	Comments
8. Lowered the bed rail near you.	___	___	_____
9. Covered the person with a bath blanket. Moved top linens to the foot of the bed.	___	___	_____
10. Positioned the person on her back.	___	___	_____
11. Positioned the waterproof pad under her buttocks.	___	___	_____
12. Draped the person.	___	___	_____
13. Raised the bed rail.	___	___	_____
14. Filled the washbasin. Water temperature was about 105° to 109° Fahrenheit (41° to 43° Celsius).	___	___	_____
15. Placed the basin on the overbed table on top of the paper towels.	___	___	_____
16. Lowered the bed rail.	___	___	_____
17. Helped the person flex her knees and spread her legs. If the person could not flex her knees, helped her spread her legs as much as possible with her knees straight.	___	___	_____
18. Put on the gloves.	___	___	_____
19. Folded the corner of the bath blanket between the person's legs onto her abdomen.	___	___	_____
20. Wet the washcloths. Squeezed out excess water before using them.	___	___	_____
21. Applied soap to a washcloth.	___	___	_____
22. Separated the labia. Cleansed downward from front to back with one stroke.	___	___	_____

Procedure—cont'd | S | U | Comments

23. Repeated steps 21 and 22 until the area was clean. Used a different part of the washcloth for each stroke. Used more than one washcloth if needed.

24. Rinsed the perineum with a clean washcloth. Separated the labia. Stroked downward from front to back. Repeated this step as necessary. Used a different part of the washcloth for each stroke. Used more than one washcloth if needed.

25. Patted the area dry with the towel.

26. Folded the blanket back between her legs.

27. Helped the person lower her legs and turn away.

28. Applied soap to a washcloth.

29. Cleansed the rectal area. Cleansed from the vagina to the anus with one stroke.

30. Repeated steps 28 and 29 until the area was clean. Used a different part of the washcloth for each stroke. Used more than one washcloth if needed.

31. Rinsed the rectal area with a washcloth. Stroked from the vagina to the anus. Repeated this step as necessary, using a different part of the washcloth for each stroke. Used more than one washcloth if needed.

32. Patted the area dry with the towel.

33. Removed and discarded the gloves.

Post-Procedure

34. Positioned the person so that she was comfortable.

35. Returned linens to their proper position and removed the bath blanket.

36. Lowered the bed to its lowest position.

37. Raised or lowered bed rails. Followed the care plan.

38. Placed the signal light within reach.

39. Emptied and cleaned the washbasin.

40. Returned the basin and supplies to their proper places.

41. Wiped off the overbed table with the paper towels and discarded them.

42. Unscreened the person.

43. Followed the center policy for dirty linen.

44. Decontaminated hands.

45. Reported observations to the nurse:
    - Any odors
    - Redness, swelling, discharge, or irritation
    - Complaints of pain, burning, or other discomfort

Giving Male Perineal Care

QUALITY OF LIFE

Remember to:
- Knock before entering the person's room
- Address the person by name
- Introduce yourself by name and title

Name: _____

Date: _____

Pre-Procedure

	S	U	Comments

1. Explained the procedure to the person.   ___ ___ _____
2. Decontaminated hands.   ___ ___ _____
3. Collected the following:
   - Soap dish with bar or liquid soap   ___ ___ _____
   - At least four washcloths   ___ ___ _____
   - Bath towel   ___ ___ _____
   - Bath blanket   ___ ___ _____
   - Waterproof pad   ___ ___ _____
   - Disposable gloves   ___ ___ _____
   - Paper towels   ___ ___ _____
4. Arranged items on the overbed table.   ___ ___ _____
5. Identified the person.   ___ ___ _____
6. Provided for privacy.   ___ ___ _____
7. Raised the bed to the best level for good body mechanics. Made sure bed rails were up.   ___ ___ _____

Procedure

8. Lowered the bed rail near you.   ___ ___ _____
9. Covered the person with a bath blanket. Moved top linens to the foot of the bed.   ___ ___ _____
10. Positioned the person on his back.   ___ ___ _____
11. Positioned the waterproof pad under his buttocks.   ___ ___ _____
12. Draped the person.   ___ ___ _____
13. Raised the bed rail.   ___ ___ _____
14. Filled the washbasin. Water temperature was about 105° to 109° Fahrenheit (41° to 43° Celsius).   ___ ___ _____
15. Placed the basin on the overbed table on top of the paper towels.   ___ ___ _____
16. Lowered the bed rail.   ___ ___ _____
17. Helped the person flex his knees and spread his legs. If the person could not flex his knees, helped him spread his legs as much as possible with his knees straight.   ___ ___ _____
18. Put on the gloves.   ___ ___ _____
19. Folded the corner of the bath blanket between the person's legs onto his abdomen.   ___ ___ _____
20. Wet the washcloths. Squeezed out excess water before using them.   ___ ___ _____
21. Applied soap to a washcloth.   ___ ___ _____
22. Retracted the foreskin, if the person was uncircumcised.   ___ ___ _____

Procedure—cont'd

	S	U	Comments
23. Grasped the penis.	___	___	_____
24. Cleansed the tip using a circular motion. Started at the urethral opening and worked outward. Repeated as necessary. Used a different part of the washcloth each time.	___	___	_____
25. Rinsed the area with another washcloth.	___	___	_____
26. Returned the foreskin to its natural position.	___	___	_____
27. Cleansed the shaft of the penis with firm downward strokes. Rinsed the area.	___	___	_____
28. Helped the person flex his knees and spread his legs. If the person could not flex his knees, helped him spread his legs as much as possible with knees straight.	___	___	_____
29. Cleansed the scrotum and rinsed well. Observed for redness and irritation in the skin folds.	___	___	_____
30. Patted dry the penis and scrotum.	___	___	_____
31. Folded the bath blanket back between his legs.	___	___	_____
32. Helped him lower his legs and turn away on his side.	___	___	_____
33. Cleansed the rectal area. Rinsed and dried well.	___	___	_____
34. Removed and discarded the gloves.	___	___	_____

Post-Procedure

	S	U	Comments
35. Positioned the person so that he was comfortable.	___	___	_____
36. Returned linens to their proper position and removed the bath blanket.	___	___	_____
37. Lowered the bed to its lowest position.	___	___	_____
38. Raised or lowered bed rails. Followed the care plan.	___	___	_____
39. Placed the signal light within reach.	___	___	_____
40. Emptied and cleaned the washbasin.	___	___	_____
41. Returned the basin and supplies to their proper places.	___	___	_____
42. Wiped off the overbed table with the paper towels and discarded them.	___	___	_____
43. Unscreened the person.	___	___	_____
44. Followed the center policy for dirty linen.	___	___	_____
45. Decontaminated hands.	___	___	_____
46. Reported observations to the nurse:			
• Any odors	___	___	_____
• Redness, swelling, discharge, or irritation	___	___	_____
• Complaints of pain, burning, or other discomfort	___	___	_____

Brushing and Combing Hair

QUALITY OF LIFE

Remember to:
- Knock before entering the person's room
- Address the person by name
- Introduce yourself by name and title

Name: _____

Date: _____

	S	U	Comments

Pre-Procedure

1. Identified the person.   _____ _____ _____
2. Explained the procedure to the person.   _____ _____ _____
3. Collected the following:
   - Comb and brush   _____ _____ _____
   - Bath towel   _____ _____ _____
   - Other toilet items as requested   _____ _____ _____
4. Arranged items on the bedside stand.   _____ _____ _____
5. Decontaminated hands.   _____ _____ _____
6. Provided for privacy.   _____ _____ _____

Procedure

7. Lowered bed rails (if used).   _____ _____ _____
8. Helped the person to the chair. (If person is in bed, raised the   _____ _____ _____
   bed to the best position for good body mechanics.) Made sure
   side rails were up. Lowered the bed rail near you and positioned
   the person in semi-Fowler's position (if allowed).
9. Placed the towel across the person's shoulders. Placed the towel   _____ _____ _____
   across the pillow, if the person was in bed.
10. Asked the person to remove eyeglasses. Put them in the eye-   _____ _____ _____
    glass case. Put the eyeglass case in the bedside stand.
11. Parted the hair into two main sections. Then divided one side   _____ _____ _____
    into two sections.
12. Brushed the hair. Started at the scalp and brushed toward the   _____ _____ _____
    hair ends.
13. Styled the hair as the person preferred.   _____ _____ _____
14. Removed the towel.   _____ _____ _____
15. Let the person put eyeglasses on.   _____ _____ _____

Post-Procedure

16. Provided for comfort.   _____ _____ _____
17. Raised or lowered bed rails. Followed the care plan.   _____ _____ _____
18. Placed the signal light within reach.   _____ _____ _____
19. Unscreened the person.   _____ _____ _____
20. Cleaned and returned equipment to its proper place.   _____ _____ _____
21. Followed center policy for dirty linen.   _____ _____ _____
22. Decontaminated hands.   _____ _____ _____

Shampooing the Person's Hair

QUALITY OF LIFE

Remember to: ● Knock before entering the person's room
              ● Address the person by name
              ● Introduce yourself by name and title

Name: _____

Date: _____

Pre-Procedure	S	U	Comments
1. Explained the procedure to the person.	___	___	_____
2. Decontaminated hands.	___	___	_____
3. Collected the following:			
• Two bath towels	___	___	_____
• Face towel or washcloth folded lengthwise	___	___	_____
• Shampoo	___	___	_____
• Hair conditioner, if requested	___	___	_____
• Bath thermometer	___	___	_____
• Pitcher or hand-held nozzle	___	___	_____
• Equipment for the shampoo in bed (if needed)	___	___	_____
• Trough	___	___	_____
• Basin or pail	___	___	_____
• Waterproof bed protector	___	___	_____
• Comb and brush	___	___	_____
• Hair dryer	___	___	_____
4. Arranged equipment where it could easily be reached.	___	___	_____
5. Identified the person.	___	___	_____
6. Provided for privacy.	___	___	_____

Procedure			
7. Positioned the person for the method to be used.	___	___	_____
8. Placed a bath towel across the shoulders or across the pillow under the person's head.	___	___	_____
9. Brushed and combed hair thoroughly.	___	___	_____
10. Raised side rails on the bed or stretcher when obtaining water.	___	___	_____
11. Obtained water. Measured water temperature with the bath thermometer. Water temperature was about 110° Fahrenheit (43° to 44° Celsius).	___	___	_____
12. Lowered the bed rail.	___	___	_____
13. Asked the person to hold the face towel or washcloth over the eyes. Made sure it did not slip down over the nose or mouth.	___	___	_____
14. Used the pitcher or nozzle to wet the hair completely.	___	___	_____
15. Used a small amount of shampoo.	___	___	_____
16. Worked up a lather with both hands. Started at the hairline and worked toward the back of the head.	___	___	_____
17. Massaged the scalp with fingertips. Did not scratch with fingernails.	___	___	_____
18. Rinsed the hair.	___	___	_____

Procedure—cont'd   S   U   Comments

19. Repeated steps 15 through 18. _____ _____ _____
20. Rinsed the hair thoroughly. _____ _____ _____
21. Applied conditioner and rinsed as directed. _____ _____ _____
22. Wrapped the person's head with a bath towel. _____ _____ _____
23. Dried the person's face with the towel or washcloth used to protect the eyes. _____ _____ _____
24. Helped the person raise his or her head, if appropriate. _____ _____ _____
25. Rubbed the hair and scalp with the towel. Used the second towel if the first towel became too wet. _____ _____ _____
26. Combed hair. Curled or rolled a woman's hair as requested. _____ _____ _____
27. Dried the hair as quickly as possible. _____ _____ _____

Post-Procedure

28. Provided for comfort. _____ _____ _____
29. Raised or lowered bed rails. Followed the care plan. _____ _____ _____
30. Placed the signal light within reach. _____ _____ _____
31. Cleaned and returned equipment to its proper place. Discarded disposable items. _____ _____ _____
32. Followed center policy for dirty linen. _____ _____ _____
33. Decontaminated hands. _____ _____ _____

Shaving a Person With a Safety Razor

QUALITY OF LIFE

Remember to:
- Knock before entering the person's room
- Address the person by name
- Introduce yourself by name and title

Name: _____

Date: _____

Pre-Procedure

	S	U	Comments
1. Followed Delegation Guidelines.	___	___	_____
2. Explained the procedure to the person.	___	___	_____
3. Decontaminated hands.	___	___	_____
4. Collected the following:			
• Washbasin	___	___	_____
• Bath towel	___	___	_____
• Face towel	___	___	_____
• Washcloth	___	___	_____
• Safety razor	___	___	_____
• Mirror	___	___	_____
• Shaving cream, soap, or lotion	___	___	_____
• Shaving brush	___	___	_____
• Aftershave lotion (men only)	___	___	_____
• Tissues	___	___	_____
• Paper towels	___	___	_____
• Gloves	___	___	_____
5. Arranged paper towels and supplies on the overbed table.	___	___	_____
6. Identified the person. Checked identification bracelet against the assignment sheet. Called the person by name.	___	___	_____
7. Provided for privacy.	___	___	_____

Procedure

	S	U	Comments
8. Raised the bed for good body mechanics. Raised bed rails, if used.	___	___	_____
9. Filled the basin with water. Measured water temperature by following agency policy.	___	___	_____
10. Placed the basin on the overbed table.	___	___	_____
11. Lowered the bed rail near you, if up.	___	___	_____
12. Positioned the person in semi-Fowler's position, if allowed, or in the supine position.	___	___	_____
13. Adjusted lighting to see the person's face clearly.	___	___	_____
14. Placed the bath towel over the chest.	___	___	_____
15. Adjusted the overbed table for easy reach.	___	___	_____
16. Tightened the razor blade to the razor.	___	___	_____
17. Washed the person's face. Did not dry.	___	___	_____

Procedure—cont'd	S	U	Comments

18. Placed a washcloth or face towel in the basin and wet thoroughly. Wrung the washcloth out. _____ _____ _____

19. Applied the washcloth or towel to the face for a few minutes. _____ _____ _____

20. Put on gloves. _____ _____ _____

21. Applied shaving cream with hands or used a shaving brush to apply lather. _____ _____ _____

22. Held the skin taut with one hand. _____ _____ _____

23. Shaved in the direction of hair growth. Used shorter strokes around the chin and lips. _____ _____ _____

24. Rinsed the razor often and wiped with tissues. _____ _____ _____

25. Applied direct pressure to any bleeding area. _____ _____ _____

26. Washed off any remaining shaving cream or soap. Dried with a towel. _____ _____ _____

27. Applied aftershave lotion. _____ _____ _____

Post-Procedure

28. Removed the towel and gloves. _____ _____ _____

29. Moved the overbed table to the side of the bed. _____ _____ _____

30. Provided comfort. _____ _____ _____

31. Placed the signal light within reach. _____ _____ _____

32. Lowered the bed to its lowest position. _____ _____ _____

33. Raised or lowered bed rails. Followed the care plan. _____ _____ _____

34. Cleaned and returned equipment and supplies to the proper place. Discarded disposable items. (Wore gloves for this step.) _____ _____ _____

35. Wiped off the overbed table with the paper towels. _____ _____ _____

36. Unscreened the person. _____ _____ _____

37. Followed center policy for dirty linen. _____ _____ _____

38. Decontaminated hands. _____ _____ _____

39. Reported any nicks or bleeding to the nurse. _____ _____ _____

Giving Nail and Foot Care

QUALITY OF LIFE

Name: _____

Date: _____

Remember to:
- Knock before entering the person's room
- Address the person by name
- Introduce yourself by name and title

Pre-Procedure

	S	U	Comments
1. Followed Delegation Guidelines.	____	____	_____
2. Explained the procedure to the person.	____	____	_____
3. Decontaminated hands.	____	____	_____
4. Collected the following:			
• Washbasin	____	____	_____
• Soap	____	____	_____
• Bath thermometer	____	____	_____
• Bath towel	____	____	_____
• Face towel	____	____	_____
• Cloth	____	____	_____
• Kidney basin	____	____	_____
• Nail clippers	____	____	_____
• Orange stick	____	____	_____
• Emery board or nail file	____	____	_____
• Lotion or petrolatum jelly	____	____	_____
• Paper towels	____	____	_____
• Disposable bath mat	____	____	_____
• Gloves	____	____	_____
5. Arranged equipment on the overbed table.	____	____	_____
6. Identified the person. Checked identification bracelet against the assignment sheet. Called the person by name.	____	____	_____
7. Provided for privacy.	____	____	_____
8. Assisted the person to the bedside chair. Placed the signal light within reach.	____	____	_____

Procedure

	S	U	Comments
9. Placed the bath mat under the person's feet.	____	____	_____
10. Filled the basin with water. Water temperature was according to center policy. (Measured with a bath thermometer or tested by dipping your elbow or inner wrist into the basin of water.)	____	____	_____
11. Placed the basin on the bathmat.			
12. Assisted the person with removing shoes and socks.	____	____	_____
13. Helped the person put his or her feet into the basin.	____	____	_____
14. Positioned the overbed table in front of the person. Filled kidney basin with water and followed the center policy for assessing water temperature.	____	____	_____
15. Placed kidney basin on top of the paper towels on the overbed table.	____	____	_____
16. Put the person's fingers into the basin.	____	____	_____

Procedure—cont'd   S   U   Comments

17. Let the feet and fingernails soak for 15 to 20 minutes. Re-warmed the water as needed.   _____ _____ _____

18. Removed the kidney basin. Dried the hands and fingers thoroughly.   _____ _____ _____

19. Put on gloves.   _____ _____ _____

20. Cleaned under fingernails with the orange stick. Used a towel to wipe the orange stick after cleaning each nail.   _____ _____ _____

21. Clipped fingernails straight across with nail clippers.   _____ _____ _____

22. Shaped nails with an emery board or nail file.   _____ _____ _____

23. Pushed cuticles back with a washcloth or orange stick.   _____ _____ _____

Post-Procedure

24. Moved the overbed table to the side.   _____ _____ _____

25. Washed the feet with soap and a washcloth. Washed between the person's toes.   _____ _____ _____

26. Rinsed the feet and between the toes.   _____ _____ _____

27. Removed the feet from the basin. Dried thoroughly, especially between the toes.   _____ _____ _____

28. Applied lotion or petrolatum jelly to the tops and soles of feet. Did not apply between the toes. Warmed the lotion before application.   _____ _____ _____

29. Removed and discarded gloves.   _____ _____ _____

30. Helped the person put on socks and shoes.   _____ _____ _____

31. Provided comfort.   _____ _____ _____

32. Placed signal light within reach.   _____ _____ _____

33. Raised or lowered bed rails. Followed the care plan.   _____ _____ _____

34. Cleaned and returned equipment and supplies to the proper place. Discarded disposable items.   _____ _____ _____

35. Unscreened the person.   _____ _____ _____

36. Followed center policy for dirty linen.   _____ _____ _____

37. Decontaminated hands.   _____ _____ _____

38. Reported observations to nurse.   _____ _____ _____

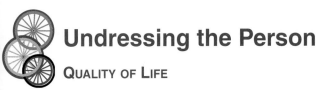

Undressing the Person

QUALITY OF LIFE

Remember to: ● Knock before entering the person's room
                 ● Address the person by name
                 ● Introduce yourself by name and title

Name: _____

Date: _____

Pre-Procedure

	S	U	Comments
1. Explained the procedure to the person.	___	___	_____
2. Decontaminated hands.	___	___	_____
3. Obtained a bath blanket.	___	___	_____
4. Identified the person.	___	___	_____
5. Provided for privacy.	___	___	_____
6. Raised the bed to a level for good body mechanics. Made sure bed rails were up.	___	___	_____
7. Lowered the bed rail on the person's weak side.	___	___	_____
8. Positioned the person supine.	___	___	_____
9. Covered the person with the bath blanket. Fanfolded linens to the foot of the bed. Did not expose the person.	___	___	_____

Procedure

10. Removed garments that open in the back:

    a. Raised the head and shoulders or turned the person onto the side away from you. ___ ___ _____

    b. Unfastened buttons, zippers, ties, or snaps. ___ ___ _____

    c. Brought the sides of garment to the person's sides. Did the following if he or she was in a sidelying position: tucked the far side under the person. Folded the near side onto the chest. ___ ___ _____

    d. Positioned the person supine. ___ ___ _____

    e. Slid the garment off the shoulder on the strong side. Removed the garment from the arm. ___ ___ _____

    f. Repeated step 10(e) for the weak side. ___ ___ _____

11. Removed garments that opened in the front:

    a. Unfastened buttons, zippers, snaps, or ties. ___ ___ _____

    b. Slid the garment off the shoulder and arm on the strong side. ___ ___ _____

    c. Raised the person's head and shoulders. Brought the garment to the weak side. Lowered the person's head and shoulders. ___ ___ _____

    d. Removed the garment from the weak side. ___ ___ _____

    e. Did the following if unable to raise the person's head and shoulders:

        (1) Turned the person toward you. Tucked the removed part under the person. ___ ___ _____

        (2) Turned the person onto the opposite side. ___ ___ _____

        (3). Pulled the side of the garment out from under the person. Made sure the person would not lie on the garment when supine. ___ ___ _____

        (4) Returned the person to the supine position. ___ ___ _____

        (5) Removed the garment from the weak side. ___ ___ _____

Procedure—cont'd	**S**	**U**	**Comments**

12. Removed pullover garments:

   a. Unfastened any buttons, zippers, ties, or snaps.

   b. Removed the garment from the strong side.

   c. Raised the person's head and shoulders or turned toward the opposite side. Brought the garment up the person's neck.

   d. Removed the garment from the weak side.

   e. Brought the garment over the person's head.

   f. Positioned the person in the supine position.

13. Removed pants or slacks:

   a. Removed footwear.

   b. Positioned the person supine.

   c. Unfastened buttons, zippers, ties, snaps, or buckles.

   d. Removed the belt, if one was worn.

   e. Asked the person to lift the buttocks off the bed. Slid the pants down over the hips and buttocks. Had the person lower the hips and buttocks.

   f. Did the following if the person could not raise hips off bed:

     (1) Turned the person toward you.

     (2) Slid the pants off the hip and buttock on the strong side.

     (3) Turned the person toward the opposite side.

     (4) Slid the pants off the hip and buttock on the weak side.

     (5) Slid the pants down the legs and over the feet.

Post-Procedure

14. Dressed the person.

15. Helped the person get out of bed if he or she was to be up.

16. Did the following for the person who would stay in bed:

   a. Covered the person and removed the bath blanket.

   b. Provided for comfort.

   c. Lowered the bed to its lowest position.

   d. Raised or lowered the bed rails. Followed the care plan.

   e. Placed the signal light within reach.

17. Unscreened the person.

18. Followed center policy for dirty linen.

19. Reported observations to the nurse.

Dressing the Person

QUALITY OF LIFE

Remember to:
- Knock before entering the person's room
- Address the person by name
- Introduce yourself by name and title

Name: _____

Date: _____

	S	U	Comments

Pre-Procedure

1. Explained the procedure to the person.   _____ _____ _____
2. Decontaminated hands.   _____ _____ _____
3. Obtained a bath blanket and necessary clothing.   _____ _____ _____
4. Identified the person.   _____ _____ _____
5. Provided for privacy.   _____ _____ _____
6. Raised the bed to the best level for good body mechanics. Made _____ _____ _____
   sure the bed rails were up.
7. Undressed the person.   _____ _____ _____
8. Lowered the bed rail on the person's strong side.   _____ _____ _____
9. Positioned the person supine.   _____ _____ _____

Procedure

10. Covered the person with the bath blanket. Fanfolded linens to   _____ _____ _____
    the foot of the bed. Did not expose the person.
11. Put on garments that open in the back:
    a. Slid the garment onto the arm and shoulder of the weak   _____ _____ _____
       side.
    b. Slid the garment onto the arm and shoulder of the strong   _____ _____ _____
       side.
    c. Raised the person's head and shoulders.   _____ _____ _____
    d. Brought the sides of the garment to the back.   _____ _____ _____
    e. Did the following if the person was in a sidelying position:
       (1) Turned the person toward you.   _____ _____ _____
       (2) Brought the side of the garment to the person's back.   _____ _____ _____
       (3) Turned the person to the opposite side.   _____ _____ _____
       (4) Brought the other side of the garment to the person's   _____ _____ _____
           back.
    f. Fastened buttons, snaps, ties, or zippers.   _____ _____ _____
    g. Positioned the person supine.   _____ _____ _____
12. Put on garments that open in the front:
    a. Slid the garment onto the arm and shoulder of the weak   _____ _____ _____
       side.
    b. Raised the head and shoulders by locking arms with the   _____ _____ _____
       person. Brought the side of the garment to the back. Low-
       ered the person to the supine position. Slid the garment onto
       the arm and shoulder of the strong arm.

Procedure—cont'd	**S**	**U**	**Comments**

c. Did the following if the person could not raise the head and shoulders:

  (1) Turned the person toward you.

  (2) Tucked the garment under the person.

  (3) Turned the person to the opposite side.

  (4) Pulled the garment out from under the person.

  (5) Turned the person back to the supine position.

  (6) Slid the garment over the arm and shoulder of the strong arm.

d. Fastened buttons, snaps, ties, or zippers.

13. Put on pullover garments:

a. Positioned the person supine.

b. Brought the neck of the garment over the head.

c. Slid the arm and shoulder of the garment onto the weak side.

d. Raised the person's head and shoulders.

e. Brought the garment down.

f. Slid the arm and shoulder of the garment onto the strong side.

g. Did the following if the person could not assume a semi-sitting position:

  (1) Turned the person toward you.

  (2) Tucked the garment under the person.

  (3) Turned the person to the opposite side.

  (4) Pulled the garment out from under the person.

  (5) Returned the person to the supine position.

  (6) Slid the arm and shoulder of the garment onto the strong side.

h. Fastened buttons, snaps, ties, or zippers.

14. Put on pants or slacks:

a. Slid the pants over the feet and up the legs.

b. Asked the person to raise the hips and buttocks off the bed.

c. Brought the pants up over the hips and buttocks.

d. Asked the person to lower the hips and buttocks.

e. Did the following if the person could not raise the hips and buttocks:

  (1) Turned the person onto the strong side.

  (2) Pulled the pants over the buttock and hip of the weak side.

  (3) Turned the person onto the weak side.

  (4) Pulled the pants over the buttock and hip of the strong side.

  (5) Positioned the person supine.

f. Fastened buttons, ties, snaps, zipper, or belt buckle.

15. Put socks and footwear on the person.

Post-Procedure

	S	U	Comments
16. Helped the person get out of bed if he or she was to be up.	_____	_____	_____
17. Did the following for the person who would stay in bed:			
a. Covered the person and removed the bath blanket.	_____	_____	_____
b. Provided for comfort.	_____	_____	_____
c. Lowered the bed to its lowest position.	_____	_____	_____
d. Raised or lowered the bed rails. Followed the care plan.	_____	_____	_____
e. Placed the signal light within reach.	_____	_____	_____
18. Unscreened the person.	_____	_____	_____
19. Followed center policy for dirty linen.	_____	_____	_____
20. Reported observations to the nurse.	_____	_____	_____

Changing the Gown of a Person With an IV

QUALITY OF LIFE

Remember to:
- Knock before entering the person's room
- Address the person by name
- Introduce yourself by name and title

Name: _____

Date: _____

Pre-Procedure

	S	U	Comments
1. Explained the procedure to the person.	___	___	_____
2. Decontaminated hands.	___	___	_____
3. Obtained a clean gown.	___	___	_____
4. Identified the person.	___	___	_____
5. Provided for privacy.	___	___	_____
6. Raised the bed to the best level for good body mechanics. Made sure the bed rails were up.	___	___	_____
7. Lowered the bed rail near you.	___	___	_____

Procedure

	S	U	Comments
8. Untied the back of the gown. Freed parts of the gown on which the person was lying.	___	___	_____
9. Removed the gown from the arm with no IV.	___	___	_____
10. Gathered up the sleeve of the arm with the IV. Slid it over the IV site and tubing. Removed the arm and hand from the sleeve.	___	___	_____
11. Kept the sleeve gathered. Slid arm along the tubing to the bag.	___	___	_____
12. Removed the IV bag from the pole. Slid the bag and tubing through the sleeve. Did not pull on tubing.	___	___	_____
13. Hung the IV on the pole.	___	___	_____
14. Gathered the sleeve of the clean gown that would go on the arm with the IV.	___	___	_____
15. Removed the bag from the pole. Quickly slipped the gathered sleeve over the bag at the shoulder part of the gown. Hung the bag on the pole.	___	___	_____
16. Slid the gathered sleeve over the tubing, hand, arm, and IV site. Slid the sleeve onto the person's shoulder.	___	___	_____
17. Put the other side of the gown on and fastened the back.	___	___	_____

Post-Procedure

	S	U	Comments
18. Provided for comfort.	___	___	_____
19. Placed the signal light within reach.	___	___	_____
20. Lowered the bed to its lowest position.	___	___	_____
21. Raised or lowered bed rails. Followed the care plan.	___	___	_____
22. Unscreened the person.	___	___	_____
23. Followed center policy for dirty linen.	___	___	_____
24. Decontaminated hands.	___	___	_____
25. Asked the nurse to check the IV flow rate.	___	___	_____

Giving the Bedpan

QUALITY OF LIFE

Remember to: ● Knock before entering the person's room
              ● Address the person by name
              ● Introduce yourself by name and title

Name: _____

Date: _____

	S	U	Comments

Pre-Procedure

1. Provided for privacy.   ____ ____ _____

2. Put on gloves.   ____ ____ _____

3. Collected the following:
   • Bedpan   ____ ____ _____
   • Bedpan cover   ____ ____ _____
   • Toilet tissue   ____ ____ _____

4. Arranged equipment on the chair or bed.   ____ ____ _____

5. Explained the procedure to the person.   ____ ____ _____

6. Raised the bed to the best level for good body mechanics. Made   ____ ____ _____
   sure the bed rails were up.

Procedure

7. Warmed and dried the bedpan, if necessary.   ____ ____ _____

8. Lowered the bed rail near you.   ____ ____ _____

9. Positioned the person supine. Raised the head of the bed   ____ ____ _____
   slightly.

10. Folded the top linens and gown out of the way. Kept the lower   ____ ____ _____
    body covered.

11. Asked the person to flex the knees and raise the buttocks by   ____ ____ _____
    pushing against the mattress with his or her feet.

12. Slid hand under the lower back and helped raise the buttocks.   ____ ____ _____

13. Slid the bedpan under the person.   ____ ____ _____

14. Did the following if the person could not assist in getting on the
    bedpan:
    a. Turned the person onto the opposite side.   ____ ____ _____
    b. Placed the bedpan firmly against the buttocks.   ____ ____ _____
    c. Pushed the bedpan down and toward the person.   ____ ____ _____
    d. Held the bedpan securely. Turned the person onto the back.   ____ ____ _____
       Made sure the bedpan was centered under the person.

15. Returned top linens to their proper position.   ____ ____ _____

16. Raised the head of the bed so that the person was in a sitting   ____ ____ _____
    position.

17. Made sure the person was correctly positioned on the bedpan.   ____ ____ _____

18. Raised the bed rail, if used.   ____ ____ _____

19. Placed the toilet tissue and signal light within reach.   ____ ____ _____

20. Asked the person to signal when done or when help was   ____ ____ _____
    needed.

21. Removed the gloves and washed hands.   ____ ____ _____

22. Left the room and closed the door.   ____ ____ _____

Procedure—cont'd   S   U   Comments

23. Returned when the person signaled. Knocked before entering.   _____   _____   _____

24. Lowered the bed rail, if used, and the head of the bed.   _____   _____   _____

25. Put on gloves.   _____   _____   _____

26. Asked the person to raise the buttocks. Removed the bedpan or held the bedpan securely and turned the person onto the opposite side.   _____   _____   _____

27. Cleansed the genital area if the person could not do so. Cleaned from front to back with toilet paper. Used fresh tissue for each wipe. Provided perineal care if necessary.   _____   _____   _____

28. Covered the bedpan. Took it to the bathroom or dirty utility room. Raised the bed rail before leaving the bedside.   _____   _____   _____

29. Noted the color, amount, and character of urine or feces.   _____   _____   _____

30. Emptied and rinsed the bedpan. Cleaned it with disinfectant.   _____   _____   _____

31. Returned the bedpan and clean cover to the bedside stand.   _____   _____   _____

32. Removed soiled gloves. Washed hands and put on clean gloves.   _____   _____   _____

33. Helped person wash hands.   _____   _____   _____

34. Removed gloves.   _____   _____   _____

Post-Procedure

35. Provided for comfort.   _____   _____   _____

36. Placed the signal light within reach.   _____   _____   _____

37. Lowered the bed to its lowest position.   _____   _____   _____

38. Raised or lowered bed rails. Followed the care plan.   _____   _____   _____

39. Unscreened the person.   _____   _____   _____

40. Followed center policy for soiled linen.   _____   _____   _____

41. Washed hands.   _____   _____   _____

42. Reported observations to the nurse.   _____   _____   _____

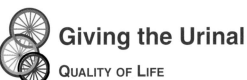

Giving the Urinal

QUALITY OF LIFE

Remember to: ● Knock before entering the person's room
              ● Address the person by name
              ● Introduce yourself by name and title

Name: _____

Date: _____

Pre-Procedure	S	U	Comments
1. Provided for privacy.	_____	_____	_____
2. Determined whether the person would stand or stay in bed.	_____	_____	_____
3. Put on gloves.	_____	_____	_____

Procedure

	S	U	Comments
4. Gave him the urinal if he was in bed. Reminded him to tilt bottom down to prevent spills.	_____	_____	_____
5. Did the following if he was going to stand:			
a. Helped him sit on the side of the bed.	_____	_____	_____
b. Put nonskid shoes or slippers on him.	_____	_____	_____
c. Assisted him to a standing position.	_____	_____	_____
d. Provided support if he was unsteady.	_____	_____	_____
e. Gave him the urinal.	_____	_____	_____
6. Positioned the urinal between his legs if necessary. Positioned his penis in the urinal if he could not hold the urinal.	_____	_____	_____
7. Covered him to provide for privacy.	_____	_____	_____
8. Placed the signal light within reach. Asked him to signal when done or when he needed help.	_____	_____	_____
9. Removed the gloves and washed hands.	_____	_____	_____
10. Left the room and closed the door.	_____	_____	_____
11. Returned when signaled. Knocked before entering.	_____	_____	_____
12. Put on gloves.	_____	_____	_____
13. Covered the urinal. Took it to the bathroom or dirty utility room.	_____	_____	_____
14. Noted the color, amount, and character of the urine.	_____	_____	_____
15. Emptied the urinal and rinsed it with cold water. Cleaned it with a disinfectant.	_____	_____	_____
16. Returned the urinal to the bedside stand.	_____	_____	_____
17. Removed soiled gloves. Washed hands and put on clean gloves.	_____	_____	_____
18. Helped the person wash his or her hands.	_____	_____	_____
19. Removed gloves.	_____	_____	_____

Post-Procedure

	S	U	Comments
20. Provided for comfort.	____	____	_____
21. Placed the signal light within reach.	____	____	_____
22. Raised or lowered bed rails. Followed the care plan.	____	____	_____
23. Unscreened the person.	____	____	_____
24. Followed center policy for soiled linen.	____	____	_____
25. Washed hands.	____	____	_____
26. Reported observations to the nurse.	____	____	_____

Helping a Person to the Commode

QUALITY OF LIFE

Remember to: ● Knock before entering the person's room
                ● Address the person by name
                ● Introduce yourself by name and title

Name: _____

Date: _____

Pre-Procedure

	S	U	Comments
1. Explained the procedure to the person.	___	___	_____
2. Provided for privacy.	___	___	_____
3. Put on gloves.	___	___	_____
4. Collected the following:			
• Commode	___	___	_____
• Toilet tissue	___	___	_____
• Bath blanket	___	___	_____

Procedure

	S	U	Comments
5. Brought the commode next to the bed. Removed the chair seat and lid from the container.	___	___	_____
6. Helped the person sit on the side of the bed.	___	___	_____
7. Helped him or her put on a robe and slippers.	___	___	_____
8. Assisted the person to the commode.	___	___	_____
9. Placed a bath blanket over his or her lap for warmth.	___	___	_____
10. Placed the toilet tissue and signal light within reach.	___	___	_____
11. Asked the person to signal when done or when help was needed. If not safe to leave the person alone, stayed with the person.	___	___	_____
12. Removed the gloves and washed hands.	___	___	_____
13. Left the room and closed the door.	___	___	_____
14. Returned when the person signaled. Knocked before entering.	___	___	_____
15. Put on gloves.	___	___	_____
16. Helped the person clean the genital area, if indicated. Removed the gloves.	___	___	_____
17. Helped the person back to bed. Removed the robe and slippers. Raised the bed rail according to the care plan.	___	___	_____
18. Put on clean gloves. Covered and removed the container from the commode. Cleaned the commode, if necessary.	___	___	_____
19. Took the container to the bathroom or dirty utility room.	___	___	_____
20. Checked urine and feces for color, amount, and character. Measured, if I&O was ordered. Collected a specimen, if one was needed.	___	___	_____
21. Cleaned and disinfected the container.	___	___	_____
22. Returned the container to the commode. Returned other supplies to their proper place.	___	___	_____
23. Returned the commode to its proper place.	___	___	_____

Procedure—cont'd   S   U   Comments

24. Removed soiled gloves. Washed hands and put on clean gloves.   _____ _____ _____

25. Helped the person wash his or her hands.   _____ _____ _____

26. Removed gloves.   _____ _____ _____

Post-Procedure

27. Provided for comfort.   _____ _____ _____

28. Placed the signal light within reach.   _____ _____ _____

29. Raised or lowered the bed rails. Followed the care plan.   _____ _____ _____

30. Unscreened the person.   _____ _____ _____

31. Followed center policy for soiled linen.   _____ _____ _____

32. Washed hands.   _____ _____ _____

33. Reported observations to the nurse.   _____ _____ _____

Giving Catheter Care

QUALITY OF LIFE

Name: _____

Date: _____

Remember to:
- ● Knock before entering the person's room
- ● Address the person by name
- ● Introduce yourself by name and title

Pre-Procedure

	S	U	Comments

1. Explained the procedure to the person. _____ _____ _____
2. Washed hands. _____ _____ _____
3. Collected the following:
   - Equipment for perineal care _____ _____ _____
   - Gloves _____ _____ _____
   - Bed linen protector _____ _____ _____
   - Blanket _____ _____ _____
4. Identified the person. _____ _____ _____
5. Provided for privacy. _____ _____ _____
6. Raised the bed to the best level for good body mechanics. Made sure bed rails were up. _____ _____ _____

Procedure

7. Lowered the bed rail near you. _____ _____ _____
8. Put on the gloves. _____ _____ _____
9. Covered the person with a bath blanket. Fanfolded top linens to the foot of the bed. _____ _____ _____
10. Draped the person for perineal care. _____ _____ _____
11. Folded back the bath blanket between the legs to expose the genital area. _____ _____ _____
12. Placed the bed protector under the buttocks. Asked the person to flex the knees and raise the buttocks off the bed by pushing against the mattress with the feet. _____ _____ _____
13. Performed perineal care. _____ _____ _____
14. Separated the labia (woman) or retracted the foreskin (uncircumcised man). Checked for crusts, abnormal drainage, or secretions. _____ _____ _____
15. Cleaned the catheter from the meatus down the catheter about 4 inches. Used soap and water and a clean washcloth. Avoided tugging or pulling on the catheter. Repeated as necessary with a clean washcloth. _____ _____ _____
16. Made sure the catheter was secured properly. Coiled and secured the tubing. _____ _____ _____
17. Removed the bed protector. _____ _____ _____
18. Covered the person and removed the bath blanket. _____ _____ _____
19. Removed the gloves. _____ _____ _____

Post-Procedure

	S	U	Comments
20. Provided for comfort.	_____	_____	_____
21. Placed the signal light within reach.	_____	_____	_____
22. Raised or lowered bed rails. Followed the care plan.	_____	_____	_____
23. Lowered the bed to its lowest position.	_____	_____	_____
24. Cleaned and returned equipment to its proper place. Discarded disposable items.	_____	_____	_____
25. Unscreened the person.	_____	_____	_____
26. Followed center policy for soiled linen.	_____	_____	_____
27. Washed hands.	_____	_____	_____
28. Reported observations to the nurse.	_____	_____	_____

Changing a Leg Bag to a Drainage Bag

QUALITY OF LIFE

Remember to:
- ● Knock before entering the person's room
- ● Address the person by name
- ● Introduce yourself by name and title

Name: _____

Date: _____

Pre-Procedure	S	U	Comments
1. Followed Delegation Guidelines.	___	___	_____
2. Explained the procedure to the person.	___	___	_____
3. Washed hands.	___	___	_____
4. Collected the following:			
• Gloves	___	___	_____
• Drainage bag and tubing	___	___	_____
• Antiseptic wipes	___	___	_____
• Bed protector	___	___	_____
• Sterile cap and plug	___	___	_____
• Catheter clamp	___	___	_____
• Paper towels	___	___	_____
• Bedpan	___	___	_____
• Bath blanket	___	___	_____
5. Arranged paper towels and equipment on the side of the bed.	___	___	_____
6. Identified the person. Checked identification bracelet against the assignment sheet. Called the person by name.	___	___	_____
7. Provided for privacy.	___	___	_____

Procedure			
8. Assisted the person to sit on the side of the bed.	___	___	_____
9. Put on gloves.	___	___	_____
10. Exposed the catheter and leg bag.	___	___	_____
11. Clamped the catheter. Prevented urine from draining from the catheter into the tubing.	___	___	_____
12. Allowed urine to drain from below the clamp site into the draining tubing, emptying the lower end of the catheter.	___	___	_____
13. Helped the person lie down.	___	___	_____
14. Raised the bed for good body mechanics. Bed rails were up, if used.	___	___	_____
15. Covered the person with a bath blanket. Exposed the catheter leg and bag.	___	___	_____
16. Placed the bed protector under the leg.	___	___	_____
17. Opened the antiseptic wipes and set them on the paper towels.	___	___	_____
18. Opened the package with the sterile cap and plug. Placed the package on the paper towels. Did not let anything touch the sterile cap or plug.	___	___	_____
19. Opened the package with the drainage bag and tubing.	___	___	_____
20. Attached the drainage bag to the bed frame.	___	___	_____

Procedure—cont'd   S   U   Comments

21. Disconnected the catheter from the drainage tubing. Did not let anything touch the ends.

22. Inserted the sterile plug into the catheter end. Touched only the end of the plug. Did not touch the part that went inside the catheter. (Wiped the catheter end with an antiseptic wipe if the end of the catheter is accidentally contaminated. Wiped the end before inserting the sterile plug.)

23. Placed the sterile cap on the end of the leg bag. (Wiped the catheter end with an antiseptic wipe if the end of the catheter is accidentally contaminated.) Wiped the end before inserting the sterile plug.

24. Removed the cap from the new drainage tubing.

25. Removed the sterile plug from the catheter.

26. Inserted the end for the drainage tubing into the catheter.

27. Removed the clamp from the catheter.

28. Looped drainage tubing on the bed. Secured the tubing into the mattress.

29. Removed the leg bag and placed it in the bedpan.

30. Removed and discarded the bed protector.

31. Covered the person. Removed the bath blanket.

32. Took the bedpan to the bathroom.

33. Removed gloves and washed hands.

Post-Procedure

34. Provided comfort.

35. Placed the signal light within reach.

36. Raised or lowered bed rails. Followed the care plan.

37. Lowered the bed to the lowest position.

38. Unscreened the person.

39. Put on clean gloves. Discarded disposable supplies.

40. Empties the drainage bag.

41. Discarded the drainage tubing and bag, following center policy. If reusable, cleaned the bag following center policy.

42. Cleaned the bedpan. Placed it in a clean cover.

43. Removed gloves.

44. Returned the bedpan and other supplies to their proper place.

45. Washed your hands.

46. Reported observations to the nurse.

47. Reversed the procedure if a leg bag is attached to the catheter.

Emptying a Urinary Drainage Bag

QUALITY OF LIFE

Name: _____

Date: _____

Remember to: ● Knock before entering the person's room
                 ● Address the person by name
                 ● Introduce yourself by name and title

Pre-Procedure

	S	U	Comments

1. Collected equipment:
   - Graduate (measuring container)   ____ ____ _____
   - Gloves   ____ ____ _____
   - Paper towels   ____ ____ _____
2. Washed hands.   ____ ____ _____
3. Explained the procedure to the person. ____ ____ _____
4. Identified the person.   ____ ____ _____
5. Provided for privacy.   ____ ____ _____

Procedure

6. Put on the gloves.   ____ ____ _____
7. Placed a paper towel on the floor. Placed the measuring container on top of the paper towel. ____ ____ _____
8. Positioned measuring container (graduate) so that urine was collected when the drain was open. ____ ____ _____
9. Opened the clamp on the bottom of the drainage bag. ____ ____ _____
10. Let all the urine drain into the graduate. Did not let the drain touch the graduate. ____ ____ _____
11. Closed the clamp. Replaced the clamped drain in the holder on the bag. ____ ____ _____
12. Measured urine.   ____ ____ _____
13. Removed and discarded paper towel.   ____ ____ _____
14. Rinsed the graduate and returned it to its proper place. ____ ____ _____
15. Removed gloves and washed hands.   ____ ____ _____
16. Recorded the time and amount on the I&O record. ____ ____ _____

Post-Procedure

17. Unscreened the person.   ____ ____ _____
18. Reported the amount and other observations to the nurse. ____ ____ _____

Applying a Condom Catheter

QUALITY OF LIFE

Remember to:
- Knock before entering the person's room
- Address the person by name
- Introduce yourself by name and title

Name: _____

Date: _____

Pre-Procedure

	S	U	Comments
1. Explained the procedure to the person.	___	___	_____
2. Washed hands.	___	___	_____
3. Collected the following:			
• Condom catheter	___	___	_____
• Elastic tape	___	___	_____
• Drainage bag or leg bag	___	___	_____
• Basin of warm water	___	___	_____
• Soap	___	___	_____
• Towel and washcloths	___	___	_____
• Bath blanket	___	___	_____
• Gloves	___	___	_____
• Bed protector	___	___	_____
• Paper towels	___	___	_____
4. Arranged paper towels and equipment on the overbed table.	___	___	_____
5. Provided for privacy.	___	___	_____
6. Raised the bed to the best level for good body mechanics. Made sure bed rails were up.	___	___	_____

Procedure

	S	U	Comments
7. Lowered the bed rail near you.	___	___	_____
8. Covered the person with a bath blanket. Brought the top linens to the foot of the bed.	___	___	_____
9. Asked the person to raise his buttocks off the bed; or turned him onto his side away from you.	___	___	_____
10. Slid the bed protector under buttocks.	___	___	_____
11. Had the person lower his buttocks or turned him on his back.	___	___	_____
12. Brought top linens up to cover knees and lower legs.	___	___	_____
13. Secured the drainage bag to the bed frame or had a leg bag ready. Closed the drain.	___	___	_____
14. Raised the bath blanket to expose genital area.			
15. Put on the gloves.	___	___	_____
16. Removed the condom catheter:			
a. Removed the tape and rolled the sheath off the penis.	___	___	_____
b. Disconnected the drainage tubing from the condom.	___	___	_____
c. Discarded the tape and condom.	___	___	_____

Procedure—cont'd	S	U	Comments

17. Provided perineal care. Observed the penis for skin breakdown or irritation.

18. Removed the protective backing from the condom.

19. Held the penis firmly. Rolled the condom onto the penis. Left a 1-inch space between the penis and the end of the catheter.

20. Secured the condom with elastic tape. Applied the tape in a spiral. Did not tape completely around the penis.

21. Connected the condom to the drainage tubing. Coiled excess tubing on the bed or attached a leg bag.

22. Removed the bed protector.

23. Removed the gloves.

24. Returned top linens and removed the bath blanket.

Post-Procedure

25. Provided for comfort.

26. Placed the signal light within reach.

27. Raised or lowered bed rails. Followed the care plan.

28. Lowered the bed to its lowest position.

29. Washed hands. Put on clean gloves.

30. Cleaned and returned the washbasin and other equipment. Returned items to their proper place.

31. Unscreened the person.

32. Measured and recorded the amount of urine in the bag. Discarded the collection bag and disposable items.

33. Removed the gloves and washed hands.

34. Reported observations to the nurse.

Collecting a Random Urine Specimen

QUALITY OF LIFE

Remember to: ● Knock before entering the person's room
               ● Address the person by name
               ● Introduce yourself by name and title

Name: _____

Date: _____

Pre-Procedure

	S	U	Comments
1. Explained the procedure to the person.	___	___	_____
2. Washed hands.	___	___	_____
3. Collected the following:			
• Bedpan and cover, urinal, or specimen pan	___	___	_____
• Specimen container and lid	___	___	_____
• Label	___	___	_____
• Gloves	___	___	_____
• Plastic bag	___	___	_____
• Supplies for perineal care	___	___	_____

Procedure

	S	U	Comments
4. Filled out the label. Put it on the container.	___	___	_____
5. Put the container and lid in the bathroom.	___	___	_____
6. Identified the person.	___	___	_____
7. Provided for privacy.	___	___	_____
8. Put on the gloves.	___	___	_____
9. Asked the person to urinate in the receptacle. Reminded him or her to put toilet tissue into the wastebasket or toilet, not in the bedpan or specimen pan.	___	___	_____
10. Took the receptacle to the bathroom.	___	___	_____
11. Measured urine if I&O was ordered.	___	___	_____
12. Poured about 120 ml (4 oz) of urine into the specimen container. Disposed of excess urine.	___	___	_____
13. Placed the lid on the specimen container. Put the container in the plastic bag.	___	___	_____
14. Cleaned and returned the receptacle to its proper place.	___	___	_____
15. Helped the person wash his or her hands.	___	___	_____
16. Removed gloves.	___	___	_____

Post-Procedure

	S	U	Comments
17. Provided for comfort.	___	___	_____
18. Placed the signal light within reach.	___	___	_____
19. Raised or lowered bed rails. Followed the care plan.	___	___	_____
20. Unscreened the person.	___	___	_____
21. Washed hands.	___	___	_____
22. Reported observations to the nurse.	___	___	_____
23. Took the specimen and the requisition to the storage area.	___	___	_____

Collecting a Midstream Specimen

Name: _____

Date: _____

Remember to:
- ● Knock before entering the person's room
- ● Address the person by name
- ● Introduce yourself by name and title

Pre-Procedure	S	U	Comments
1. Explained the procedure to the person.	_____	_____	_____
2. Washed hands.	_____	_____	_____
3. Collected the following:			
• Clean-voided specimen kit with sterile specimen container	_____	_____	_____
• Label	_____	_____	_____
• Antiseptic solution	_____	_____	_____
• Disposable gloves	_____	_____	_____
• Sterile gloves (if not part of the kit)	_____	_____	_____
• Bedpan, urinal, or commode (if the person cannot use the bedpan)	_____	_____	_____
• Plastic bag	_____	_____	_____
• Supplies for perineal care	_____	_____	_____
4. Labeled the container with the requested information.	_____	_____	_____
5. Identified the person.	_____	_____	_____
6. Provided for privacy.	_____	_____	_____

Procedure			
7. Let the person complete perineal care if able. Placed the signal light within reach.	_____	_____	_____
8. Provided perineal care if the person could not.	_____	_____	_____
9. Opened the sterile kit using sterile technique.	_____	_____	_____
10. Put on the sterile gloves.	_____	_____	_____
11. Poured the antiseptic solution over the cotton balls.	_____	_____	_____
12. Opened the sterile specimen container. Did not touch the inside of the container or lid. Set the lid so that the inside was up.	_____	_____	_____
13. Cleaned the perineum with cotton balls, if the person could not.			
a. Female:			
(1) Spread the labia. Used nondominant hand.	_____	_____	_____
(2) Cleaned down the urethral area from front to back. Used a clean cotton ball for each stroke.	_____	_____	_____
(3) Kept the labia separated to collect the urine specimen.	_____	_____	_____
b. Male:			
(1) Held the penis with nondominant hand.	_____	_____	_____
(2) Cleaned the penis starting at the meatus. Used a cotton ball and cleaned in a circular motion.	_____	_____	_____
(3) Kept holding the penis until the specimen was collected.	_____	_____	_____

Procedure—cont'd	**S**	**U**	**Comments**
14. Asked the person to start urinating into the toilet, bedpan, commode, or urinal.	_____	_____	_____
15. Passed the specimen container into the stream of urine. Kept the labia separated.	_____	_____	_____
16. Collected about 30 to 60 ml of urine (1 to 2 oz).	_____	_____	_____
17. Removed the specimen container before the person stopped urinating.	_____	_____	_____
18. Released the labia or penis.	_____	_____	_____
19. Let the person finish urinating into the toilet, bedpan, commode, or urinal.	_____	_____	_____
20. Placed the lid on the specimen container. Touched only the outside of the container or lid.	_____	_____	_____
21. Wiped the outside of the container.	_____	_____	_____
22. Placed the container in a plastic bag.	_____	_____	_____
23. Provided toilet tissue after the person finished urinating.	_____	_____	_____
24. Removed and emptied the bedpan, commode container, or urinal.	_____	_____	_____
25. Cleaned the bedpan, urinal, or commode container, and other equipment. Returned equipment to its proper place.	_____	_____	_____
26. Removed soiled gloves. Washed hands and put on clean gloves.	_____	_____	_____
27. Let the person wash his or her hands.	_____	_____	_____
28. Removed the gloves.	_____	_____	_____

Post-Procedure

	S	**U**	**Comments**
29. Provided for comfort.	_____	_____	_____
30. Placed the signal light within reach.	_____	_____	_____
31. Raised or lowered bed rails. Followed the care plan.	_____	_____	_____
32. Unscreened the person.	_____	_____	_____
33. Washed hands.	_____	_____	_____
34. Reported observations to the nurse.	_____	_____	_____
35. Took the specimen and the requisition to the storage area.	_____	_____	_____

Collecting a Double-Voided Specimen

QUALITY OF LIFE

Name: _____

Date: _____

Remember to:
- ● Knock before entering the person's room
- ● Address the person by name
- ● Introduce yourself by name and title

Pre-Procedure	S	U	Comments
1. Explained the procedure to the person.	____	____	_____
2. Washed hands.	____	____	_____
3. Collected the following:			
• Bedpan, urinal, commode, or disposable specimen pan	____	____	_____
• Two specimen containers	____	____	_____
• Testing equipment	____	____	_____
• Gloves	____	____	_____
4. Identified the person.	____	____	_____
5. Provided for privacy.	____	____	_____

Procedure

	S	U	Comments
6. Put on the gloves.	____	____	_____
7. Offered the bedpan or urinal or assisted the person to the bathroom or commode.	____	____	_____
8. Asked the person to urinate.	____	____	_____
9. Took the receptacle to the bathroom.	____	____	_____
10. Measured urine if I&O was ordered. Poured some urine into the specimen container.	____	____	_____
11. Tested the specimen in case a second specimen was not obtained.	____	____	_____
12. Cleaned the receptacle. Removed the gloves.	____	____	_____
13. Returned the receptacle to its proper place.	____	____	_____
14. Helped the person wash the hands.	____	____	_____
15. Asked the person to drink an 8-ounce glass of water.	____	____	_____
16. Made sure the person was comfortable, the bed rails were up (if needed), and the signal light was within reach.	____	____	_____
17. Unscreened the person.	____	____	_____
18. Washed hands.	____	____	_____
19. Returned to the room in 20 to 30 minutes.	____	____	_____
20. Repeated steps 5 through 18.	____	____	_____
21. Reported the results of the second test and any observations to the nurse.	____	____	_____

Collecting a 24-Hour Urine Specimen

QUALITY OF LIFE

Name: _____

Date: _____

Remember to:
- Knock before entering the person's room
- Address the person by name
- Introduce yourself by name and title

Pre-Procedure

	S	U	Comments
1. Reviewed the procedure with the nurse.	____	____	_____
2. Explained the procedure to the person.	____	____	_____
3. Washed hands.	____	____	_____
4. Collected the following:			
• Urine container for a 24-hour collection	____	____	_____
• Preservative from the laboratory, if needed	____	____	_____
• Bucket with ice, if needed	____	____	_____
• Two 24-hour urine specimen labels	____	____	_____
• Funnel	____	____	_____
• Bedpan, urinal, commode, or specimen pan	____	____	_____
• Gloves	____	____	_____
• Measuring containers	____	____	_____

Procedure

	S	U	Comments
5. Labeled the specimen container.	____	____	_____
6. Identified the person.	____	____	_____
7. Arranged equipment in the person's bathroom or dirty utility room.	____	____	_____
8. Placed one 24-hour specimen label in the bathroom or dirty utility room. Placed the other near the bed.	____	____	_____
9. Put on the gloves.	____	____	_____
10. Offered the bedpan or urinal or assisted the person to the bathroom or bedside commode.	____	____	_____
11. Asked the person to void.	____	____	_____
12. Discarded the specimen and noted the time. Recognized that this started the 24-hour collection period.	____	____	_____
13. Cleaned the bedpan, urinal, commode, or specimen pan.	____	____	_____
14. Removed the gloves. Washed hands.	____	____	_____
15. Marked the time the test began and the time it ended on the room and bathroom labels. Also marked the specimen container.	____	____	_____
16. Asked the person to use the bedpan, urinal, commode, or specimen pan when voiding during the next 24 hours. Told the person to signal after voiding. Reminded him or her not to have a bowel movement at the same time and not to put toilet tissue in the receptacle.	____	____	_____
17. Put on the gloves.			
18. Measured all urine if I&O was ordered.	____	____	_____

Procedure—cont'd

S   U   Comments

19. Poured urine into the specimen container using the funnel. Did not spill any urine. Knew to restart the test if urine was spilled or discarded. _____ _____ _____

20. Cleaned the bedpan, urinal, commode, or specimen pan. Removed the gloves and washed hands. _____ _____ _____

21. Added ice to the bucket as necessary. _____ _____ _____

22. Asked the person to void at the end of the 24-hour period. Poured the urine into the specimen container. _____ _____ _____

23. Thanked the person for cooperating. _____ _____ _____

Post-Procedure

24. Provided for comfort. _____ _____ _____

25. Placed the signal light within reach. _____ _____ _____

26. Raised or lowered bed rails. Followed the care plan. _____ _____ _____

27. Removed the labels from the room and bathroom. Cleaned and returned equipment to its proper place. Discarded disposable items. _____ _____ _____

28. Washed hands. _____ _____ _____

29. Reported observations to the nurse. _____ _____ _____

30. Took the specimen and requisition slip to the storage area. _____ _____ _____

Testing Urine With Reagent Strips

QUALITY OF LIFE

Remember to:
- ● Knock before entering the person's room
- ● Address the person by name
- ● Introduce yourself by name and title

Name: _____

Date: _____

	S	U	Comments

Pre-Procedure

1. Explained the procedure to the person.   ___ ___ _____
2. Washed hands.   ___ ___ _____
3. Identified the person.   ___ ___ _____

Procedure

4. Put on the gloves.   ___ ___ _____
5. Collected the following:
   - Urine specimen (routine specimen for pH and occult blood, double-voided specimen for sugar and ketones)   ___ ___ _____
   - Reagent strip as ordered   ___ ___ _____
   - Gloves   ___ ___ _____
6. Removed a strip from the bottle. Put the cap back on immediately. Made sure it was tight.   ___ ___ _____
7. Dipped the strip test areas into the specimen.   ___ ___ _____
8. Removed the strip after the correct amount of time.   ___ ___ _____
9. Tapped the strip gently against the container to remove excess urine.   ___ ___ _____
10. Waited the required amount of time.   ___ ___ _____
11. Compared the strip with the color chart on the bottle. Read the results.   ___ ___ _____
12. Discarded disposable items and the specimen.   ___ ___ _____

Post-Procedure

13. Cleaned and returned equipment to its proper place.   ___ ___ _____
14. Removed the gloves and washed hands.   ___ ___ _____
15. Reported the results and other observations to the nurse.   ___ ___ _____

Straining Urine

QUALITY OF LIFE

Remember to: ● Knock before entering the person's room
               ● Address the person by name
               ● Introduce yourself by name and title

Name: _____

Date: _____

	S	U	Comments

Pre-Procedure

1. Explained the procedure to the person.
2. Washed hands.
3. Collected the following:
   - Strainer or 4 × 4 gauze
   - Specimen container
   - Urinal, bedpan, commode, or specimen pan
   - Two labels stating that all urine is strained
   - Gloves
   - Plastic bag
4. Identified the person.

Procedure

5. Arranged items in the person's bathroom.
6. Placed one label in the bathroom. Placed the other near the bed.
7. Put on the gloves.
8. Offered the bedpan or urinal or assisted the person to the bed-side commode or bathroom.
9. Provided for privacy and removed the gloves.
10. Told the person to signal after voiding.
11. Put on gloves.
12. Placed the strainer or gauze into the specimen container.
13. Poured urine into the specimen container. Urine passed through the strainer or gauze.
14. Removed the strainer and discarded the urine.
15. Placed the strainer or gauze in the container if any crystals, stones, or particles appeared.
16. Helped the person clean the perineal area, if necessary.
17. Cleaned and returned equipment to its proper place.
18. Removed soiled gloves. Washed hands and put on clean gloves.
19. Helped the person wash his or her hands.
20. Removed the gloves.

Post-Procedure

21. Provided for comfort.
22. Placed the signal light within reach.
23. Unscreened the person.

Post-Procedure—cont'd

	S	U	Comments
24. Labeled the specimen container with the requested information. Placed the container in the plastic bag. (Wore gloves for this step.)	_____	_____	_____
25. Washed hands.	_____	_____	_____
26. Reported observations to the nurse.	_____	_____	_____
27. Took the specimen and requisition slip to the storage area.	_____	_____	_____

Changing a Ureterostomy Pouch

QUALITY OF LIFE

Name: _____

Remember to: ● Knock before entering the person's room   Date: _____
                ● Address the person by name
                ● Introduce yourself by name and title

Pre-Procedure	S	U	Comments
1. Explained the procedure to the person.	___	___	_____
2. Washed hands.	___	___	_____
3. Collected the following:			
• Clean pouch with skin barrier	___	___	_____
• Skin barrier (if not part of the pouch)	___	___	_____
• Pouch clamp, clip, or wire closure	___	___	_____
• Clean ostomy belt (if used)	___	___	_____
• Skin barrier as ordered	___	___	_____
• Four to eight gauze squares	___	___	_____
• Adhesive remover	___	___	_____
• Cotton balls	___	___	_____
• Bedpan with cover	___	___	_____
• Waterproof pad	___	___	_____
• Bath blanket	___	___	_____
• Toilet tissue	___	___	_____
• Washbasin	___	___	_____
• Bath thermometer	___	___	_____
• Prescribed soap or cleansing agent	___	___	_____
• Pouch deodorant	___	___	_____
• Paper towels	___	___	_____
• Gloves	___	___	_____
• Disposable bag	___	___	_____
4. Arranged the work area.	___	___	_____
5. Identified the person.	___	___	_____
6. Provided for privacy.	___	___	_____
7. Raised the bed to the best level for good body mechanics. Made sure bed rails were up.	___	___	_____

Procedure

	S	U	Comments
8. Lowered the bed rail near you.	___	___	_____
9. Covered the person with a bath blanket. Fanfolded linens to the foot of the bed.	___	___	_____
10. Placed the waterproof pad under the buttocks.	___	___	_____
11. Put on the gloves.	___	___	_____
12. Disconnected the pouch from the belt, if one was worn. Removed the belt.	___	___	_____
13. Removed the pouch gently. Gently pushed the skin down and away from the skin barrier. Placed the pouch in the bedpan.	___	___	_____

Procedure—cont'd   S   U   Comments

14. Placed one or two gauze squares over the stoma to absorb urine.   _____ _____ _____

15. Wiped around the stoma with toilet tissue or a gauze square. Placed soiled tissue or gauze in the bedpan.   _____ _____ _____

16. Moistened a cotton ball with adhesive remover. Cleaned around the stoma to remove any remaining skin barrier. Cleaned from the stoma outward.   _____ _____ _____

17. Covered the bedpan and took it to the bathroom. Raised the bed rail before leaving the bedside.   _____ _____ _____

18. Measured urine. Asked the nurse to observe abnormal urine. Emptied the pouch and bedpan into the toilet. Noted the color, amount, clarity, and odor of urine. Put the pouch in the disposable bag.   _____ _____ _____

19. Removed the gloves. Washed hands and put on clean gloves.   _____ _____ _____

20. Filled the washbasin with warm water. Placed the basin on the overbed table on top of the paper towels. Lowered the bed rail near you.   _____ _____ _____

21. Cleansed the skin around the stoma with water. Rinsed and patted dry. Used soap or other cleansing agent as directed by the nurse.   _____ _____ _____

22. Observed the stoma and skin around the stoma. Reported any irritation or skin breakdown to the nurse.   _____ _____ _____

23. Applied the skin barrier if it was a separate device.   _____ _____ _____

24. Put a clean ostomy belt on the person, if a belt was worn.   _____ _____ _____

25. Added deodorant to the new pouch.   _____ _____ _____

26. Removed the gauze square used to absorb urine from the stoma.   _____ _____ _____

27. Removed adhesive backing on the pouch.   _____ _____ _____

28. Centered the pouch over the stoma. Made sure the drain pointed downward.   _____ _____ _____

29. Pressed around the skin barrier so that the pouch sealed to the skin. Applied gentle pressure from the stoma outward.   _____ _____ _____

30. Maintained pressure for 1 to 2 minutes.   _____ _____ _____

31. Connected the belt to the pouch (if a belt was worn).   _____ _____ _____

32. Removed the waterproof pad.   _____ _____ _____

33. Covered the person. Removed the bath blanket.   _____ _____ _____

Post-Procedure	S	U	Comments
34. Provided for comfort.	_____	_____	_____
35. Raised or lowered the bed rails. Followed the care plan.	_____	_____	_____
36. Lowered the bed to its lowest position.	_____	_____	_____
37. Placed the signal light within reach.	_____	_____	_____
38. Unscreened the person.	_____	_____	_____
39. Cleaned the bedpan, washbasin, and other equipment.	_____	_____	_____
40. Returned equipment to its proper place.	_____	_____	_____
41. Discarded the disposable bag and followed center policy for soiled linen.	_____	_____	_____
42. Removed the gloves and washed hands.	_____	_____	_____
43. Reported observations to the nurse.	_____	_____	_____

Giving a Cleansing Enema

QUALITY OF LIFE

Remember to:
- Knock before entering the person's room
- Address the person by name
- Introduce yourself by name and title

Name: _____

Date: _____

Pre-Procedure

	S	U	Comments

1. Followed Delegation Guidelines.

2. Explained the procedure to the person.

3. Decontaminated hands.

4. Collected the following:
   - Disposable enema kit (enema bag, tube, clamp, and water-proof pad) as directed by the nurse.
   - Bath thermometer
   - Waterproof pad
   - Water-soluble lubricant
   - Gloves
   - Material for enema solution: 5 ml (1 teaspoon) castile soap or 2 teaspoons of salt
   - Toilet tissue
   - Bath blanket
   - IV pole
   - Robe and nonskid footwear
   - Bedpan or commode
   - Paper towels

5. Identified the person. Checked identification bracelet against the assignment sheet. Called the person by name.

6. Provided for privacy.

7. Raised the bed for good body mechanics. Bed rails were up, if used.

Procedure

8. Lowered the bed rail near you, if up.

9. Covered the person with a bath blanket. Fan-folded top linens to the foot of the bed.

10. Positioned the IV pole so that the enema bag was 12 inches above the anus or to a height directed by the nurse.

11. Raised the bed rail (if used).

Procedure—cont'd   **S**   **U**   **Comments**

12. Prepared the enema:

    a. Closed the clamp on the tube.   _____ _____ _____

    b. Adjusted water flow until it was lukewarm.   _____ _____ _____

    c. Filled the enema bag for the amount ordered.   _____ _____ _____

    d. Measured water temperature. For adults, water was 105° F   _____ _____ _____
        (40.5° C) or as instructed by nurse.

    e. Prepared the enema solution:

        • Saline enema: added 2 teaspoons salt.   _____ _____ _____

        • Soapsuds enema: added 5 ml (1 teaspoon) of castile soap.   _____ _____ _____

        • Tap-water enema: added nothing to the water.   _____ _____ _____

    f. Stirred the solution with the bath thermometer. Scooped off   _____ _____ _____
        any suds (SSE).

    g. Sealed the bag.   _____ _____ _____

    h. Hung the bag on the IV pole.   _____ _____ _____

13. Lowered the bed rail, if up.   _____ _____ _____

14. Positioned the person in the left Sims' position or in a left side-   _____ _____ _____
    lying position.

15. Placed a waterproof pad under the buttocks.   _____ _____ _____

16. Put on the gloves.   _____ _____ _____

17. Exposed the anal area.   _____ _____ _____

18. Placed the bedpan behind the person.   _____ _____ _____

19. Positioned the enema tube in the bedpan. Opened the clamp. Let   _____ _____ _____
    solution flow through the tube to remove air. Clamped the tube.

20. Lubricated the tube 3 to 4 inches from the tip.   _____ _____ _____

21. Separated the buttocks to expose the anus.   _____ _____ _____

22. Asked the person to take a deep breath through the mouth.   _____ _____ _____

23. Inserted the tube gently 3 to 4 inches into the rectum when the   _____ _____ _____
    person exhaled. Stopped if the person complained of pain or if
    resistance was felt.

24. Checked the quantity of solution in the bag.   _____ _____ _____

25. Unclamped the tube. Administered solution slowly.   _____ _____ _____

26. Asked the person to take slow deep breaths.   _____ _____ _____

27. Clamped the tube if the person needed to defecate, had abdom-   _____ _____ _____
    inal cramping, or started to expel solution. Unclamped when
    symptoms subsided.

28. Gave the amount of solution ordered. Stopped if the person   _____ _____ _____
    could not tolerate the procedure.

29. Clamped the tube before it emptied.   _____ _____ _____

30. Held toilet tissue around the tube and against the anus. Re-   _____ _____ _____
    moved the tube.

31. Discarded the soiled toilet tissue into the bedpan.   _____ _____ _____

32. Wrapped the tubing tip with paper towels and placed it inside   _____ _____ _____
    the enema bag.

Procedure—cont'd   S   U   **Comments**

33. Helped the person onto the bedpan. Raised the head of the bed,   _____   _____   _____
    and raised the bed rail, if used, or assisted the person to the
    bathroom or commode. The person wore a robe and nonskid
    footwear while up. The bed was in the lowest position.

34. Placed the signal light and toilet tissue within reach. Reminded   _____   _____   _____
    the person not to flush the toilet.

35. Discarded disposable items.   _____   _____   _____

36. Removed the gloves and decontaminated hands.   _____   _____   _____

37. Left the room, if the person could be left alone.   _____   _____   _____

38. Returned when the person signaled. Knocked before entering.   _____   _____   _____
    Decontaminated your hands and lowered bed rail, if up.

39. Put on the gloves.   _____   _____   _____

40. Observed enema results for amount, color, consistency, and   _____   _____   _____
    odor. Called nurse to observe results.

41. Provided perineal care as needed.   _____   _____   _____

42. Removed the bed protector.   _____   _____   _____

43. Emptied, cleaned, and disinfected the bedpan or commode.   _____   _____   _____
    Flushed the toilet after the nurse observed the results. Returned
    items to their proper place. Removed gloves and decontami-
    nated hands.

44. Assisted the person with hand hygiene. (Wore gloves, if   _____   _____   _____
    necessary.)

45. Returned top linens and removed the bath blanket.   _____   _____   _____

Post-Procedure

46. Provided for comfort.   _____   _____   _____

47. Placed the signal light within reach.   _____   _____   _____

48. Lowered the bed to its lowest position.   _____   _____   _____

49. Raised or lowered bed rails. Followed the care plan.   _____   _____   _____

50. Unscreened the person.   _____   _____   _____

51. Followed center policy for soiled linen and used supplies.   _____   _____   _____

52. Decontaminated hands.   _____   _____   _____

53. Reported observations to the nurse.   _____   _____   _____

Giving a Commercial Enema

QUALITY OF LIFE

Remember to:
- Knock before entering the person's room
- Address the person by name
- Introduce yourself by name and title

Name: _____

Date: _____

Pre-Procedure

	S	U	Comments
1. Followed Delegation Guidelines.	_____	_____	_____
2. Explained the procedure to the person.	_____	_____	_____
3. Decontaminated hands.	_____	_____	_____
4. Collected the following:			
• Commercial enema	_____	_____	_____
• Bedpan or commode	_____	_____	_____
• Waterproof pad	_____	_____	_____
• Toilet tissue	_____	_____	_____
• Gloves	_____	_____	_____
• Robe and nonskid footwear	_____	_____	_____
• Bath blanket	_____	_____	_____
5. Identified the person. Checked the identification bracelet against the assignment sheet. Called the person by name.	_____	_____	_____
6. Provided for privacy.	_____	_____	_____
7. Raised the bed for good body mechanics. Bed rails were up, if used.	_____	_____	_____

Procedure

	S	U	Comments
8. Lowered the bed rail near you, if up.	_____	_____	_____
9. Covered the person with a bath blanket. Fanfolded top linens to the foot of the bed.	_____	_____	_____
10. Positioned the person in the left Sims' or left sidelying position.	_____	_____	_____
11. Placed the waterproof pad under the buttocks.	_____	_____	_____
12. Put on the gloves.	_____	_____	_____
13. Exposed the anal area.	_____	_____	_____
14. Positioned the bedpan near the person.	_____	_____	_____
15. Removed the cap from the enema.	_____	_____	_____
16. Separated the buttocks to see the anus.	_____	_____	_____
17. Asked the person to take a deep breath through the mouth.	_____	_____	_____
18. Gently inserted the enema tip 2 inches into the rectum when the person was exhaling.	_____	_____	_____
19. Squeezed and rolled the bottle gently. Released pressure on the bottle after tip was removed from the rectum.	_____	_____	_____
20. Placed the bottle into the box, tip first.	_____	_____	_____

Procedure—cont'd   S   U   **Comments**

21. Helped the person onto the bedpan; raised the head of the bed,   ____ ____ _____
    or assisted the person to the bathroom or commode. The person
    wore a robe and nonskid footwear when up. The bed was in the
    lowest position.

22. Placed the signal light and toilet tissue within reach. Reminded   ____ ____ _____
    the person not to flush the toilet.

23. Discarded used disposable items. Removed the gloves and de-   ____ ____ _____
    contaminated your hands.

24. Left the room, if the person could be left alone.   ____ ____ _____

25. Returned when the person signaled. Knocked before entering.   ____ ____ _____
    Decontaminated hands, and lowered the bed rail, if up.

26. Put on gloves.   ____ ____ _____

27. Observed enema results for amount, color, consistency,   ____ ____ _____
    and odor.

28. Helped the person clean the perineal area.   ____ ____ _____

29. Removed the bed protector.   ____ ____ _____

30. Emptied, cleaned, and disinfected the bedpan or commode.   ____ ____ _____
    Flushed the toilet after the nurse observed results. Returned
    equipment to its proper place. Removed the gloves and decon-
    taminated hands.

31. Assisted the person hand hygiene. (Wore gloves if necessary.)   ____ ____ _____

Post-Procedure

32. Provided for comfort.   ____ ____ _____

33. Placed the signal light within reach.   ____ ____ _____

34. Lowered the bed to its lowest position.   ____ ____ _____

35. Raised or lowered bed rails. Followed the care plan.   ____ ____ _____

36. Unscreened the person.   ____ ____ _____

37. Followed center policy for soiled linen and used supplies.   ____ ____ _____

38. Decontaminated hands.   ____ ____ _____

39. Reported observations to the nurse.   ____ ____ _____

Giving an Oil-Retention Enema

QUALITY OF LIFE

Remember to:
- Knock before entering the person's room
- Address the person by name
- Introduce yourself by name and title

Name: _____

Date: _____

Pre-Procedure

	S	U	Comments
1. Followed Delegation Guidelines.	____	____	_____
2. Explained the procedure to the person.	____	____	_____
3. Decontaminated hands.	____	____	_____
4. Collected the following:			
• Commercial oil-retention enema	____	____	_____
• Waterproof pad	____	____	_____
• Gloves	____	____	_____
• Bath blanket	____	____	_____
5. Identified the person. Checked the identification bracelet against the assignment sheet. Called the person by name.	____	____	_____
6. Provided for privacy.	____	____	_____
7. Raised the bed for good body mechanics. Bed rails were up, if used.	____	____	_____

Procedure

	S	U	Comments
8. Lowered the bed rail near you, if up.	____	____	_____
9. Covered the person with a bath blanket. Fanfolded top linens to the foot of the bed.	____	____	_____
10. Positioned the person in the left Sims' or left sidelying position.	____	____	_____
11. Placed a waterproof pad under the buttocks.	____	____	_____
12. Put on the gloves.	____	____	_____
13. Exposed the anal area.	____	____	_____
14. Removed the cap from the enema.	____	____	_____
15. Separated the buttocks to see the anus.	____	____	_____
16. Asked the person to take a deep breath through the mouth.	____	____	_____
17. Gently inserted the tip 2 inches into the rectum when the person was exhaling.	____	____	_____
18. Squeezed and rolled the bottle slowly and gently. Released pressure on the bottle after tip was removed from rectum.	____	____	_____
19. Placed the bottle in the box, tip first.	____	____	_____
20. Covered the person. Left the person in Sims' or left sidelying position.	____	____	_____
21. Encouraged the person to retain the enema for the time ordered.	____	____	_____
22. Placed additional waterproof pads on the bed, if needed.	____	____	_____
23. Removed the gloves.	____	____	_____

Procedure—cont'd   S   U   Comments

24. Lowered the bed to its lowest position.   _____ _____ _____
25. Raised or lowered bed rails. Followed the care plan. _____ _____ _____
26. Provided for comfort.   _____ _____ _____
27. Placed the signal light within reach.   _____ _____ _____
28. Checked the person often. Observed results.   _____ _____ _____

Post-Procedure

29. Provided for comfort.   _____ _____ _____
30. Placed the signal light within reach.   _____ _____ _____
31. Lowered the bed to its lowest position.   _____ _____ _____
32. Raised or lowered bed rails. Followed the care plan. _____ _____ _____
33. Unscreened the person.   _____ _____ _____
34. Followed center policy for soiled linen and used supplies. _____ _____ _____
35. Decontaminated hands.   _____ _____ _____
36. Reported observations to the nurse.   _____ _____ _____

Inserting a Rectal Tube

QUALITY OF LIFE

Remember to: ● Knock before entering the person's room
               ● Address the person by name
               ● Introduce yourself by name and title

Name: _____

Date: _____

Pre-Procedure

	S	U	Comments
1. Followed Delegation Guidelines.	___	___	_____
2. Explained the procedure to the person.	___	___	_____
3. Decontaminated hands.	___	___	_____
4. Collected the following:			
• Disposable rectal tube with flatus bag	___	___	_____
• Water-soluble lubricant	___	___	_____
• Tape	___	___	_____
• Gloves	___	___	_____
• Waterproof pad	___	___	_____
5. Identified the person. Checked the identification bracelet against the assignment sheet. Called the person by name.	___	___	_____
6. Provided for privacy.	___	___	_____
7. Raised the bed for good body mechanics. Bed rails were up, if used.	___	___	_____

Procedure

	S	U	Comments
8. Lowered the bed rail near you.	___	___	_____
9. Positioned the person in the left Sims' or left sidelying position.	___	___	_____
10. Placed the waterproof pad under the buttocks.	___	___	_____
11. Put on the gloves.	___	___	_____
12. Exposed the anal area.	___	___	_____
13. Lubricated 4 inches from the tip of the tube.	___	___	_____
14. Separated the buttocks to expose the anus.	___	___	_____
15. Asked the person to take a deep breath through the mouth.	___	___	_____
16. Gently inserted the tube 4 inches into the rectum when the person was exhaling. Stopped if the person complained of pain or resistance was felt.	___	___	_____
17. Taped the rectal tube to the buttocks.	___	___	_____
18. Positioned the flatus bag so that it rested on the bed protector.	___	___	_____
19. Covered the person.	___	___	_____
20. Left the tube in place for the time specified by the nurse, not longer than 30 minutes.	___	___	_____
21. Lowered the bed to its lowest position. Placed the signal light within reach. Raised or lowered bed rails. Followed the care plan.	___	___	_____

Procedure—cont'd   S   U   Comments

22. Removed the gloves and decontaminated hands.   _____ _____ _____

23. Left the room. Checked the person often. Knocked before en-   _____ _____ _____
    tering room.

24. Returned to the room when time to remove tube. Knocked be-   _____ _____ _____
    fore entering the room.

25. Decontaminated hands, put on gloves, and removed the tube.   _____ _____ _____
    Wiped the rectal area.

26. Wrapped the rectal tube and flatus bag in the bed protector. Re-   _____ _____ _____
    moved bed protector and gloves. Decontaminated your hands.

27. Asked the person about the amount of gas expelled.   _____ _____ _____

Post-Procedure

28. Provided for comfort.   _____ _____ _____

29. Placed the signal light within reach.   _____ _____ _____

30. Unscreened the person.   _____ _____ _____

31. Discarded disposable items. Followed center policy for soiled   _____ _____ _____
    linen. (Wore gloves.)

32. Reported observations to the nurse.   _____ _____ _____

Changing an Ostomy Pouch

QUALITY OF LIFE

Name: _____

Date: _____

Remember to:
- Knock before entering the person's room
- Address the person by name
- Introduce yourself by name and title

Pre-Procedure

	S	U	Comments
1. Followed Delegation Guidelines.	___	___	_____
2. Explained the procedure to the person.	___	___	_____
3. Decontaminated hands.	___	___	_____
4. Collected the following:			
• Clean pouch with skin barrier	___	___	_____
• Skin barrier (if not part of the pouch)	___	___	_____
• Pouch clamp, clip, or wire closure	___	___	_____
• Clean ostomy belt (if used)	___	___	_____
• Skin barrier as ordered	___	___	_____
• Gauze squares or washcloths	___	___	_____
• Adhesive remover	___	___	_____
• Cotton balls	___	___	_____
• Bedpan with cover	___	___	_____
• Waterproof pad	___	___	_____
• Bath blanket	___	___	_____
• Toilet tissue	___	___	_____
• Washbasin	___	___	_____
• Bath thermometer	___	___	_____
• Prescribed soap or cleansing agent	___	___	_____
• Pouch deodorant	___	___	_____
• Paper towels	___	___	_____
• Gloves	___	___	_____
• Disposable bag	___	___	_____
5. Arranged work area.	___	___	_____
6. Identified the person. Checked identification bracelet against the assignment sheet. Called the person by name.	___	___	_____
7. Provided for privacy.	___	___	_____
8. Raised the bed for good body mechanics. Made sure bed rails were up, if used.	___	___	_____

Procedure	S	U	Comments
9. Lowered the bed rail near you, if up.	_____	_____	_____
10. Covered the person with a bath blanket. Fanfolded linens to the foot of the bed.	_____	_____	_____
11. Placed the waterproof pad under the buttocks.	_____	_____	_____
12. Put on the gloves.	_____	_____	_____
13. Disconnected the pouch from the belt, if one was worn. Removed the belt.	_____	_____	_____
14. Removed the pouch, gently. Gently pushed the skin down and away from the skin barrier. Placed the pouch in the bedpan.	_____	_____	_____
15. Wiped around the stoma with toilet tissue or a gauze square. Placed soiled tissue or gauze in the bedpan.	_____	_____	_____
16. Moistened a cotton ball with adhesive remover. Cleaned around the stoma to remove any remaining skin barrier. Cleaned from stoma outward.	_____	_____	_____
17. Covered the bedpan and took it to the bathroom. (Raised the bed rail before leaving, if used.)	_____	_____	_____
18. Measured feces as directed by nurse. Asked nurse to observe abnormal feces. Emptied the pouch and bedpan in the toilet. Noted the color, amount, consistency, and odor of feces. Placed pouch in the disposable bag.	_____	_____	_____
19. Removed gloves and decontaminated hands. Put on clean gloves.	_____	_____	_____
20. Filled the washbasin with warm water. Placed the basin on the overbed table on top of the paper towels. Lowered the bed rail near you, if up.	_____	_____	_____
21. Cleaned the skin around the stoma with water. Rinsed and patted dry. Used soap or other cleansing agent as directed by the nurse.	_____	_____	_____
22. Applied the skin barrier if a separate device.	_____	_____	_____
23. Put a clean ostomy belt on the person, if worn.	_____	_____	_____
24. Added deodorant to the new pouch.	_____	_____	_____
25. Removed adhesive backing on the pouch.	_____	_____	_____
26. Centered the pouch over the stoma with the drain pointed downward.	_____	_____	_____
27. Pressed around the skin barrier so that the pouch sealed to the skin. Applied gentle pressure from the stoma outward.	_____	_____	_____
28. Maintained pressure for 1 to 2 minutes.	_____	_____	_____
29. Connected the belt to the pouch (if worn).	_____	_____	_____
30. Removed the waterproof pad.	_____	_____	_____
31. Removed the gloves.	_____	_____	_____
32. Covered the person. Removed the bath blanket.	_____	_____	_____

Post-Procedure

	S	U	Comments
33. Provided for comfort.	_____	_____	_____
34. Raised or lowered bed rails. Followed the care plan.	_____	_____	_____
35. Lowered the bed to its lowest position.	_____	_____	_____
36. Placed the signal light within reach.	_____	_____	_____
37. Unscreened the person.	_____	_____	_____
38. Cleaned the bedpan, washbasin, and other equipment. (Wore gloves.)	_____	_____	_____
39. Returned equipment to its proper place.	_____	_____	_____
40. Discarded the disposable bag according to center policy. Followed center policy for soiled linen.	_____	_____	_____
41. Removed the gloves and decontaminated hands.	_____	_____	_____
42. Reported observations to the nurse.	_____	_____	_____

Collecting a Stool Specimen

QUALITY OF LIFE

Remember to: ● Knock before entering the person's room
                ● Address the person by name
                ● Introduce yourself by name and title

Name: _____

Date: _____

Pre-Procedure

	S	U	Comments
1. Followed Delegation Guidelines.	___	___	_____
2. Explained the procedure to the person.	___	___	_____
3. Decontaminated hands.	___	___	_____
4. Collected the following:			
• Bedpan and cover or commode	___	___	_____
• Urinal (or bedpan with cover) for voiding	___	___	_____
• Specimen pan for the toilet or commode	___	___	_____
• Specimen container and lid	___	___	_____
• Tongue blade	___	___	_____
• Disposable bag	___	___	_____
• Gloves	___	___	_____
• Toilet tissue	___	___	_____
• Laboratory requisition slip	___	___	_____
• Plastic bag	___	___	_____

Procedure

	S	U	Comments
5. Labeled the container.	___	___	_____
6. Identified the person. Checked identification bracelet with the requisition slip. Called the person by name.	___	___	_____
7. Provided for privacy.	___	___	_____
8. Asked the person to urinate. Provided the bedpan or urinal.	___	___	_____
9. Placed the specimen pan under the toilet seat.	___	___	_____
10. Assisted the person onto the bedpan or to the toilet or commode. The person wore a robe and nonskid footwear when up.	___	___	_____
11. Asked the person not to put toilet tissue in the bedpan, commode, or specimen pan. Provided a disposable bag for toilet tissue.	___	___	_____
12. Placed the signal light and toilet tissue within reach. Raised or lowered bed rails. Followed the care plan.	___	___	_____
13. Decontaminated hands and left the room.	___	___	_____
14. Returned when the person signaled. Knocked before entering. Decontaminated your hands.	___	___	_____
15. Lowered the bed rail near you, if up.	___	___	_____
16. Put on the gloves. Provided perineal care, if necessary.	___	___	_____
17. Used a tongue blade to take about 2 tablespoons of feces. Placed in the specimen container.	___	___	_____

	S	U	Comments
Procedure—cont'd			
18. Placed the lid on the specimen container. Did not touch the inside of the lid or container. Placed the container in the plastic bag.	_____	_____	_____
19. Placed the tongue blade in the disposable bag.	_____	_____	_____
20. Emptied, cleaned, and disinfected equipment. Removed the gloves and decontaminated hands.	_____	_____	_____
21. Returned equipment to its proper place.	_____	_____	_____
22. Helped the person with hand hygiene. (Wore gloves, if necessary.)	_____	_____	_____

Post-Procedure

23. Provided for comfort.	_____	_____	_____
24. Placed the signal light within reach.	_____	_____	_____
25. Lowered the bed to its lowest position.	_____	_____	_____
26. Raised or lowered bed rails. Followed the care plan.	_____	_____	_____
27. Unscreened the person.	_____	_____	_____
28. Took the specimen and requisition slip to the nurse.	_____	_____	_____
29. Decontaminated hands.	_____	_____	_____
30. Reported observations to the nurse.	_____	_____	_____

Testing a Stool Specimen for Blood

QUALITY OF LIFE

Remember to:
- Knock before entering the person's room
- Address the person by name
- Introduce yourself by name and title

Name: _____

Date: _____

Pre-Procedure

	S	U	Comments

1. Followed Delegation Guidelines.
2. Explained the procedure to the person.
3. Decontaminated hands.

Procedure

4. Collected a stool specimen.
5. Collected the following:
   - Paper towel
   - Hemoccult test kit (includes developer)
   - Tongue blades
   - Gloves
6. Put on the gloves.
7. Opened the test kit.
8. Used a tongue blade to obtain a small amount of stool.
9. Applied a thin smear of stool on box "A" on the test paper.
10. Used another tongue blade to obtain some feces from another part of the specimen.
11. Applied a thin smear of stool on box "B" on the test paper.
12. Closed the test packet.
13. Turned the test packet to the other side. Opened the flap. Applied developer to boxes "A" and "B."
14. Waited the amount of time noted in the manufacturer's instructions.
15. Noted and recorded the color changes. Followed the manufacturer's instructions.
16. Disposed of the test packet.
17. Discarded the tongue blade.
18. Disposed of the specimen.

Post-Procedure

19. Removed the gloves and decontaminated hands.
20. Reported the test results and observations to the nurse.

Measuring Intake and Output

QUALITY OF LIFE

Remember to:
- Knock before entering the person's room
- Address the person by name
- Introduce yourself by name and title

Name: _____

Date: _____

Pre-Procedure

	S	U	Comments

1. Followed Delegation Guidelines. _____ _____ _____
2. Explained the procedure to the person. _____ _____ _____
3. Decontaminated hands. _____ _____ _____
4. Collected the following:
   - Intake and output (I&O) record _____ _____ _____
   - Graduate _____ _____ _____
   - Gloves _____ _____ _____

Procedure

5. Measured intake as follows:
   a. Put on gloves. _____ _____ _____
   b. Poured liquid remaining in a container into the graduate. _____ _____ _____
   c. Measured the amount at eye level. _____ _____ _____
   d. Checked the amount of the serving on the I&O record. _____ _____ _____
   e. Subtracted the remaining amount from the full-serving amount. Recorded the amount. _____ _____ _____
   f. Repeated the same for each liquid. Added the amounts from each liquid together. Recorded the amount and time on the I&O record. _____ _____ _____
6. Measured the output as follows:
   a. Decontaminated hands. _____ _____ _____
   b. Put on gloves. _____ _____ _____
   c. Poured fluid into the graduate. Avoided spills. _____ _____ _____
   d. Measured the amount at eye level. Kept the container level. _____ _____ _____
   e. Disposed of fluid in the toilet. Avoided splashes. _____ _____ _____
   f. Rinsed the graduate. Discarded rinse into the toilet. Returned the graduate to its proper place. _____ _____ _____
   g. Cleaned and rinsed the bedpan, urinal, emesis basin, or other drainage container. Discarded the rinse into the toilet. Returned the items to their proper place. _____ _____ _____
   h. Removed the gloves and decontaminated hands. _____ _____ _____
   i. Recorded the amount on the I&O record. _____ _____ _____

Post-Procedure

7. Reported and recorded observations. _____ _____ _____

Preparing the Person for Meals

QUALITY OF LIFE

Remember to:
- Knock before entering the person's room
- Address the person by name
- Introduce yourself by name and title

Name: _____

Date: _____

Pre-Procedure	S	U	Comments

1. Followed Delegation Guidelines.
2. Explained to the person that it was mealtime.
3. Decontaminated hands.
4. Collected the following:
   - Equipment for oral hygiene
   - Bedpan or urinal and toilet tissue
   - Washbasin
   - Soap
   - Washcloth
   - Towel
   - Gloves
5. Provided for privacy.

Procedure

6. Made sure the person's eyeglasses and hearing aids were in place.
7. Assisted with oral hygiene using Standard Precautions. Made sure dentures were in place.
8. Assisted the person with elimination. Made sure the incontinent person was clean and dry. (Followed Standard Precautions.)
9. Helped the person with hand hygiene.
10. Did the following for persons eating in bed:
    a. Raised the head of the bed to a comfortable sitting position.
    b. Adjusted the overbed table in front of the person. Clean the table.
    c. Placed the signal light within reach.
    d. Unscreened the person.
11. Did the following for persons who could sit in a chair:
    a. Positioned the person in a chair or wheelchair.
    b. Removed items from the overbed table. Cleaned the table.
    c. Adjusted the overbed table in front of the person.
    d. Placed the signal light within reach.
    e. Unscreened the person.
12. Assisted the person to the correct dining area. Followed center procedure for dining programs.

Post-Procedure	S	U	Comments
13. Returned to the room.	_____	_____	_____
14. Cleaned and returned equipment to its proper place. (Followed Standard and the Bloodborne Pathogen Standard.)	_____	_____	_____
15. Straightened the room. Eliminated unpleasant noise, odors, or equipment.	_____	_____	_____
16. Decontaminated hands.	_____	_____	_____

Serving Meal Trays

QUALITY OF LIFE

Remember to: ● Knock before entering the person's room
                ● Address the person by name
                ● Introduce yourself by name and title

Name: _____

Date: _____

Pre-Procedure

	`S	U	Comments
1. Followed Delegation Guidelines.	___	___	_____
2. Decontaminated hands.	___	___	_____

Procedure

3. Made sure the tray was complete. Checked items on the tray with the dietary card. Included adaptive equipment, if used. ___ ___ _____

4. Identified the person. Checked the identification bracelet with the dietary card. Called the person by name. ___ ___ _____

5. Placed the tray within the person's reach. Adjusted the overbed table as needed. ___ ___ _____

6. Removed food covers. Opened cartons, cut meat, and buttered bread as needed. ___ ___ _____

7. Placed the napkin, clothes protector, adaptive equipment, and silverware within reach. ___ ___ _____

8. Measured and recorded intake, if ordered. Noted the amount and type of foods eaten. ___ ___ _____

9. Checked for and removed any food in the mouth. (Wore gloves.) ___ ___ _____

10. Removed the tray. ___ ___ _____

11. Cleaned any spills and changed soiled linen. ___ ___ _____

12. Helped the person to bed, if indicated. ___ ___ _____

Post-Procedure

13. Assisted with oral hygiene and with hand hygiene. ___ ___ _____

14. Provided for comfort. ___ ___ _____

15. Removed the gloves and decontaminated hands. ___ ___ _____

16. Placed the signal light within reach. ___ ___ _____

17. Raised or lowered bed rails. Followed the care plan. ___ ___ _____

18. Followed center policy for soiled linen. ___ ___ _____

19. Decontaminated hands. ___ ___ _____

20. Reported and recorded observations. ___ ___ _____

Feeding a Person

QUALITY OF LIFE

Name: _____

Date: _____

Remember to:
- Knock before entering the person's room
- Address the person by name
- Introduce yourself by name and title

Pre-Procedure

	S	U	Comments

1. Explained the procedure to the person.
2. Decontaminated hands.
3. Positioned the person in a comfortable sitting position.
4. Brought the tray into the room or the dining room. Placed tray on the overbed table or dining table.

Procedure

5. Identified the person.
6. Draped a napkin across the person's chest and underneath the chin.
7. Prepared the food for eating.
8. Told the person what foods were on the tray.
9. Served foods in the order the person preferred. Alternated between solid and liquid foods. Used a spoon. Allowed enough time for chewing. Did not rush the person.
10. Used straws for liquids if the person could not drink out of a glass or cup. Had one straw for each liquid. Provided a short straw for weak persons. Did not use a straw for persons with dysphagia. Gave thickened liquids with a spoon.
11. Pleasantly conversed with the person.
12. Encouraged the person to eat as much as possible.
13. Wiped the person's mouth with a napkin as needed.
14. Noted how much and which foods were eaten when the person was done eating.
15. Measured and recorded intake, if ordered.
16. Removed the tray.
17. Took the person back to his or her room.
18. Provided oral hygiene. Wore gloves.

Post-Procedure

	S	U	Comments
19. Provided for comfort.	_____	_____	_____
20. Placed the signal light within reach.	_____	_____	_____
21. Raised or lowered bed rails if the person was in bed. Followed the care plan.	_____	_____	_____
22. Decontaminated hands	_____	_____	_____
23. Reported observations to the nurse:			
• The amount and kind of food eaten	_____	_____	_____
• Complaints of nausea or dysphagia	_____	_____	_____
• Signs of aspiration	_____	_____	_____

Performing Range-of-Motion Exercises

QUALITY OF LIFE

Name: _____

Date: _____

Remember to:
- Knock before entering the person's room
- Address the person by name
- Introduce yourself by name and title

Pre-Procedure

	S	U	Comments
1. Followed Delegation Guidelines.	___	___	_____
2. Identified the person. Checked the identification bracelet against the assignment sheet. Called the person by name.	___	___	_____
3. Explained the procedure to the person.	___	___	_____
4. Decontaminated hands.	___	___	_____
5. Obtained a bath blanket.	___	___	_____
6. Provided for privacy.	___	___	_____
7. Raised the bed for good body mechanics. Made sure bed rails were up, if used.	___	___	_____

Procedure

	S	U	Comments
8. Lowered the bed rail near you if up.	___	___	_____
9. Positioned the person supine.	___	___	_____
10. Covered the person with a bath blanket. Fan folded top linens to the foot of the bed.	___	___	_____
11. Exercised the neck *if allowed and if the RN instructed you to:*			
a. Placed your hands over the person's ears and supported the head.	___	___	_____
b. Performed flexion—brought the head forward. Chin touched chest.	___	___	_____
c. Performed extension—straightened the head.	___	___	_____
d. Performed hyperextension—brought the head backward until chin pointed up.	___	___	_____
e. Performed rotation—turned the head side to side, chin to shoulder, chin to other shoulder.	___	___	_____
f. Performed lateral flexion—moved head to the right and to the left, ear to shoulder, ear to other shoulder.	___	___	_____
g. Repeated flexion, extension, hyperextension, rotation, and lateral flexion five times or the number of times stated in the care plan.	___	___	_____
12. Exercised the shoulder:			
a. Grasped the wrist with one hand and the elbow with the other.	___	___	_____
b. Performed flexion—raised the arm straight in front and over the head.	___	___	_____
c. Performed extension—brought the arm down to the side.	___	___	_____
d. Performed hyperextension—moved the arm behind the body. (Performed this movement if person was seated in a straight-backed chair or was standing.)	___	___	_____

Procedure—cont'd	S	U	Comments

12. Exercised the shoulder—cont'd

e. Performed abduction—moved the straight arm away from the side of the body. _____ _____ _____

f. Performed adduction—moved the straight arm to the side of the body. _____ _____ _____

g. Performed internal rotation—bent the elbow and placed it at the same level as the shoulder. Moved the forearm down toward the body. _____ _____ _____

h. Performed external rotation— moved the forearm toward the head. _____ _____ _____

i. Repeated flexion, extension, hyperextension, abduction, adduction, and internal and external rotation five times or the number of times stated in the care plan. _____ _____ _____

13. Exercised the elbow:

a. Grasped the person's wrist with one hand and the elbow with the other. _____ _____ _____

b. Performed flexion—bent the arm to touch the shoulder on the same side. _____ _____ _____

c. Performed extension—straightened the arm. _____ _____ _____

d. Repeated each flexion and extension five times or the number of times stated in the care plan. _____ _____ _____

14. Exercised the forearm:

a. Performed pronation—turned the hand palm down. _____ _____ _____

b. Performed supination—turned the hand palm up. _____ _____ _____

c. Repeated pronation and supination five times or the number of times stated in the care plan. _____ _____ _____

15. Exercised the wrist:

a. Held the wrist with both hands. _____ _____ _____

b. Performed flexion—bent the hand down. _____ _____ _____

c. Performed extension—straightened the hand. _____ _____ _____

d. Performed hyperextension—bent the hand back. _____ _____ _____

e. Performed radial flexion—turned the hand toward the thumb. _____ _____ _____

f. Performed ulnar flexion—turned the hand toward the little finger. _____ _____ _____

g. Repeated flexion, extension, hyperextension, radial flexion, and ulnar flexion five times or the number of times stated in the care plan. _____ _____ _____

16. Exercised the thumb:

a. Held the person's hand with one hand and the thumb with the other hand. _____ _____ _____

b. Performed abduction—moved the thumb away from the inner part of the index finger. _____ _____ _____

c. Performed adduction—moved the thumb back next to the index finger. _____ _____ _____

d. Performed opposition—touched each fingertip with the thumb. _____ _____ _____

Procedure—cont'd   S   U   Comments

16. Exercised the thumb—cont'd

    e. Performed flexion—bent the thumb into the hand.   _____ _____ _____

    f. Performed extension—moved the thumb out to the side of the fingers.   _____ _____ _____

    g. Repeated abduction, adduction, opposition, flexion, and extension five times or the number of times stated in the care plan.   _____ _____ _____

17. Exercised the fingers:

    a. Performed abduction—spread the fingers and the thumb apart.   _____ _____ _____

    b. Performed adduction—brought the fingers and the thumb together.   _____ _____ _____

    c. Performed extension—straightened the fingers so that the fingers, hand, and arm were straight.   _____ _____ _____

    d. Performed flexion—made a fist.   _____ _____ _____

    e. Repeated abduction, adduction, extension, and flexion five times or the number of times stated in the care plan.   _____ _____ _____

18. Exercised the hip:

    a. Placed one hand under the knee and the other under the ankle to support the leg.   _____ _____ _____

    b. Performed flexion—raised the leg.   _____ _____ _____

    c. Performed extension—straightened the leg.   _____ _____ _____

    d. Performed abduction—moved the leg away from the body.   _____ _____ _____

    e. Performed adduction—moved the leg toward the other leg.   _____ _____ _____

    f. Performed internal rotation—turned the leg inward.   _____ _____ _____

    g. Performed external rotation—turned the leg outward.   _____ _____ _____

    h. Repeated flexion, extension, abduction, adduction, and internal and external rotation five times or the number of times stated in the care plan.   _____ _____ _____

19. Exercised the knee:

    a. Placed one hand under the knee and the other under the ankle to support the leg.   _____ _____ _____

    b. Performed flexion—bent the leg.   _____ _____ _____

    c. Performed extension—straightened the leg.   _____ _____ _____

    d. Repeated flexion and extension five times or the number of times stated in the care plan.   _____ _____ _____

20. Exercised the ankle:

    a. Placed one hand under the foot and the other under the ankle to support the part.   _____ _____ _____

    b. Performed dorsiflexion—pulled the foot forward, and pushed down on the heel at the same time.   _____ _____ _____

    c. Performed plantar flexion—pushed the foot downward, or pointed the toes.   _____ _____ _____

    d. Repeated dorsiflexion and plantar flexion five times or the number of times stated in the care plan.   _____ _____ _____

Procedure—cont'd	**S**	**U**	**Comments**

21. Exercised the foot:

    a. Performed pronation—turned the outside of the foot up and the inside down.   ____ ____ _____

    b. Performed supination—turned the inside of the foot up and the outside down.   ____ ____ _____

    c. Repeated pronation and supination five times or the number of times stated in the care plan.   ____ ____ _____

22. Exercised the toes:

    a. Performed flexion—curled the toes.   ____ ____ _____

    b. Performed extension—straightened the toes.   ____ ____ _____

    c. Performed abduction—spread the toes apart.   ____ ____ _____

    d. Performed adduction—pulled the toes together.   ____ ____ _____

    e. Repeated flexion, extension, abduction, and adduction five times or the number of times stated in the care plan.   ____ ____ _____

23. Covered the leg and raised the bed rail, if used.   ____ ____ _____

24. Went to the other side. Lowered the bed rail near you, if used.   ____ ____ _____

25. Repeated exercises on other side of body.

    a. Exercised the shoulder:

      (1) Grasped the wrist with one hand and the elbow with the other.   ____ ____ _____

      (2) Performed flexion—raised the arm straight in front and over the head.   ____ ____ _____

      (3) Performed extension—brought the arm down to the side.   ____ ____ _____

      (4) Performed hyperextension—moved the arm behind the body. (Performed this movement if person was seated in straight-backed chair or was standing.)   ____ ____ _____

      (5) Performed abduction—moved the straight arm away from the side of the body.   ____ ____ _____

      (6) Performed adduction—moved the straight arm to the side of the body.   ____ ____ _____

      (7) Performed internal rotation—bent the elbow and placed it at the same level as the shoulder. Moved the forearm down toward the body.   ____ ____ _____

      (8) Performed external rotation—moved the forearm toward the head.   ____ ____ _____

      (9) Repeated flexion, extension, hyperextension, abduction, adduction, and internal and external rotation five times or the number of times stated in the care plan.   ____ ____ _____

    b. Exercised the elbow:

      (1) Grasped the person's wrist with one hand and the elbow with the other.   ____ ____ _____

      (2) Performed flexion—bent the arm to touch the shoulder on the same side.   ____ ____ _____

      (3) Performed extension—straightened the arm.   ____ ____ _____

      (4) Repeated each flexion and extension five times or the number of times stated in the care plan.   ____ ____ _____

Procedure—cont'd	**S**	**U**	**Comments**

25. Repeated exercises on other side of body—cont'd

   c. Exercised the forearm:

      (1) Performed pronation—turned the hand palm down.

      (2) Performed supination—turned the hand palm up.

      (3) Repeated pronation and supination five times or the number of times stated in the care plan.

   d. Exercised the wrist:

      (1) Held the wrist with both hands.

      (2) Performed flexion—bent the hand down.

      (3) Performed extension—straightened the hand.

      (4) Performed hyperextension—bent the hand back.

      (5) Performed radial flexion—turned the hand toward the thumb.

      (6) Performed ulnar flexion—turned the hand toward the little finger.

      (7) Repeated flexion, extension, hyperextension, radial flexion, and ulnar flexion five times or the number of times stated in the care plan.

   e. Exercised the thumb:

      (1) Held the person's hand with one hand and the thumb with the other hand.

      (2) Performed abduction—moved the thumb away from the inner part of the index finger.

      (3) Performed adduction—moved the thumb back next to the index finger.

      (4) Performed opposition—touched each fingertip with the thumb.

      (5) Performed flexion—bent the thumb into the hand.

      (6) Performed extension—moved the thumb out to the side of the fingers.

      (7) Repeated abduction, adduction, opposition, and flexion and extension five times or the number of times stated in the care plan.

   f. Exercised the fingers:

      (1) Performed abduction—spread the fingers and the thumb apart.

      (2) Performed adduction—brought the fingers and the thumb together.

      (3) Performed extension—straightened the fingers so that the fingers, hand, and arm were straight.

      (4) Performed flexion—made a fist.

      (5) Repeated abduction, adduction, extension, and flexion five times or the number of times stated in the care plan.

Procedure—cont'd   **S**   **U**   **Comments**

25. Repeated exercises on other side of body—cont'd

    g. Exercised the hip:

        (1) Placed one hand under the knee and the other under the ankle to support the leg.

        (2) Performed flexion—raised the leg.

        (3) Performed extension—straightened the leg.

        (4) Performed abduction—moved the leg away from the body.

        (5) Performed adduction—moved the leg toward the other leg.

        (6) Performed internal rotation—turned the leg inward.

        (7) Performed external rotation—turned the leg outward.

        (8) Repeated flexion, extension, abduction, adduction, and internal and external rotation five times or the number of times stated in the care plan.

    h. Exercised the knee:

        (1) Placed one hand under the knee and the other under the ankle to support the leg.

        (2) Performed flexion—bent the leg.

        (3) Performed extension—straightened the leg.

        (4) Repeated flexion and extension five times or the number of times stated in the care plan.

    i. Exercised the ankle:

        (1) Placed one hand under the foot and the other under the ankle to support the part.

        (2) Performed dorsiflexion—pulled the foot forward and pushed down on the heel at the same time.

        (3) Performed plantar flexion—pushed the foot downward or pointed the toes.

        (4) Repeated dorsiflexion and plantar flexion five times or the number of times stated in the care plan.

    j. Exercised the foot:

        (1) Performed pronation—turned the outside of the foot up and the inside down.

        (2) Performed supination—turned the inside of the foot up and the outside down.

        (3) Repeated pronation and supination five times or the number of times stated in the care plan.

    k. Exercised the toes:

        (1) Performed flexion—curled the toes.

        (2) Performed extension—straightened the toes.

        (3) Performed abduction—spread the toes apart.

        (4) Performed adduction—pulled the toes together.

        (5) Repeated flexion, extension, abduction, and adduction five times or the number of times stated in the care plan.

    l. Covered the leg and raised the bed rail, if used.

Post-Procedure	S	U	Comments
26. Provided for comfort.	_____	_____	_____
27. Covered the person. Removed the bath blanket.	_____	_____	_____
28. Raised or lowered bed rails. Followed the care plan.	_____	_____	_____
29. Lowered the bed to its lowest level.	_____	_____	_____
30. Placed the signal light within reach.	_____	_____	_____
31. Unscreened the person.	_____	_____	_____
32. Returned the bath blanket to its proper place.	_____	_____	_____
33. Decontaminated hands.	_____	_____	_____
34. Reported and recorded observations.	_____	_____	_____

Helping the Person to Walk

QUALITY OF LIFE

Remember to:
- ● Knock before entering the person's room
- ● Address the person by name
- ● Introduce yourself by name and title

Name: _____

Date: _____

	S	U	Comments

Pre-Procedure

1. Followed Delegation Guidelines.   _____ _____ _____
2. Explained the procedure to the person.   _____ _____ _____
3. Decontaminated hands.   _____ _____ _____
4. Collected the following:
   - Robe and nonskid shoes   _____ _____ _____
   - Paper or sheet to protect bottom linens   _____ _____ _____
   - Gait (transfer or safety) belt   _____ _____ _____
5. Identified the person. Checked identification bracelet against the assignment sheet. Called the person by name.   _____ _____ _____
6. Provided for privacy.   _____ _____ _____

Procedure

7. Lowered the bed to its lowest position. Locked the bed wheels.   _____ _____ _____
8. Fan-folded top linens to the foot of the bed.   _____ _____ _____
9. Placed the paper or sheet under the person's feet (protected linen). Put shoes on the person.   _____ _____ _____
10. Helped the person to dangle.   _____ _____ _____
11. Helped the person put on the robe.   _____ _____ _____
12. Applied the gait belt.   _____ _____ _____
13. Helped the person stand. Grasped the gait belt on each side, or placed your arms under the person's arms around to the shoulder blades.   _____ _____ _____
14. Stood at the person's side while he or she gained balance. Held the gait belt at the side and back, or had one arm around the back to support the person.   _____ _____ _____
15. Encouraged the person to stand erect with head up and back straight.   _____ _____ _____
16. Assisted the person to walk. Walked at side and slightly behind the person. Provided support with gait belt, or placed one arm around the back to support the person.   _____ _____ _____
17. Encouraged the person to walk normally. The heels struck the floor first. Discouraged shuffling, sliding, or walking on tiptoes.   _____ _____ _____
18. Walked the required distance if the person could tolerate the activity. Did not rush the person.   _____ _____ _____
19. Helped the person return to bed.   _____ _____ _____
20. Lowered the head of the bed. Helped the person to the center of the bed.   _____ _____ _____
21. Removed the footwear, and removed the paper or sheet over the bottom sheet.   _____ _____ _____

Post-Procedure

	S	U	Comments
22. Provided for comfort. Covered the person.	_____	_____	_____
23. Placed the signal light within reach.	_____	_____	_____
24. Raised or lowered bed rails. Followed the care plan.	_____	_____	_____
25. Returned the robe and footwear to their proper places.	_____	_____	_____
26. Unscreened the person.	_____	_____	_____
27. Decontaminated hands.	_____	_____	_____
28. Reported and recorded your observations.	_____	_____	_____

Helping the Falling Person

QUALITY OF LIFE

Name: _____

Date: _____

Remember to:
- Knock before entering the person's room
- Address the person by name
- Introduce yourself by name and title

Procedure	S	U	Comments
1. Stood with feet apart. Kept back straight.	____	____	_____
2. Brought the person close to the body as quickly as possible. Used the gait belt, or wrapped arms around the person's waist, or held person under the arms.	____	____	_____
3. Moved your leg so that the person's buttocks rested on it. Moved the leg near the person.	____	____	_____
4. Lowered the person to the floor. Let the person slide down your leg to the floor. Bent at the hips and knees as you lowered the person.	____	____	_____
5. Called a nurse to check the person.	____	____	_____
6. Helped the nurse return the person to bed. Obtained other help as necessary.	____	____	_____
7. Reported the following to the nurse:			
• How the fall occurred	____	____	_____
• How far the person walked	____	____	_____
• How the activity was tolerated before the fall	____	____	_____
• Any complaints before the fall	____	____	_____
• Amount of assistance needed by the person while walking	____	____	_____
8. Completed an incident report.	____	____	_____

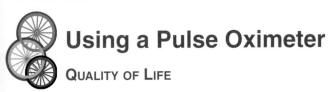

Using a Pulse Oximeter

QUALITY OF LIFE

Remember to:
- Knock before entering the person's room
- Address the person by name
- Introduce yourself by name and title

Name: _____

Date: _____

Pre-Procedure

	S	U	Comments
1. Followed Delegation Guidelines.	___	___	_____
2. Reviewed the procedure with the nurse.	___	___	_____
3. Explained the procedure to the person.	___	___	_____
4. Decontaminated your hands.	___	___	_____
5. Collected the following:			
• Oximeter and sensor	___	___	_____
• Nail polish remover	___	___	_____
• Cotton balls	___	___	_____
• Saturation pulse oxygen (SpO_2) flow sheet	___	___	_____
• Tape (if needed)	___	___	_____
• Towel	___	___	_____
6. Provided for privacy.	___	___	_____

Procedure

	S	U	Comments
7. Provided for comfort.	___	___	_____
8. Removed nail polish with a cotton ball.	___	___	_____
9. Dried the site with a towel.	___	___	_____
10. Clipped or taped the sensor to the site.	___	___	_____
11. Attached the sensor cables to the oximeter.	___	___	_____
12. Turned on the oximeter.	___	___	_____
13. Set the high and low alarm limits for SpO_2 and pulse rate. Turned on the audio and visual alarms.	___	___	_____
14. Checked the person's pulse (apical or radial) with the pulse on the display. Told the nurse if they were not equal.	___	___	_____
15. Read the SpO_2 and the pulse rate on the display and noted them on the flow sheet.	___	___	_____
16. Left the sensor in place for continuous monitoring or turned off the device and removed the sensor as directed by the nurse.	___	___	_____

Post-Procedure

	S	U	Comments
17. Provided for comfort.	___	___	_____
18. Placed the signal light within reach.	___	___	_____
19. Raised or lowered bed rails. Followed care plan.	___	___	_____
20. Unscreened the person.	___	___	_____
21. Returned the device to its proper place when monitoring discontinued.	___	___	_____
22. Decontaminated your hands.	___	___	_____
23. Reported the SpO_2 and pulse rate to the nurse and any other observations.	___	___	_____

Collecting a Sputum Specimen

QUALITY OF LIFE

Remember to:
- Knock before entering the person's room
- Address the person by name
- Introduce yourself by name and title

Name: _____

Date: _____

Pre-Procedure

	S	U	Comments
1. Followed Delegation Guidelines.	____	____	_____
2. Explained the procedure to the person.	____	____	_____
3. Decontaminated your hands.	____	____	_____
4. Collected the following:			
• Sputum specimen container and label	____	____	_____
• Laboratory requisition	____	____	_____
• Disposable bag	____	____	_____
• Gloves	____	____	_____
• Tissues	____	____	_____

Procedure

	S	U	Comments
5. Labeled the container.	____	____	_____
6. Identified the person. Checked the identification bracelet with the requisition slip. Called the person by name.	____	____	_____
7. Provided for privacy. If able, the person used the bathroom to obtain specimen.	____	____	_____
8. Asked the person to rinse the mouth out with clear water.	____	____	_____
9. Put on gloves.	____	____	_____
10. Had the person hold the container. Touched only the outside of the container.	____	____	_____
11. Asked the person to cover mouth and nose with tissue while coughing.	____	____	_____
12. Asked the person to take two or three deep breaths and coughed up sputum.	____	____	_____
13. Had the person expectorate into the container. The sputum did not touch the outside.	____	____	_____
14. Collected 1 to 2 tablespoons of sputum or as instructed by the nurse.	____	____	_____
15. Placed the lid on the container.	____	____	_____
16. Placed the container in the bag and attached the requisition to the bag.	____	____	_____
17. Removed gloves.	____	____	_____

Post-Procedure   S   U   **Comments**

18. Decontaminated your hands.   ____ ____ _____
19. Provided for comfort.   ____ ____ _____
20. Placed the signal light within reach.   ____ ____ _____
21. Unscreened the person.   ____ ____ _____
22. Took the bag to the storage area.   ____ ____ _____
23. Decontaminated your hands.   ____ ____ _____
24. Reported and recorded your observations.   ____ ____ _____

Assisting With Coughing and Deep Breathing Exercises

Name: _____

Date: _____

QUALITY OF LIFE

Remember to: ● Knock before entering the person's room
              ● Address the person by name
              ● Introduce yourself by name and title

Pre-Procedure	S	U	Comments
1. Followed Delegation Guidelines.	___	___	_____
2. Explained the procedure to the person.	___	___	_____
3. Identified the person. Checked the identification bracelet against the assignment sheet. Called the person by name.	___	___	_____
4. Decontaminated your hands.	___	___	_____
5. Provided for privacy.	___	___	_____

Procedure

	S	U	Comments
6. Helped the person to a comfortable sitting position: dangling, semi-Fowler's, or Fowler's.	___	___	_____
7. Had the person deep breathe:			
a. Had the person place his or her hands over the rib cage.	___	___	_____
b. Asked the person to exhale. Explained that the ribs should move as far down as possible.	___	___	_____
c. Had the person take a deep breath. Reminded the person to inhale through the nose as deep as possible.	___	___	_____
d. Asked the person to hold breath for 3 seconds.	___	___	_____
e. Asked the person to exhale slowly through pursed lips. The ribs moved as far down as possible.	___	___	_____
f. Had the person repeat the inhale-exhale exercise four more times.	___	___	_____
8. Asked the person to cough:			
a. Had the person support the incision by interlaced fingers over the site. Held a small pillow or folded towel over the incision.	___	___	_____
b. Had the person take a deep breath though the nose.	___	___	_____
c. Asked the person to cough strongly twice with the mouth open.	___	___	_____

Post-Procedure

	S	U	Comments
9. Provided for comfort.	___	___	_____
10. Raised or lowered bed rails. Followed the care plan.	___	___	_____
11. Placed the signal light within reach.	___	___	_____
12. Unscreened the person.	___	___	_____
13. Reported and recorded your observations.	___	___	_____

Setting Up for Oxygen Administration

QUALITY OF LIFE

Name: _____

Date: _____

Remember to:
- Knock before entering the person's room
- Address the person by name
- Introduce yourself by name and title

Pre-Procedure

                                                      S   **U**   **Comments**

1. Followed Delegation Guidelines.
2. Decontaminated your hands.
3. Collected the following:
   - Oxygen administration device with tubing
   - Flowmeter
   - Humidifier (if ordered)
   - Distilled water (if using humidifier)
4. Identified the person. Checked the identification bracelet against the assignment sheet. Called the person by name.
5. Explained to the person what you are doing.

Procedure

6. Made sure the flowmeter was in the "off" position.
7. Attached the flowmeter to the wall outlet or to the tank.
8. Filled the humidifier with distilled water.
9. Attached the humidifier to the bottom of the flowmeter.
10. Attached the oxygen administration device and the connecting tubing to the humidifier. (Did not set the flowmeter or apply the oxygen administration device on the person.)

Post-Procedure

11. Discarded packaging.
12. Secured cap on the distilled water and stored it according to center policy.
13. Provided for comfort.
14. Placed the signal light within reach.
15. Decontaminated your hands.
16. Told the nurse when you finished set up. (The nurse: turned on the oxygen and set rate; applied the oxygen administration device on the person.)

Taking a Temperature With a Glass Thermometer

QUALITY OF LIFE

Remember to: ● Knock before entering the person's room
             ● Address the person by name
             ● Introduce yourself by name and title

Name: _____

Date: _____

Pre-Procedure

	S	U	Comments

1. Followed Delegation Guidelines. ___ ___ _____

2. Explained the procedure to the person. For an oral temperature, asked the person not to eat, drink, smoke, or chew gum for at least 15 to 20 minutes. ___ ___ _____

3. Collected the following:

   • Oral or rectal thermometer and holder ___ ___ _____

   • Tissues ___ ___ _____

   • Plastic covers, if used ___ ___ _____

   • Gloves ___ ___ _____

   • Toilet tissue (rectal temperature) ___ ___ _____

   • Water-soluble lubricant (rectal temperature) ___ ___ _____

   • Towel (axillary temperature) ___ ___ _____

4. Decontaminated hands. ___ ___ _____

5. Identified the person. Checked the identification bracelet against the assignment sheet. Called the person by name. ___ ___ _____

6. Provided for privacy. ___ ___ _____

Procedure

7. Put on the gloves. ___ ___ _____

8. Rinsed the thermometer in cold water, if it was soaking in a disinfectant solution. Dried it with tissues. ___ ___ _____

9. Checked the thermometer for breaks or chips. ___ ___ _____

10. Shook down thermometer below 95° Fahrenheit or 35° Celsius. ___ ___ _____

11. Inserted the thermometer into plastic cover, if used. ___ ___ _____

12. For an *oral temperature:*

    a. Asked the person to moisten the lips. ___ ___ _____

    b. Placed the bulb end of the thermometer under the tongue. ___ ___ _____

    c. Asked the person to close the lips around the thermometer. ___ ___ _____

    d. Asked the person not to talk. Reminded the person not to bite down on the thermometer. ___ ___ _____

    e. Left the thermometer in place for 2 to 3 minutes or as required by center policy. ___ ___ _____

13. For a *rectal temperature:*

    a. Positioned the person in Sims' position. ___ ___ _____

    b. Applied a small amount of lubricant on a tissue. Lubricated the bulb end of the thermometer. ___ ___ _____

Procedure—cont'd	S	U	Comments

Procedure—cont'd

c. Folded back top linens and exposed the anal area.

d. Raised the upper buttock and exposed the anus.

e. Inserted the thermometer 1 inch into the rectum. Did not force the thermometer.

f. Held the thermometer in place for 2 minutes or as required by center policy.

14. For an *axillary temperature:*

a. Assisted the person to remove an arm from the gown. Did not expose the person.

b. Dried the axilla with the towel.

c. Placed the bulb end of the thermometer in the center of the axilla.

d. Asked the person to place the arm across the chest to hold the thermometer in place. Held the thermometer and the arm, if person needed assistance.

e. Left the thermometer in place for 5 to 10 minutes or as required by center policy.

15. Removed the thermometer.

16. Used tissues to remove the plastic cover. Wiped the thermometer with a tissue from the stem to the bulb end, if no cover was used.

17. For a *rectal temperature:*

a. Placed used toilet tissue on a paper towel and placed the thermometer on clean toilet tissue.

b. Wiped the anal area. Removed excess lubricant and feces. Covered the person.

18. For an *axillary temperature:*

a. Helped the person put gown back on.

19. Read the thermometer.

20. Recorded the person's name and temperature. Wrote an "R" for rectal temperature; wrote an "A" for axillary temperature.

21. Shook down the thermometer.

22. Cleaned the thermometer according to center policy.

23. Discarded tissue.

24. Removed gloves and decontaminated hands.

Post-Procedure

25. Provided for comfort.

26. Placed the signal light within reach.

27. Unscreened the person.

28. Reported an abnormal temperature to the nurse. Recorded temperature in the proper place.

Taking a Temperature With an Electronic Thermometer

Name: _____

Date: _____

QUALITY OF LIFE

Remember to: ● Knock before entering the person's room
                 ● Address the person by name
                 ● Introduce yourself by name and title

Pre-Procedure	S	U	Comments

1. Followed Delegation Guidelines.   _____ _____ _____

2. Explained the procedure to the person. For an oral temperature, asked the person not to eat, drink, smoke, or chew gum for at least 15 to 20 minutes.   _____ _____ _____

3. Collected the following:
   - Thermometer (electronic or tympanic membrane   _____ _____ _____
   - Probe (blue for an oral or axillary temperature, red for rectal temperature)   _____ _____ _____
   - Probe covers   _____ _____ _____
   - Toilet tissue (for a rectal temperature)   _____ _____ _____
   - Water-soluble lubricant (for rectal temperature)   _____ _____ _____
   - Gloves   _____ _____ _____
   - Towel (for axillary temperature)   _____ _____ _____

4. Plugged the probe into the thermometer (not done when tympanic thermometer was used).   _____ _____ _____

5. Decontaminated hands.   _____ _____ _____

6. Identified the person. Checked the identification bracelet against the assignment sheet. Called the person by name.   _____ _____ _____

Procedure

7. Provided for privacy. Positioned the person for an oral, rectal, axillary, or tympanic membrane temperature.   _____ _____ _____

8. Put on the gloves, if possible contact with body fluids.   _____ _____ _____

9. Inserted the probe into a probe cover.   _____ _____ _____

10. For an *oral temperature:*
    a. Asked the person to open the mouth and raise the tongue.   _____ _____ _____
    b. Placed the covered probe at the base of the tongue.   _____ _____ _____
    c. Asked the person to lower the tongue and close the mouth.   _____ _____ _____

11. For a *rectal temperature:*
    a. Applied lubricant on a tissue and lubricated the end of the covered probe.   _____ _____ _____
    b. Exposed the anal area.   _____ _____ _____
    c. Raised the upper buttock.   _____ _____ _____
    d. Inserted the probe $1/2$ inch into the rectum.   _____ _____ _____

Procedure—cont'd   S   U   Comments

12. For an *axillary temperature:*

   a. Assisted the person to remove an arm from the gown. Did _____ _____ _____
      not expose the person.

   b. Dried the axilla with the towel. _____ _____ _____

   c. Placed the covered probe in the axilla. _____ _____ _____

   d. Placed the person's arm across the chest. _____ _____ _____

13. For a *tympanic membrane temperature:*

   a. Asked the person to turn his or her head until the ear is in _____ _____ _____
      front of you.

   b. Inserted the covered probe. Pulled back on the ear; straight- _____ _____ _____
      ened the ear canal.

14. Started the thermometer. _____ _____ _____

15. Held the probe in place until tone was heard or light (steady or _____ _____ _____
     flashing) was seen.

16. Read the temperature on the display. _____ _____ _____

17. Removed the probe and pressed the eject button that discarded _____ _____ _____
     the probe cover.

18. Noted the person's name, temperature, and temperature site on _____ _____ _____
     assignment sheet or note pad.

19. Returned the probe to the holder. _____ _____ _____

20. Provided for comfort. Assisted the person to put gown back on, _____ _____ _____
     if axillary temperature.

     For a *rectal temperature:*

   a. Wiped the anal area with tissue. _____ _____ _____

   b. Covered the person. _____ _____ _____

   c. Discarded used toilet tissue. _____ _____ _____

   d. Removed the gloves. Decontaminated hands. _____ _____ _____

Post-Procedure

21. Placed the signal light within reach. _____ _____ _____

22. Unscreened the person. _____ _____ _____

23. Returned the thermometer to the charging unit. _____ _____ _____

24. Decontaminated hands. _____ _____ _____

25. Reported an abnormal temperature and recorded temperature _____ _____ _____
     and site in proper place.

Taking a Radial Pulse

QUALITY OF LIFE

Name: _____

Date: _____

Remember to:
- Knock before entering the person's room
- Address the person by name
- Introduce yourself by name and title

Pre-Procedure

	S	U	Comments
1. Followed Delegation Guidelines.	____	____	_____
2. Decontaminated your hands.	____	____	_____
3. Identified the person. Checked the identification bracelet against the assignment sheet. Called the person by name.	____	____	_____
4. Explained the procedure to the person.	____	____	_____
5. Provided for privacy.	____	____	_____

Procedure

	S	U	Comments
6. Had the person sit or lie down.	____	____	_____
7. Located the radial pulse with your first two or three middle fingers.	____	____	_____
8. Noted if the pulse was strong or weak and regular or irregular.	____	____	_____
9. Counted the pulse for 30 seconds. Multiplied the number of beats by two, or counted the pulse for 1 minute as directed by the nurse or if required by center policy.	____	____	_____
10. Counted the pulse for 1 minute, if irregular.	____	____	_____
11. Noted the person's name and pulse rate. Also noted strength and regular or irregular.	____	____	_____

Post-Procedure

	S	U	Comments
12. Provided for comfort.	____	____	_____
13. Placed the signal light within reach.	____	____	_____
14. Unscreened the person.	____	____	_____
15. Decontaminated your hands.	____	____	_____
16. Reported and recorded the pulse rate and observations in the proper place.	____	____	_____

Taking an Apical Pulse

QUALITY OF LIFE

Remember to:
- Knock before entering the person's room
- Address the person by name
- Introduce yourself by name and title

Name: _____

Date: _____

	S	U	Comments

Pre-Procedure

1. Followed Delegation Guidelines. ____ ____ _____
2. Collected a stethoscope and alcohol wipes. ____ ____ _____
3. Decontaminated your hands. ____ ____ _____
4. Identified the person. Checked the identification bracelet against the assignment sheet. Called the person by name. ____ ____ _____
5. Explained the procedure to the person. ____ ____ _____
6. Provided for privacy. ____ ____ _____

Procedure

7. Cleaned the earpieces and diaphragm with alcohol wipes. ____ ____ _____
8. Had the person sit or lie down. ____ ____ _____
9. Exposed the nipple area of the left chest. ____ ____ _____
10. Warmed the diaphragm in your hand. ____ ____ _____
11. Placed the earpieces in your ears. ____ ____ _____
12. Found the apical pulse. Placed the diaphragm 2 to 3 inches to the left of the breastbone and below the left nipple. ____ ____ _____
13. Counted the pulse for 1 minute; noted if pulse was regular or irregular. ____ ____ _____
14. Covered the person. Removed earpieces. ____ ____ _____
15. Noted the person's name and pulse rate and whether pulse was regular or irregular. ____ ____ _____

Post-Procedure

16. Provided for comfort. ____ ____ _____
17. Placed the signal light within reach. ____ ____ _____
18. Unscreened the person. ____ ____ _____
19. Cleaned the earpieces and diaphragm with alcohol wipes. ____ ____ _____
20. Returned the stethoscope to the proper place. ____ ____ _____
21. Decontaminated your hands. ____ ____ _____
22. Reported and recorded observations. Recorded the pulse rate with "Ap" for apical. ____ ____ _____

Taking an Apical-Radial Pulse

QUALITY OF LIFE

Remember to:
- Knock before entering the person's room
- Address the person by name
- Introduce yourself by name and title

Name: _____

Date: _____

Pre-Procedure

	S	U	Comments
1. Followed Delegation Guidelines.	___	___	_____
2. Asked a nurse or nursing assistant to assist.	___	___	_____
3. Collected a stethoscope and alcohol wipes.	___	___	_____
4. Decontaminated your hands.	___	___	_____
5. Identified the person. Checked the identification bracelet against the assignment sheet. Called the person by name.	___	___	_____
6. Explained the procedure to the person.	___	___	_____
7. Provided for privacy.	___	___	_____

Procedure

	S	U	Comments
8. Wiped the earpieces and diaphragm with the alcohol wipes.	___	___	_____
9. Had the person sit or lie down.	___	___	_____
10. Warmed the diaphragm in your hand.	___	___	_____
11. Exposed the left nipple area of the chest.	___	___	_____
12. Placed the earpieces in your ears.	___	___	_____
13. Found the apical pulse. Co-worker found radial pulse.	___	___	_____
14. Gave the signal to begin counting.	___	___	_____
15. Counted the pulses for 1 minute.	___	___	_____
16. Gave the signal to stop counting.	___	___	_____
17. Covered the person. Removed the earpieces.	___	___	_____
18. Noted the person's name and the apical and radial pulses. Subtracted the radial pulse from the apical pulse for the pulse deficit.	___	___	_____

Post-Procedure

	S	U	Comments
19. Provided for comfort.	___	___	_____
20. Placed the signal light within reach.	___	___	_____
21. Unscreened the person.	___	___	_____
22. Cleaned the earpieces and diaphragm with alcohol wipes.	___	___	_____
23. Returned the stethoscope to the proper place.	___	___	_____
24. Decontaminated your hands.	___	___	_____
25. Reported and recorded the following:			
• The apical and radial pulse rates	___	___	_____
• The pulse deficit	___	___	_____

Counting Respirations

QUALITY OF LIFE

Remember to:
- Knock before entering the person's room
- Address the person by name
- Introduce yourself by name and title

Name: _____

Date: _____

Pre-Procedure

	S	U	Comments
1. Followed Delegation Guidelines.	____	____	_____
2. Continued to hold the wrist after taking the radial pulse, or kept the stethoscope in place if apical pulse.	____	____	_____
3. Did not tell the person you were counting respirations.	____	____	_____
4. Began counting as the chest rose. Counted each rise and fall of the chest as one respiration.	____	____	_____
5. Observed if respirations were regular and if both sides of the chest rose equally. Noted depth of respiration and difficulty.	____	____	_____
6. Counted respiration for 30 seconds. Multiplied the number by two.	____	____	_____
7. Counted respiration for 1 minute if abnormal, irregular, or center policy.	____	____	_____
8. Noted person's name, respiratory rate, and other observations.	____	____	_____

Post-Procedure

	S	U	Comments
9. Provided for comfort.	____	____	_____
10. Placed the signal light within reach.	____	____	_____
11. Decontaminated your hands.	____	____	_____
12. Reported and recorded your observations.	____	____	_____

Measuring Blood Pressure

QUALITY OF LIFE

Remember to: ● Knock before entering the person's room
              ● Address the person by name
              ● Introduce yourself by name and title

Name: _____

Date: _____

Pre-Procedure

	S	U	Comments
1. Followed Delegation Guidelines.	___	___	_____
2. Collected the following:			
• Sphygmomanometer (blood pressure cuff)	___	___	_____
• Stethoscope	___	___	_____
• Alcohol wipes	___	___	_____
3. Decontaminated your hands.	___	___	_____
4. Identified the person. Checked the identification bracelet against the assignment sheet. Called the person by name.	___	___	_____
5. Explained the procedure to the person.	___	___	_____
6. Provided for privacy.	___	___	_____

Procedure

	S	U	Comments
7. Wiped the stethoscope earpieces and diaphragm with alcohol wipes.	___	___	_____
8. Had the person sit or lie down.			
9. Positioned the person's arm level with the heart with the palm up.	___	___	_____
10. Stood no more than 3 feet away from the sphygmomanometer. (Mercury model was vertical, on a flat surface, and at eye level. Aneroid type was directly in front.)	___	___	_____
11. Exposed the upper arm.	___	___	_____
12. Squeezed the cuff to expel any air. Closed the valve on the bulb.	___	___	_____
13. Found the brachial artery at the inner aspect of the elbow.	___	___	_____
14. Placed the arrow on the cuff over the brachial artery. Wrapped the cuff around the upper arm at least 1 inch above the elbow. The cuff was even and snug.	___	___	_____
15. *Method 1:*			
a. Placed the stethoscope earpieces in your ears.	___	___	_____
b. Located the radial artery. Inflated the cuff until no longer felt the pulse then inflated the cuff 30 mm Hg beyond the point at which pulse was last felt.	___	___	_____

Procedure—cont'd   S   U   Comments

16. *Method 2:*

    a. Located the radial artery. Inflated the cuff until no longer felt the pulse.

    b. Deflated the cuff slowly. Noted the point where last felt the pulse.

    c. Waited 30 seconds.

    d. Placed the earpieces in your ears.

    e. Inflated the cuff 30 mm Hg beyond the point at which you felt the pulse return.

17. Positioned the diaphragm over the brachial artery.

18. Deflated the cuff at an even rate of 2 to 4 millimeters per second. Turned the valve counterclockwise to deflate the cuff.

19. Noted the point on the scale at which you heard the first sound (systolic reading; near the point at which the radial pulse disappeared).

20. Continued to deflate the cuff. Noted the point at which the sound disappeared (diastolic reading).

21. Deflated the cuff completely. Removed it from the person's arm. Removed the stethoscope.

22. Noted the person's name and blood pressure reading.

23. Returned the cuff to case or wall holder.

Post-Procedure

24. Provided for comfort.

25. Placed the signal light within reach.

26. Unscreened the person.

27. Cleaned the earpieces and diaphragm with alcohol wipes.

28. Returned the equipment to the proper place.

29. Decontaminated your hands.

30. Reported and recorded the blood pressure.

Preparing the Person for an Examination

QUALITY OF LIFE

Remember to:
- Knock before entering the person's room
- Address the person by name
- Introduce yourself by name and title

Name: _____

Date: _____

Pre-Procedure	S	U	Comments
1. Explained the procedure to the person.	___	___	_____
2. Decontaminated hands.	___	___	_____
3. Assembled the following items on a tray at the bedside or in the examination room:			
• Flashlight	___	___	_____
• Sphygmomanometer	___	___	_____
• Stethoscope	___	___	_____
• Thermometer	___	___	_____
• Tongue depressors (blades)	___	___	_____
• Laryngeal mirror	___	___	_____
• Ophthalmoscope	___	___	_____
• Otoscope	___	___	_____
• Nasal speculum	___	___	_____
• Percussion (reflux) hammer	___	___	_____
• Tuning fork	___	___	_____
• Tape measure	___	___	_____
• Gloves	___	___	_____
• Water-soluble lubricant	___	___	_____
• Vaginal speculum	___	___	_____
• Cotton-tipped applicators	___	___	_____
• Specimen containers and lids	___	___	_____
• Disposable bag	___	___	_____
• Emesis basin	___	___	_____
• Towel	___	___	_____
• Bath blanket	___	___	_____
• Tissues	___	___	_____
• Drape	___	___	_____
• Paper towels	___	___	_____
• Cotton balls	___	___	_____
• Waterproof bed protector	___	___	_____
• Eye chart	___	___	_____
• Slides	___	___	_____
• Gown	___	___	_____
• Alcohol wipes	___	___	_____
• Wastebasket	___	___	_____
• Container for soiled instruments	___	___	_____
• Marking pencils or pens	___	___	_____

Pre-Procedure—cont'd   S   U   Comments

4. Identified the person.

5. Provided for privacy.

6. Asked the person to put on the gown. Instructed the person to remove all clothes. Assisted as necessary.

7. Asked the person to urinate. If the person was not ambulatory, offered the bedpan or urinal. Provided privacy.

8. Transported the person to the examination room.

9. Weighed and measured the person.

10. Helped the person get on the examination table.

11. Positioned the person as directed. Raised the bed to its highest level. Raised the bed rails if the person was in bed.

12. Draped the person.

13. Placed a bed protector under the buttocks.

14. Arranged for adequate lighting.

15. Put the signal light on for the nurse or examiner. Did not leave the person unattended.

Preparing the Person's Room

QUALITY OF LIFE

Remember to:
- Knock before entering the person's room
- Address the person by name
- Introduce yourself by name and title

Name: _____

Date: _____

Pre-Procedure

	S	U	Comments

1. Followed Delegation Guidelines.   _____ _____ _____
2. Knew which room and bed to prepare. Found out if the person was to arrive by wheelchair or stretcher.   _____ _____ _____
3. Decontaminated your hands.   _____ _____ _____
4. Collected the following:
   - Personal care items: bath basin, pitcher, glass, bedpan, and urinal (if male)   _____ _____ _____
   - Admission checklist   _____ _____ _____
   - Sphygmomanometer   _____ _____ _____
   - Stethoscope   _____ _____ _____
   - Gown or pajamas, towel, and washcloth   _____ _____ _____
   - IV pole, if needed   _____ _____ _____
   - Other equipment as directed by the nurse   _____ _____ _____

Procedure

5. For the person arriving by stretcher:
   a. Made a surgical bed.   _____ _____ _____
   b. Raised the bed to its highest level.   _____ _____ _____
6. For the person who is ambulatory or arriving by wheelchair:
   a. Left the bed closed.   _____ _____ _____
   b. Lowered the bed to its lowest level.   _____ _____ _____
7. Attached the signal light to the bed linens.   _____ _____ _____
8. Placed the sphygmomanometer, stethoscope, and admission checklist on the overbed table.   _____ _____ _____
9. Placed the gown or pajamas, towel, washcloth, and personal care items in the bedside stand.   _____ _____ _____
10. Placed the water pitcher and glass on the bedside stand or overbed table. (Omitted if person was NPO.)   _____ _____ _____
11. Decontaminated your hands.   _____ _____ _____

Measuring Height and Weight

QUALITY OF LIFE

Remember to:
- Knock before entering the person's room
- Address the person by name
- Introduce yourself by name and title

Name: _____

Date: _____

Pre-Procedure

	S	U	Comments
1. Explained the procedure to the person.	____	____	_____
2. Asked the person to urinate.	____	____	_____
3. Decontaminated hands.	____	____	_____
4. Collected the following:			
• Scale	____	____	_____
• Paper towels	____	____	_____
5. Identified the person.	____	____	_____
6. Provided for privacy.	____	____	_____

Procedure

7. Standing scale:

	S	U	Comments
a. Placed the paper towels on the scale platform.	____	____	_____
b. Raised the height measurement rod.	____	____	_____
c. Asked the person to remove the robe and slippers. Assisted if necessary.	____	____	_____
d. Helped the person stand on the scale platform with the arms to the sides.	____	____	_____
e. Moved the weights until the balance pointer was in the middle.	____	____	_____
f. Recorded the name and weight.	____	____	_____
g. Asked the person to stand as straight as possible.	____	____	_____
h. Lowered the height measurement rod until it rested on the person's head.	____	____	_____
i. Recorded the height.	____	____	_____

8. Chair scale:

	S	U	Comments
a. Helped the person transfer from the wheelchair to the chair scale.	____	____	_____
b. Placed the person's feet on the foot platform.	____	____	_____
c. Moved the weights until the balance pointer was in the middle.	____	____	_____
d. Recorded the weight.	____	____	_____

Procedure—cont'd   S   U   Comments

9. Lift scale:

   a. Attached the sling and chains to the lift.   _____ _____ _____

   b. Placed both weights on zero.   _____ _____ _____

   c. Leveled and balanced the scale.   _____ _____ _____

   d. Removed the sling from the scale.   _____ _____ _____

   e. Placed the person on the sling and attached it to the lift.   _____ _____ _____
Raised the person about 4 inches off the bed.

   f. Moved the weights until the balance pointer was in the   _____ _____ _____
middle.

   g. Recorded the weight.   _____ _____ _____

   h. Lowered the person to the bed.   _____ _____ _____

   i. Removed the sling.   _____ _____ _____

Post-Procedure

10. Helped the person put on robe and slippers or clothing if he or   _____ _____ _____
she would be up. Assisted the person back to bed.

11. Provided for comfort.   _____ _____ _____

12. Placed the signal light within reach.   _____ _____ _____

13. Raised or lowered side rails. Followed the care plan.   _____ _____ _____

14. Unscreened the person.   _____ _____ _____

15. Returned the scale to its proper place.   _____ _____ _____

16. Decontaminated hands.   _____ _____ _____

17. Reported the height and weight to the nurse. Recorded measure-   _____ _____ _____
ments in the proper place.

Measuring Height: the Person Is in Bed

QUALITY OF LIFE

Remember to:
- Knock before entering the person's room
- Address the person by name
- Introduce yourself by name and title

Name: _____

Date: _____

Pre-Procedure

	S	U	Comments
1. Explained the procedure to the person.	___	___	_____
2. Decontaminated hands.	___	___	_____
3. Collected a measuring tape and ruler.	___	___	_____
4. Obtained a helper.	___	___	_____
5. Identified the person.	___	___	_____
6. Provided for privacy.	___	___	_____

Procedure

	S	U	Comments
7. Positioned the person supine, if allowed.	___	___	_____
8. Had helper hold the end of the measuring tape at the person's heel.	___	___	_____
9. Pulled the measuring tape alongside the person's body until it extended past the head.	___	___	_____
10. Placed the ruler flat across the top of the head; it extended from the person's head to the measuring tape. Made sure the ruler was level.	___	___	_____
11. Recorded the height.	___	___	_____
12. Provided for comfort. Assisted the person back to the wheelchair, if appropriate.	___	___	_____
13. Raised or lowered side rails if the person stayed in bed. Followed the care plan.	___	___	_____
14. Placed the signal light within reach.	___	___	_____
15. Unscreened the person.	___	___	_____
16. Returned equipment to its proper location.	___	___	_____
17. Decontaminated hands.	___	___	_____
18. Reported the height to the nurse. Recorded the measurement in the proper place.	___	___	_____

Transferring the Person to Another Nursing Unit

QUALITY OF LIFE

Name: _____

Remember to:
- Knock before entering the person's room
- Address the person by name
- Introduce yourself by name and title

Date: _____

Pre-Procedure

	S	U	Comments

1. Found out where the person was going. Found out whether you needed to use the bed, a wheelchair, or a stretcher.   _____ _____ _____
2. Explained the procedure to the person.   _____ _____ _____
3. Got a stretcher or wheelchair, bath blanket, and utility cart (if needed).   _____ _____ _____

Procedure

4. Decontaminated hands.   _____ _____ _____
5. Identified the person.   _____ _____ _____
6. Put the person's personal belongings and bedside equipment on the utility cart.   _____ _____ _____
7. Assisted the person to the wheelchair or stretcher. Covered the person with a bath blanket.   _____ _____ _____
8. Transported the person to the assigned place.   _____ _____ _____
9. Introduced the person to the receiving nurse.   _____ _____ _____
10. Helped the nurse transfer the person from the wheelchair or stretcher into bed. Helped position the person (or made sure he or she was comfortable in a chair).   _____ _____ _____
11. Brought the person's personal belongings and equipment to the new room. Helped put them away.   _____ _____ _____
12. Reported the following to the nurse:
    a. How the person tolerated the transfer   _____ _____ _____
    b. That a nurse would bring the person's chart, plan, and medications   _____ _____ _____

Post-Procedure

13. Returned the wheelchair or stretcher and utility cart to the storage area.   _____ _____ _____
14. Decontaminated hands.   _____ _____ _____
15. Stripped the bed, cleaned the unit, and made a closed bed.   _____ _____ _____

Discharging the Person

QUALITY OF LIFE

Remember to:
- Knock before entering the person's room
- Address the person by name
- Introduce yourself by name and title

Name: _____

Date: _____

Pre-Procedure	S	U	Comments
1. Made sure the person was to be discharged. Found out whether transportation arrangements had been made.	____	____	_____
2. Explained the procedure to the person.	____	____	_____
3. Decontaminated hands.	____	____	_____
4. Identified the person.	____	____	_____
5. Provided for privacy.	____	____	_____
6. Helped the person dress, if needed.	____	____	_____
7. Helped the person pack. Checked all drawers and closets.	____	____	_____
8. Checked off clothing list. Asked the person or responsible party to sign the form.	____	____	_____
9. Told the nurse that the person was ready for the final visit. The nurse:			
a. Gave prescriptions written by the doctor.	____	____	_____
b. Provided discharge instructions.	____	____	_____
c. Secured valuables from the safe.	____	____	_____
10. Got a wheelchair and a utility cart for the person's belongings. Asked a co-worker for help.	____	____	_____
11. Assisted the person into the wheelchair.	____	____	_____
12. Took the person to the exit area. Locked the wheels of the wheelchair. Helped the person out of the wheelchair and into the car.	____	____	_____
13. Helped put the belongings into the car.	____	____	_____
14. Returned the wheelchair and utility cart to the storage area.	____	____	_____
15. Decontaminated hands.	____	____	_____
16. Reported the following to the nurse:			
a. The time of discharge	____	____	_____
b. How the person was transported	____	____	_____
c. Who accompanied the person	____	____	_____
d. The person's destination	____	____	_____
e. Any other observations	____	____	_____
17. Stripped the bed, cleaned the person's unit, and made a closed bed.	____	____	_____
18. Decontaminated hands.	____	____	_____

Applying Elastic Stockings

QUALITY OF LIFE

Remember to:
- Knock before entering the person's room
- Address the person by name
- Introduce yourself by name and title

Name: _____

Date: _____

	S	U	Comments

Pre-Procedure

1. Explained the procedure to the person.   _____ _____ _____
2. Decontaminated hands.   _____ _____ _____
3. Obtained elastic stockings in the correct size.   _____ _____ _____
4. Identified the person.   _____ _____ _____
5. Provided for privacy.   _____ _____ _____
6. Raised the bed to the best position for good body mechanics. Made sure bed rails were up.   _____ _____ _____
7. Lowered the bed rail near you.   _____ _____ _____

Procedure

8. Positioned the person supine.   _____ _____ _____
9. Exposed the legs. Fanfolded the linens toward the person.   _____ _____ _____
10. Turned the stocking inside out down to the heel.   _____ _____ _____
11. Slipped the foot of the stocking over the toes, foot, and heel.   _____ _____ _____
12. Grasped the stocking top. Slipped it over the foot and heel and pulled it up the leg. Stocking was even and snug.   _____ _____ _____
13. Made sure the stocking was not twisted and had no creases or wrinkles.   _____ _____ _____
14. Repeated steps 10 through 13 for the other leg.   _____ _____ _____

Post-Procedure

15. Returned top linens to their proper position.   _____ _____ _____
16. Provided for comfort.   _____ _____ _____
17. Lowered the bed to its lowest position.   _____ _____ _____
18. Raised or lowered the side rails. Followed the care plan.   _____ _____ _____
19. Placed the signal light within reach.   _____ _____ _____
20. Unscreened the person.   _____ _____ _____
21. Decontaminated hands.   _____ _____ _____
22. Told the nurse that the stockings were applied.   _____ _____ _____

Applying Elastic Bandages

QUALITY OF LIFE

Name: _____

Date: _____

Remember to:
- Knock before entering the person's room
- Address the person by name
- Introduce yourself by name and title

Pre-Procedure

	S	U	Comments
1. Explained the procedure to the person.	____	____	_____
2. Decontaminated hands.	____	____	_____
3. Collected the following:			
• Elastic bandage as directed by the nurse	____	____	_____
• Tape, metal clips, or safety pins	____	____	_____
4. Identified the person.	____	____	_____
5. Provided for privacy.	____	____	_____
6. Raised the bed to the best level for good body mechanics. Made sure the bed rails were up.	____	____	_____

Procedure

	S	U	Comments
7. Lowered the bed rail near you.	____	____	_____
8. Helped the person to a comfortable position. Exposed the part to be bandaged.	____	____	_____
9. Made sure the area was clean and dry.	____	____	_____
10. Held the bandage so that the roll was up and the loose end was on the bottom.	____	____	_____
11. Applied the bandage to the smallest part of the extremity.	____	____	_____
12. Made two circular turns around the part.	____	____	_____
13. Made overlapping spiral turns in an upward direction. Each turn overlapped about two thirds of the previous turn.	____	____	_____
14. Applied the bandage smoothly with firm, even pressure. The bandage was not tight.	____	____	_____
15. Pinned, taped, or clipped the end of the bandage to hold it in place. Made sure the pin or clip was not under the part.	____	____	_____
16. Checked the fingers or toes for coldness or cyanosis. Also checked for complaints of pain, numbness, or tingling. Removed the bandage if any were noted. Reported observations to the nurse.	____	____	_____

Post-Procedure

	S	U	Comments
17. Provided for comfort.	_____	_____	_____
18. Placed the signal light within reach.	_____	_____	_____
19. Lowered the bed.	_____	_____	_____
20. Raised or lowered side rails. Followed the care plan.	_____	_____	_____
21. Unscreened the person.	_____	_____	_____
22. Decontaminated hands.	_____	_____	_____
23. Reported the following to the nurse:			
• The time the bandage was applied	_____	_____	_____
• The site of the application	_____	_____	_____
• Any other observations	_____	_____	_____

Applying a Dry Nonsterile Dressing

QUALITY OF LIFE

Name: _____

Date: _____

Remember to:
- Knock before entering the person's room
- Address the person by name
- Introduce yourself by name and title

Pre-Procedure

	S	U	Comments
1. Followed Delegation Guidelines.	___	___	_____
2. Explained the procedure to the person.	___	___	_____
3. Allowed time for pain medication to take effect.	___	___	_____
4. Provided for the person's fluid and elimination needs.	___	___	_____
5. Decontaminated hands.	___	___	_____
6. Collected the following:			
• Gloves	___	___	_____
• Personal protective equipment as needed	___	___	_____
• Tape or Montgomery ties	___	___	_____
• Dressing as directed by the nurse	___	___	_____
• Adhesive remover	___	___	_____
• Scissors	___	___	_____
• Plastic bag	___	___	_____
• Bath blanket	___	___	_____
7. Identified the person. Checked identification bracelet against the assignment sheet. Called the person by name.	___	___	_____
8. Provided for privacy.	___	___	_____
9. Arranged work area.	___	___	_____
10. Raised the bed for body mechanics. Bed rails were up, if used.	___	___	_____

Procedure

	S	U	Comments
11. Lowered the bed rail near you, if up.	___	___	_____
12. Helped the person to a comfortable position.	___	___	_____
13. Covered the person with a bath blanket. Fanfolded top linens to the foot of the bed.	___	___	_____
14. Exposed the affected body part.	___	___	_____
15. Made a cuff on the plastic bag and placed it within reach.	___	___	_____
16. Put on a gown and mask, if needed.	___	___	_____
17. Put on gloves.	___	___	_____
18. Unfastened Montgomery ties or removed tape.			
a. Montgomery ties: folded ties away from the wound.	___	___	_____
b. Tape: held the skin down and gently pulled the tape toward the wound.	___	___	_____
19. Removed adhesive from skin. Wet 4 × 4 gauze dressing with the adhesive remover. Cleaned away from the wound.	___	___	_____

Procedure—cont'd   S   U   Comments

20. Removed gauze dressings. Started with the top dressing. The
    soiled side was out of the person's sight. Put dressings in the
    bag. (Soiled dressings did not touch the outside of the bag.)

21. Gently removed the dressing directly over the wound.

22. Observed the wound drainage.

23. Removed gloves. Put them in bag.

24. Decontaminated your hands. (Raised the bed rails, if used, when
    you left the bedside; lowered them when you returned.)

25. Put on clean gloves.

26. Opened the dressings.

27. Cut the length of tape needed.

28. Applied dressings as directed by nurse.

29. Secured the dressings in place. Used tape or Montgomery ties.

30. Removed gloves and placed them in the bag.

Post-Procedure

31. Provided comfort. Covered the person, and removed the bath
    blanket.

32. Placed signal light within reach.

33. Lowered the bed to its lowest position.

34. Raised or lowered bed rails. Followed the care plan.

35. Unscreened the person.

36. Discarded supplies into the bag. Tied the bag closed. Discarded
    the bag according to center policy.

37. Cleaned work surface. Followed the Bloodborne Pathogen
    Standard.

38. Decontaminated hands.

39. Reported any observations to the nurse.

Applying Hot Compresses

QUALITY OF LIFE

Remember to:
- Knock before entering the person's room
- Address the person by name
- Introduce yourself by name and title

Name: _____

Date: _____

Pre-Procedure

	S	U	Comments
1. Explained the procedure to the person.	____	____	_____
2. Decontaminated hands.	____	____	_____
3. Collected the following:			
• Basin	____	____	_____
• Bath thermometer	____	____	_____
• Small towel, washcloth, or gauze squares	____	____	_____
• Plastic wrap or Aquathermia pad	____	____	_____
• Ties, tape, or rolled gauze	____	____	_____
• Bath towel	____	____	_____
• Waterproof bed protector	____	____	_____
4. Identified the person.	____	____	_____
5. Provided for privacy.	____	____	_____

Procedure

	S	U	Comments
6. Placed the protector under the body part.	____	____	_____
7. Filled the basin one-half to two-thirds full with hot water as directed.	____	____	_____
8. Placed the compress in the water.	____	____	_____
9. Wrung out the compress.	____	____	_____
10. Applied the compress to the area. Noted the time.	____	____	_____
11. Covered the compress quickly. Did one of the following as directed by the nurse:			
a. Covered the compress with plastic wrap and then with a bath towel. Secured the towel in place.	____	____	_____
b. Covered the compress with an Aquathermia pad.	____	____	_____
12. Placed the signal light within reach. Raised or lowered the bed rails. Followed the care plan.	____	____	_____
13. Checked the area every 5 minutes. Checked for redness and complaints of pain, discomfort, or numbness. Removed the compress if any occurred. Told the nurse immediately.	____	____	_____
14. Changed the compress if cooling occurred.	____	____	_____
15. Removed the compress after 20 minutes or as directed by the nurse. Patted the area dry with a towel.	____	____	_____

Post-Procedure

	S	U	Comments
16. Provided for comfort.	_____	_____	_____
17. Unscreened the person.	_____	_____	_____
18. Raised or lowered bed rails. Followed the care plan.	_____	_____	_____
19. Placed the signal light within reach.	_____	_____	_____
20. Cleaned equipment. Discarded disposable items.	_____	_____	_____
21. Followed center policy for soiled linen.	_____	_____	_____
22. Decontaminated hands.	_____	_____	_____
23. Reported the following to the nurse:			
• Time, site, and length of the application	_____	_____	_____
• Observations of the skin	_____	_____	_____
• The person's response	_____	_____	_____
• Ties, tape, or rolled gauze	_____	_____	_____

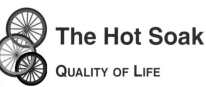

The Hot Soak

Quality of Life

Remember to:
- Knock before entering the person's room
- Address the person by name
- Introduce yourself by name and title

Name: _____

Date: _____

Pre-Procedure

	S	U	Comments

1. Explained the procedure to the person.
2. Decontaminated hands.
3. Collected the following:
   - Water basin or an arm bath or footbath
   - Bath thermometer
   - Bath blanket
   - Waterproof pads
4. Identified the person.
5. Provided for privacy.

Procedure

6. Positioned the person for the treatment. Placed the signal light within reach.
7. Placed a waterproof pad under the area.
8. Filled the container one-half full with hot water as directed. Measured water temperature.
9. Exposed the area. Avoided unnecessary exposure.
10. Placed the body part into the water. Padded the edge of the container with a towel. Noted the time.
11. Covered the person with a bath blanket for extra warmth.
12. Checked the area every 5 minutes. Checked for redness and complaints of pain, numbness, or discomfort. Removed the part from the soak if any of these complications occurred. Wrapped the part in a towel and told the nurse immediately.
13. Checked water temperature every 5 minutes. Changed water as necessary. Wrapped the part in a towel while changing water.
14. Removed the body part from the water in 15 to 20 minutes. Patted dry with a towel.

Post-Procedure   S   U   **Comments**

15. Provided for comfort.   _____   _____   _____

16. Unscreened the person.   _____   _____   _____

17. Raised or lowered bed rails. Followed the care plan. _____   _____   _____

18. Placed the signal light within reach.   _____   _____   _____

19. Cleaned equipment. Discarded disposable items.   _____   _____   _____

20. Followed center policy for soiled linen.   _____   _____   _____

21. Decontaminated hands.   _____   _____   _____

22. Reported the following to the nurse:

    • Time, site, and length of the application   _____   _____   _____

    • Observations of the skin   _____   _____   _____

    • The person's response   _____   _____   _____

Assisting the Person to Take a Sitz Bath

QUALITY OF LIFE

Name: _____

Date: _____

Remember to:
- Knock before entering the person's room
- Address the person by name
- Introduce yourself by name and title

Pre-Procedure	S	U	Comments
1. Explained the procedure to the person.	____	____	_____
2. Decontaminated hands.	____	____	_____
3. Collected the following:			
• Disposable sitz bath or wheelchair if the built-in sitz bath was used	____	____	_____
• Bath thermometer	____	____	_____
• Large water container	____	____	_____
• Two bath blankets, bath towels, and a clean gown	____	____	_____
• Footstool (if the person is short)	____	____	_____
• Disinfectant solution	____	____	_____
• Utility gloves	____	____	_____
4. Identified the person.	____	____	_____
5. Provided for privacy.	____	____	_____

Procedure	S	U	Comments
6. Did one of the following:			
a. Placed the disposable sitz bath on the toilet seat.	____	____	_____
b. Transported the person by wheelchair to the sitz bath room.	____	____	_____
7. Filled the sitz bath two-thirds full with water as directed by the nurse. Measured water temperature.	____	____	_____
8. Used bath towels to pad the metal parts that would have contact with the person.	____	____	_____
9. Raised the gown and secured it above the waist.	____	____	_____
10. Helped the person sit in the sitz bath.	____	____	_____
11. Placed a bath blanket around the shoulders. Placed another over the legs for warmth.	____	____	_____
12. Provided a footstool if the edge of the sitz bath caused pressure under the knees.	____	____	_____
13. Placed the signal light within reach and provided comfort.	____	____	_____
14. Stayed with a person that was weak or unsteady.	____	____	_____
15. Checked the person every 5 minutes for complaints of weakness, faintness, and drowsiness. Checked for a rapid pulse. If any complaints occurred, got assistance to help the person back to bed.	____	____	_____
16. Helped the person out of the sitz bath after 20 minutes or as directed.	____	____	_____
17. Assisted the person with drying and dressing.	____	____	_____
18. Assisted the person back to bed.	____	____	_____

Post-Procedure

	S	U	Comments
19. Provided for comfort.	_____	_____	_____
20. Unscreened the person.	_____	_____	_____
21. Placed the signal light within reach.	_____	_____	_____
22. Raised or lowered bed rails. Followed care plan.	_____	_____	_____
23. Cleaned the sitz bath with disinfectant solution. Wore utility gloves.	_____	_____	_____
24. Returned reusable items to their proper places. Followed center policy for soiled linen.	_____	_____	_____
25. Decontaminated hands.	_____	_____	_____
26. Reported observations to the nurse.	_____	_____	_____

Applying a Hot Pack

QUALITY OF LIFE

Remember to:
- Knock before entering the person's room
- Address the person by name
- Introduce yourself by name and title

Name: _____

Date: _____

Pre-Procedure

	S	U	Comments
1. Followed Delegation Guidelines.	_____	_____	_____
2. Explained the procedure to the person.	_____	_____	_____
3. Decontaminated hands.	_____	_____	_____
4. Collected the following:			
• Commercial pack	_____	_____	_____
• Towel	_____	_____	_____
• Pack cover	_____	_____	_____
• Ties, tape, or rolled gauze (if needed)	_____	_____	_____
• Bed protector	_____	_____	_____
• Waterproof pad	_____	_____	_____
5. Heated the pack following the manufacturer's instructions.	_____	_____	_____
6. Put the pack in the cover.	_____	_____	_____
7. Identified the person. Checked identification bracelet against the assignment sheet. Called the person by name.	_____	_____	_____
8. Provided for privacy.	_____	_____	_____

Procedure

	S	U	Comments
9. Placed the pad under the body part.	_____	_____	_____
10. Applied the pack quickly. Noted the time.	_____	_____	_____
11. Secured the pack in place with ties, tape, or rolled gauze. (Some have Velcro straps.)	_____	_____	_____
12. Placed the signal light within reach.	_____	_____	_____
13. Raised or lowered the bed rails. Followed care plan.	_____	_____	_____
14. Checked area every 5 minutes. Checked for redness and complaints of pain, numbness, or discomfort. Removed pack if any complaints occurred. Told the nurse immediately.	_____	_____	_____
15. Changed the pack if cooling occurred.	_____	_____	_____
16. Removed pack after 20 minutes or as directed by the nurse. Patted the area dry. Lowered the bed rail, if up.	_____	_____	_____

Post-Procedure

	S	U	Comments
17. Provided for comfort.	___	___	_____
18. Unscreened the person.	___	___	_____
19. Raised or lowered the bed rails. Followed the care plan.	___	___	_____
20. Placed the signal light within reach.	___	___	_____
21. Cleaned the equipment. Discarded disposable items.	___	___	_____
22. Followed center policy for soiled linens.	___	___	_____
23. Decontaminated hands.	___	___	_____
24. Reported and recorded:			
• Time, sight, and length of application	___	___	_____
• Observations of the skin	___	___	_____
• The person's response	___	___	_____

Applying an Aquathermia Pad

QUALITY OF LIFE

Name: _____

Date: _____

Remember to:
- Knock before entering the person's room
- Address the person by name
- Introduce yourself by name and title

Pre-Procedure	S	U	Comments
1. Explained the procedure to the person.	____	____	_____
2. Decontaminated hands.	____	____	_____
3. Collected the following:			
• Aquathermia pad and heating unit	____	____	_____
• Distilled water	____	____	_____
• Flannel cover, pillowcase, or towel	____	____	_____
• Ties, tape, or rolled gauze	____	____	_____
4. Identified the person.	____	____	_____
5. Provided for privacy.	____	____	_____

Procedure

	S	U	Comments
6. Filled the heating unit to the "fill" line with distilled water.	____	____	_____
7. Removed air bubbles.	____	____	_____
8. Set the temperature as instructed by the nurse (usually 105° Fahrenheit, or 40.5° Celsius). Removed the key.	____	____	_____
9. Placed the pad in the cover.	____	____	_____
10. Plugged in the unit. Let water warm to the desired temperature.	____	____	_____
11. Set the heating unit on the bedside stand. Kept the pad and connecting hoses level with the unit.	____	____	_____
12. Applied the pad to the part. Noted the time.	____	____	_____
13. Secured the pad in place. Did not use pins.	____	____	_____
14. Unscreened the person. Placed the signal light within reach.	____	____	_____
15. Raised or lowered the bed rails. Followed the care plan.	____	____	_____
16. Checked the skin for redness, swelling, and blisters. Asked about pain, discomfort, or decreased sensation. Removed the pad if any occurred. Told the nurse immediately.	____	____	_____
17. Removed the pad at the specified time.	____	____	_____

Post-Procedure   S   U   Comments

18. Provided for comfort.   _____   _____   _____

19. Unscreened the person.   _____   _____   _____

20. Raised or lowered bed rails. Followed the care plan.   _____   _____   _____

21. Placed the signal light within reach.   _____   _____   _____

22. Cleaned equipment. Discarded disposable items. _____   _____   _____

23. Followed center policy for soiled linen.   _____   _____   _____

24. Decontaminated hands.   _____   _____   _____

25. Reported the following to the nurse:

    • Time, site, and length of the application   _____   _____   _____

    • Observations of the skin   _____   _____   _____

    • The person's response   _____   _____   _____

Applying an Ice Bag, Ice Collar, Ice Glove, or Dry Cold Pack

Name: _____

Date: _____

QUALITY OF LIFE

Remember to: ● Knock before entering the person's room
              ● Address the person by name
              ● Introduce yourself by name and title

Pre-Procedure

	S	U	Comments
1. Explained the procedure to the person.	___	___	_____
2. Decontaminated hands.	___	___	_____
3. Collected a disposable cold pack or the following:			
• Ice bag or collar	___	___	_____
• Crushed ice	___	___	_____
• Flannel cover, towel, or pillowcase	___	___	_____
• Paper towels	___	___	_____
4. Applied an ice bag or collar:			
a. Filled the ice bag with water. Put in the stopper. Checked for leaks.	___	___	_____
b. Emptied the bag.	___	___	_____
c. Filled the bag one-half to two-thirds full with crushed ice or ice chips.	___	___	_____
d. Removed excess air.	___	___	_____
e. Placed the cap or stopper on securely.	___	___	_____
f. Dried the bag with paper towels.	___	___	_____
g. Placed the bag in the cover.	___	___	_____
5. Applied a disposable cold pack:			
a. Squeezed, kneaded, or struck the cold pack as directed.	___	___	_____
b. Placed the bag in the cover.	___	___	_____
6. Identified the person.	___	___	_____
7. Provided for privacy.	___	___	_____

Procedure

	S	U	Comments
8. Applied the ice bag. Secured it in place. Noted the time.	___	___	_____
9. Placed the signal light within reach. Raised or lowered the bed rails. Followed the care plan.	___	___	_____
10. Checked the skin every 10 minutes. Checked for blisters; pale, white, or gray skin; cyanosis; and shivering. Asked about numbness, pain, or burning. Removed the bag if any complaints occurred. Told the nurse immediately.	___	___	_____
11. Removed the bag after 20 minutes or as directed.	___	___	_____

Post-Procedure   S   U   Comments

12. Provided for comfort.   _____ _____ _____

13. Unscreened the person.   _____ _____ _____

14. Raised or lowered bed rails. Followed the care plan. _____ _____ _____

15. Placed the signal light within reach.   _____ _____ _____

16. Cleaned equipment. Discarded disposable items.   _____ _____ _____

17. Followed center policy for soiled linen.   _____ _____ _____

18. Decontaminated hands.   _____ _____ _____

19. Reported the following to the nurse:

    • Time, site, and length of the application   _____ _____ _____

    • Observations of the skin   _____ _____ _____

    • The person's response   _____ _____ _____

Applying Cold Compresses

QUALITY OF LIFE

Name: _____

Date: _____

Remember to:
- Knock before entering the person's room
- Address the person by name
- Introduce yourself by name and title

Pre-Procedure

	S	U	Comments
1. Explained the procedure to the person.	___	___	_____
2. Decontaminated hands.	___	___	_____
3. Collected the following:			
• Large basin with ice	___	___	_____
• Small basin with cold water	___	___	_____
• Gauze squares, washcloths, or small towels	___	___	_____
• Waterproof pad	___	___	_____
• Bath towel	___	___	_____
4. Identified the person.	___	___	_____
5. Provided for privacy.	___	___	_____

Procedure

	S	U	Comments
6. Placed the small basin with cold water into the large basin with ice.	___	___	_____
7. Placed the compresses into the cold water.	___	___	_____
8. Placed a bed protector under the affected body part. Exposed the area.	___	___	_____
9. Wrung out a compress so that water was not dripping.	___	___	_____
10. Applied the compress to the part. Noted the time.	___	___	_____
11. Checked the skin every 10 minutes. Checked for blisters; pale, white, or gray skin; cyanosis; and shivering. Asked about numbness, pain or burning. Removed the bag if any complaints occurred. Told the nurse immediately.	___	___	_____
12. Changed the compress when it warmed.	___	___	_____
13. Removed the compress after 20 minutes or as directed.	___	___	_____
14. Patted the area dry with the bath towel.	___	___	_____

Post-Procedure

	S	U	Comments
15. Provided for comfort.	___	___	_____
16. Unscreened the person.	___	___	_____
17. Raised or lowered bed rails. Followed the care plan.	___	___	_____
18. Placed the signal light within reach.	___	___	_____
19. Cleaned equipment. Discarded disposable items.	___	___	_____
20. Followed center policy for soiled linen.	___	___	_____
21. Decontaminated hands.	___	___	_____

22. Reported the following to the nurse:

	S	U	Comments
• Time, site, and length of the application	___	___	_____
• Observations of the skin	___	___	_____
• The person's response	___	___	_____

Adult CPR—One Rescuer

QUALITY OF LIFE

Remember to:
- Knock before entering the person's room
- Address the person by name
- Introduce yourself by name and title

Name: _____

Date: _____

Procedure	S	U	Comments
1. Checked for unresponsiveness.	____	____	_____
2. Called for help. Activated the emergency medical service (EMS) system.	____	____	_____
3. Positioned the person supine on hard, flat surface. Logrolled the person. Placed the person's arms alongside the body.	____	____	_____
4. Opened the airway. Used the head-tilt/chin-tilt maneuver.	____	____	_____
5. Checked for breathlessness.	____	____	_____
6. Gave two breaths, $1\frac{1}{2}$ to 2 seconds in length. Let the person's chest deflate between breaths.	____	____	_____
7. Checked for pulselessness. Checked the pulse for 5 to 10 seconds. Used the other hand to keep the airway open with the head-tilt maneuver.	____	____	_____
8. Gave chest compressions at a rate of 80 to 100 per minute. Gave 15 compressions, then two breaths.	____	____	_____
a. Established a rhythm and counted out loud.	____	____	_____
b. Opened the airway and gave two breaths.	____	____	_____
c. Repeated this step until four cycles of 15 compressions and two breaths are given.	____	____	_____
9. Checked for a carotid pulse (3 to 5 seconds).	____	____	_____
10. Continued CPR if the person had no pulse. Began with chest compressions.	____	____	_____
11. Continued the cycle of 15 compressions and two breaths. Checked for a pulse every few minutes.	____	____	_____
12. Repeated steps 10 and 11 as long as necessary.	____	____	_____

Adult CPR—Two Rescuers

Name: _____

Remember to: ● Knock before entering the person's room
               ● Address the person by name   Date: _____
               ● Introduce yourself by name and title

Procedure	S	U	Comments
1. Performed one-person CPR until a helper arrived.	___	___	_____
2. Continued chest compressions.	___	___	_____
3. Indicated that help was needed. Asked that the EMS system be activated, if not already done.	___	___	_____
4. Did not stop chest compressions. Began procedure after completing a cycle of 15 compressions and two breaths.	___	___	_____
5. Stopped compressions for 3 to 5 seconds. Helper checked for carotid pulse. Started two-rescuer procedure after completing a cycle of 15 compressions and two breaths.	___	___	_____
6. Performed two-person CPR as follows:			
a. Helper gave two breaths.	___	___	_____
b. Gave chest compressions at a rate of 80 to 100 per minute. Counted out loud in a rhythm.	___	___	_____
c. Helper gave a breath immediately after the fifth compression. Paused for the breath. Continued chest compressions after the breath.	___	___	_____
d. A breath was given after every fifth compression.	___	___	_____
7. Stopped compressions after 1 minute. Helper checked for a carotid pulse. After the first minute, compressions were stopped every few minutes to check for breathing and circulation. Compressions were stopped for only 5 seconds.	___	___	_____
8. Called for a switch in position when tired.	___	___	_____
9. Changed positions quickly as follows:			
a. Helper gave a breath after the fifth compression.	___	___	_____
b. Helper moved down to kneel at the person's shoulder and found proper hand position.	___	___	_____
c. Moved to the person's head after giving the fifth compression.	___	___	_____
d. Checked for a pulse (3 to 5 seconds).	___	___	_____
e. Said, "No pulse."	___	___	_____
f. Gave one breath before helper started chest compression.	___	___	_____
10. Gave one breath after every fifth compression.	___	___	_____
11. Switched positions when the person giving compressions was tired. Checked for a pulse and breathing at every position change.	___	___	_____

FBAO—The Responsive Adult

QUALITY OF LIFE

Remember to:
- Knock before entering the person's room
- Address the person by name
- Introduce yourself by name and title

Name: _____

Date: _____

Pre-Procedure   S   U   **Comments**

1. Asked the person whether he or she was choking.   ___ ___ _____

2. Determined whether the person could cough or speak.   ___ ___ _____

3. Performed the Heimlich maneuver, if the person was standing or sitting:

   a. Stood behind the person.   ___ ___ _____

   b. Wrapped arms around the person's waist.   ___ ___ _____

   c. Made a fist with one hand.   ___ ___ _____

   d. Placed the thumb side of the fist against the abdomen above the navel and below the end of the sternum.   ___ ___ _____

   e. Grasped fist with other hand.   ___ ___ _____

   f. Pressed fist and hand into the person's abdomen with a quick, upward thrust.   ___ ___ _____

   g. Repeated the abdominal thrust until the object was expelled or the person lost consciousness.   ___ ___ _____

4. Positioned the person in the supine position.   ___ ___ _____

5. Activated the EMS system.   ___ ___ _____

6. Did the finger sweep maneuver to check for a foreign object:

   a. Opened the person's mouth. Used the tongue-jaw lift method:

   - Grasped the tongue and lower jaw with thumb and fingers.   ___ ___ _____

   - Lifted the lower jaw upward.   ___ ___ _____

   b. Inserted other index finger into the mouth along the side of the cheek and deep into the throat.   ___ ___ _____

   c. Formed a hook with index finger.   ___ ___ _____

   d. Tried to dislodge and remove the object. Did not push it deeper into the throat.   ___ ___ _____

   e. Grasped and removed the object if it was within reach.   ___ ___ _____

7. Opened the airway with the head-tilt/chin-lift maneuver.   ___ ___ _____

8. Gave one or two breaths.   ___ ___ _____

9. Repositioned the person's head if chest did not rise. Gave one or two breaths.   ___ ___ _____

10. Gave up to five abdominal thrusts.   ___ ___ _____

11. Repeated steps 6 through 10 (finger sweeps, rescue breathing, and abdominal thrusts) until the object was expelled or EMS personnel arrived.   ___ ___ _____

FBAO—The Unresponsive Adult

QUALITY OF LIFE

Remember to:
- Knock before entering the person's room
- Address the person by name
- Introduce yourself by name and title

Name: _____

Date: _____

Procedure	S	U	Comments
1. Checked for unresponsiveness.	____	____	_____
2. Called for help. Activated EMS system or the center's response system.	____	____	_____
3. Logrolled the person to the supine position, face up, and arms at side.	____	____	_____
4. Opened the airway. Used the head-tilt/chin-lift maneuver.	____	____	_____
5. Checked for breathing.	____	____	_____
6. Gave one to two slow rescue breaths. Repositioned the person's head, and opened the airway if chest did not rise and gave one or two rescue breaths.	____	____	_____
7. Gave five abdominal thrusts, if person was not ventilated.	____	____	_____
a. Straddled the person's thighs.	____	____	_____
b. Placed the heel of one hand against the person's abdomen in the middle above the navel and below the end of the breastbone.	____	____	_____
c. Placed your second hand on top of your first hand.	____	____	_____
d. Pressed both hands into the abdomen. Used a quick, upward thrust, five times.	____	____	_____
8. Performed the finger sweep maneuver, checked for a foreign object.	____	____	_____
9. Repeated two rescue breaths. Repositioned the head to open airway, gave two rescue breaths and five abdominal thrusts, and performed a finger sweep until rescue breathing was effective. Started CPR, if necessary.	____	____	_____

Assisting With Postmortem Care

QUALITY OF LIFE

Remember to: ● Knock before entering the person's room
                ● Address the person by name
                ● Introduce yourself by name and title

Name: _____

Date: _____

Pre-Procedure

	S	U	Comments
1. Decontaminated hands.	___	___	_____
2. Collected the following:			
• Postmortem kit if used (shroud, gown, two tags, gauze squares, and safety pins)	___	___	_____
• Valuables list	___	___	_____
• Waterproof bed protectors	___	___	_____
• Washbasin	___	___	_____
• Bath towels	___	___	_____
• Washcloth	___	___	_____
• Tape	___	___	_____
• Dressing	___	___	_____
• Gloves	___	___	_____
• Cotton balls	___	___	_____
3. Provided for privacy.	___	___	_____
4. Raised the bed to the best possible level for good body mechanics.	___	___	_____

Procedure

	S	U	Comments
5. Made sure the bed was flat.	___	___	_____
6. Put on the gloves.	___	___	_____
7. Positioned the body supine.	___	___	_____
8. Closed the eyes. Applied moistened cotton balls gently over eyelids, if the eyes would not stay closed.	___	___	_____
9. Inserted dentures or put them in a labeled container.	___	___	_____
10. Closed the mouth. Placed a rolled towel under the chin to support the mouth, if necessary.	___	___	_____
11. Followed center policy about jewelry. Listed all jewelry that was removed.	___	___	_____
12. Placed a cotton ball over rings and secured in place with tape.	___	___	_____
13. Removed drainage bottles, bags, and containers. Left tubes and catheters in place if an autopsy was to be performed. Asked nurse for direction.	___	___	_____
14. Bathed soiled areas with plain water. Dried thoroughly.	___	___	_____
15. Placed a bed protector under the buttocks.	___	___	_____
16. Removed soiled dressings and replaced with clean ones.	___	___	_____
17. Put a clean gown on the body. Made sure the body is positioned supine.	___	___	_____

Procedure—cont'd   S   U   Comments

18. Brushed and combed the hair if necessary.   _____   _____   _____

19. Filled out identification tags. Tied one to an ankle or to the right big toe.   _____   _____   _____

20. Covered the body to the shoulder with a sheet if the family would be viewing the body.   _____   _____   _____

21. Collected the person's belongings. Placed them in a bag labeled with the person's name.   _____   _____   _____

22. Removed all supplies, equipment, and linens except the shroud and the other identification tag. Made sure the room was neat. Adjusted the lighting so that it was soft.   _____   _____   _____

23. Removed the gloves and decontaminated hands.   _____   _____   _____

24. Let the family view the body. Provided for privacy. Gave the person's belongings to the family.   _____   _____   _____

25. Put on another pair of gloves.   _____   _____   _____

26. Placed the body on the shroud or covered the body with a sheet after the family left. Applied the shroud:

    a. Brought the top down over the head.   _____   _____   _____

    b. Folded the bottom up over the feet.   _____   _____   _____

    c. Folded the sides over the body.   _____   _____   _____

27. Secured the shroud in place with safety pins or tape.   _____   _____   _____

28. Attached the second identification tag to the shroud.   _____   _____   _____

29. Left the body on the bed for the funeral director. Left the denture cup with the body.   _____   _____   _____

30. Pulled the privacy curtain around the bed or closed the door.   _____   _____   _____

31. Removed the gloves and Decontaminated hands.   _____   _____   _____

Post-Procedure

32. Put on gloves.   _____   _____   _____

33. Stripped the person's unit after the body was removed.   _____   _____   _____

34. Removed the gloves and decontaminated hands.   _____   _____   _____

35. Reported the following to the nurse:

    a. The time the body was taken by the funeral director   _____   _____   _____

    b. What was done with jewelry and personal belongings   _____   _____   _____

    c. What was done with dentures   _____   _____   _____